Paroxysmal Nocturnal Hemoglobinuria

Yuzuru Kanakura • Taroh Kinoshita
Jun-ichi Nishimura
Editors

Paroxysmal Nocturnal Hemoglobinuria

From Bench to Bedside

Springer

Editors
Yuzuru Kanakura
Department of Hematology and Oncology
Osaka University Graduate School of Medicine
Suita, Osaka, Japan

Jun-ichi Nishimura
Department of Hematology and Oncology
Osaka University Graduate School of Medicine
Suita, Osaka, Japan

Taroh Kinoshita
Research Institute for Microbial Diseases
Osaka University
Suita, Osaka, Japan

WPI Immunology Frontier Research Center
Osaka University
Suita, Osaka, Japan

ISBN 978-4-431-56001-2 ISBN 978-4-431-56003-6 (eBook)
DOI 10.1007/978-4-431-56003-6

Library of Congress Control Number: 2016961209

Printed on acid-free paper

This Springer imprint is published by Springer Nature
The registered company is Springer Japan KK
The registered company address is: Chiyoda First Bldg. East, 3-8-1 Nishi-Kanda, Chiyoda-ku, Tokyo 101-0065, Japan

Preface

On this occasion we hereby publish the only book in the world that focuses on paroxysmal nocturnal hemoglobinuria (PNH). PNH arises as a consequence of clonal expansion of hematopoietic stem cells that have acquired a somatic mutation in the phosphatidylinositol glycan class A (*PIGA*) gene. The resulting hematopoietic cells are deficient in glycosylphosphatidylinositol (GPI)-anchored proteins, including the complement regulatory proteins CD55 and CD59; this accounts for the intravascular hemolysis that is the primary clinical manifestation of PNH.

The *PIGA* gene was identified by our group at Osaka University in 1993, and understanding of the pathophysiology of PNH has made remarkable progress since then. To this day, we Japanese researchers have made a significant contribution and have led the world in PNH research, together with colleagues worldwide.

PNH is an ultra-rare disease with a frequency of a few people in 100,000, and for a long time there was no established significant treatment. In 2004, 10 years after the discovery of the *PIGA* gene, a humanized anti-C5 monoclonal antibody, eculizumab, was developed as a therapeutic for hemolysis in PNH due to the extraordinary leadership of Dr. Peter Hillmen. Eculizumab showed not only remarkable suppression of hemolysis, but also improvement in patient quality of life and life prognosis. In the succeeding years, PNH has become a disease that has attracted more attention.

While the clinical significance of eculizumab has been established in a variety of ways, several challenges remain such as management of the insufficient effect of eculizumab, including the manifestation of extravascular hemolysis by eculizumab treatment, management for pregnancy and childbirth, perioperative management, and other problems. In addition, because poor responders to eculizumab have been identified in Japan, intensive efforts are currently being made to develop a novel therapeutic.

Twenty years after the discovery of the *PIGA* gene and 10 years after the development of eculizumab, we have a great opportunity to pause and summarize the knowledge that has accumulated to date and to assess the challenges remaining in the future. We would like to thank the leading basic and clinical experts in PNH worldwide who kindly contributed their writing. This book consists of two sections:

Part I for basic science and Part II for clinical science. We were very pleased to invite two legends who have made great achievement in this area: Dr. Wendell Rosse handed down the history of PNH research in Chap. 1 and Dr. Lucio Luzzatto enthusiastically discussed the clonal origin and clonal selection in PNH in Chap. 12. It was also extremely helpful to obtain the cooperation of the core members of the international PNH interest group and the Japan PNH study group. Our hope here is that this book may facilitate future clinical work and basic research in PNH.

Suita, Osaka, Japan

Yuzuru Kanakura
Taroh Kinoshita
Jun-ichi Nishimura

Contents

Chapter 1
A History of Research of PNH: Defining a Disease

Wendell Franklyn Rosse

Abstract Historically, a principal reason Western medicine has progressed to the degree it has is the epistemology used to define disease. Diseases are distinguished by two main methods: (1) assembly of defining characteristics (symptoms, physical descriptions both direct and derived from imaging techniques, and laboratory findings and clinical course) that recur so as to form a clinical template and (2) assessment of cause and effects of the clinically defined disease. The method was first clearly established in the nineteenth century with the definition of microbial diseases and received its second great impetus with the development of molecular genetics. Although the pattern has been altered in more recent times with the development of science leading to the definition of disease, a study of the classical methodology has a clear place in the study of disease.

The history of the development of understanding of paroxysmal nocturnal hemoglobinuria is an excellent example of this methodology at work. In the present paper, I will emphasize the investigation of the causes and effects and show how these investigations have played a crucial role in the definition of the disease and the understanding of the clinical manifestations.

Keywords Paroxysmal nocturnal hemoglobinuria • Aplastic anemia • Thrombosis • Glycosylphosphatidylinositol anchor • Eculizumab

1.1 Early Clinical Descriptions and Investigations

The first defining clinical accounts are those of Gull in 1866 [1] and of Strubing in 1884 [2]. They noted the unusual appearance of dark red to brown urine that was periodic, although neither commented on the nocturnal occurrence of this phenomenon. Strubing also noted a number of other symptoms (fatigue, shortness of breath, esophageal spasm, and chest pain, etc.) and distinguished the cause of the dark urine

W.F. Rosse, M.D. (✉)
Medicine Emeritus, Duke University, 2212 Elba St, Durham, NC 27705, USA
e-mail: Wendell.rosse@duke.edu

Y. Kanakura et al. (eds.), *Paroxysmal Nocturnal Hemoglobinuria*,
DOI 10.1007/978-4-431-56003-6_1

from other known causes, including march hemoglobinuria and paroxysmal cold hemoglobinuria. Gull thought that the pigment in the urine was hematin which had just been defined, but Strubing correctly said that it was hemoglobin.

Gull did little else other than the clinical case report which runs for a number of pages. Strubing, however, looked more carefully. He noted that the blood plasma was also discolored by hemoglobin and concluded that the pigment was not generated in the kidneys. He surmised that it was generated by the intravascular destruction of red cells much as in incompatible red blood cell transfusion experiments of a colleague, Langlois.

In 1911, Hijmans van den Bergh, a Dutch physician, reported a case and investigated the red cells more thoroughly [3]. He noted that they were lysed in vitro by both the patient's serum and the serum of compatible normal individuals when cells and serum were incubated in an atmosphere containing CO_2. This proved that it was the cells that were abnormal, not something in the serum. Van den Bergh thought that perhaps complement was responsible for the lysis, as had been shown in incompatibility experiments, but could not prove it.

1.2 The Role of Complement

Complement was known as a "principle" in normal, unheated serum that augmented the effects of specific antibody in some immune reactions such as bacteriocide and lysis of red cells by incompatible serum. By 1930, it had been shown to consist of at least four components which reacted in the order C1, C4, C2, and C3 [4]. It became involved in the understanding of PNH in 1938, when three laboratories (Thomas Hale Ham in Boston [5], John Dacie in London [6], and F.L.J. Jordan, a student of van den Bergh in Utrecht [7]) almost simultaneously found, as had van den Bergh, that PNH red cells were lysed when incubated with acidified normal serum. The reaction was abrogated by heating the serum or removing divalent cations, reactions characteristic of complement. Further, PNH red cells were more readily lysed by other reactions where complement was activated, such as by blood group antibodies. Dacie in particular was puzzled, however, as no antibody could be demonstrated in the normal or patient's serum as was thought necessary to initiate the activation of complement. This problem was solved a few years later by the demonstration of Pillemer of the alternative pathway (or as he called it "the properdin pathway") of the activation [8] of complement that bypassed the initial steps of the "classical" pathway and thus did not require antibody for activation [9].

The peculiar sensitivity to the hemolytic action of complement in lysis of PNH red cells was quantified by Rosse and Dacie in 1964, using carefully measured gradients of serum to lyse red cells maximally sensitized by cold agglutinins [10]. These studies showed that the red cells usually consisted of two populations, one apparently normal (mistakenly called "PNH I") and one lysed by as little as 1/25 the concentration of serum required to lyse normal red cells (PNH III cells). Later, red cells of intermediate sensitivity were found in some patients (called "PNH II cells")

[11]. The two types of abnormal cells were found to be present in proportion ranging from 1 % to nearly 100 %. Uncommonly, both PNH II and PNH III cells were present in the blood of the patient.

The reason for the exceptional sensitivity of the cells to lysis unfolded as complement became better understood. No matter how complement was activated (by antibody, by acidification of serum, by cobra venom factor, etc.), much larger quantities of the third component (newly defined as a single protein, C3) were affixed to the membrane of PNH red cells than to that of normal red cells [12]. The linchpin of the alternative pathway of activation was the enzyme complex consisting the activated form of C3, C3b, which was bound to the cellular membrane, and activated factor B (Bb), a serine protease bound to C3b by Mg^{++}. This convertase complex was then able to activate the terminal steps of complement, resulting in lysis of the cell to which it was attached. When equal numbers of convertase complexes were established on normal and PNH red cells, those on PNH cells processed tenfold as many C3 molecules (the substrate of the enzyme) as normal cells [13]. The reason for this became apparent from the studies of Nicholson-Weller: PNH red cells lacked a membrane protein, decay-accelerating factor (DAF, later called CD55), whose function is to disrupt the convertase complex [14] and thus protect the cell from the action of complement.

When the lysis of PNH red cells was examined further, it became apparent that something else must be defective because the amount of lysis per affixed, C3b was far greater for the PNH cells [15]. This as explained by the studies of Parker and his associates, who demonstrated that another protein was missing, one that normally controlled the effectiveness of the so-called membrane attack complex that consisted of C5b, C6 C7 C8, and C9 [16]. The lack of this protein, originally called "membrane inhibitor of reactive lysis" (MIRL, later protectin or CD59), accounts for most of the increased effectiveness of complement on PNH cell [17].

At about this time, flow cytometry was invented that allowed evaluation of the external proteins on individual cells through the use of monoclonal antibodies [18]. Using this technique, a number of other proteins were found to be missing on a portion red cells as well as granulocytes, platelets, monocytes, and lymphocytes of blood from patients with PNH. This provided a tool for the more accurate diagnosis of the disease as well as a far greater insight into its characteristics.

1.3 Why Are the Proteins Missing?

The two complement defense proteins are not the first to be found deficient on PNH cells. Acetylcholinesterase was found to be totally lacking on PNH III red cells and present in diminished amounts on PNH II red cells [19]. Alkaline phosphatase had been found lacking on a proportion of PNH granulocytes [20].

The reason for the lack of all these proteins became apparent with the finding in the early 1980s by Lowe of the glycosylphosphatidylinositol (GPI) anchor that attaches proteins to the external membrane of all cells [21]. This moiety is used by almost all organisms as an alternative to the insertion of a hydrophobic sequence of amino acids through the lipid bilayer. It is constructed in and on the endoplasmic reticulum by a series of steps involving one or more proteins or enzymes. Since two of the proteins known to be missing in PNH (alkaline phosphatase and acetylcholinesterase) were found to be attached by the GPI anchor, Nussenzweig and his associates concluded that lack of the anchor was the problem in PNH and showed that CD55 was also attached by this anchor [22].

A series of lymphocyte cell lines were developed which did not exhibit GPI-linked proteins and which differed from each other as shown by fusion complementation studies; these were labeled A through H. PNH cells from a number of patients did not complement the cells of class A, indicating that they shared a defect in GPI anchor synthesis with that class of lymphocytes. Again using complementation studies, Kinoshita and his group were able to demonstrate that the defective gene in PNH was the so-called PIG-A gene which was located on the short arm of the X chromosome [23]. Since that time, the abnormal hematopoietic cells of all patients with PNH have been found, when tested, to have one of a great variety of mutations in this gene, most resulting in no gene product as seen in PNH III cells, others in reduced gene product as seen in PNH II cells.

1.4 Why Is Only a Proportion of PNH Cells Abnormal?

The studies of Rosse and Dacie [10] demonstrated that, in most cases, only a portion of the red cells in PNH are abnormal. The reason for this depended upon an understanding of hematopoiesis that began with the definition by Till and McCullough of the stem cell from which all the cells of the blood are derived. Studies of polycythemia rubra vera and chronic granulocytic leukemia showed that all the cell lines in the blood, not only the red cells in the former and the granulocytes in the latter, were abnormal. This was interpreted to mean that the abnormality originated in a hematopoietic stem cell and was transmitted by clonal expansion to all cell lines.

This appeared to be true of PNH as well. Enright and Aster first demonstrated that granulocytes and platelets, like red cells, were sensitive to the hemolytic action of complement [24], and their abnormality was later confirmed by flow cytometry (see above). Using this technique, an accurate evaluation of the proportion of abnormal cells in each cell line could be made. It became apparent that the abnormal cells were a clone derived from a single abnormal hematopoietic stem cell and the normal cells were residual.

1.5 Thrombosis in PNH

Thrombosis was noted in several early series of reports of PNH. Its importance was emphasized by Crosby in the early 1950s. Hartmann emphasized the occurrence of hepatic and other intra-abdominal thrombosis, and it became clear that such thromboses were a major cause of mortality in the disease [25].

The cause of this thrombophilia was not and is not yet clear. Crosby in the early 1950s had some fanciful theories about a relationship between the activation of complement and that of the coagulation system [26]. It has been suggested that hemolysis itself may contribute to the problem but no proof is offered. More recently, attention has focused on the abnormality of platelets as playing a major role. It was shown that platelets respond to the deposition of C5b-9 (membrane attack) complexes by gathering them into rafts and removing them by exocytosis [27]. The resulting microvesicles are very thrombogenic, as are microvesicles from granulocytes and monocytes. As many membrane attack complex (MAC) are deposited on PNH platelets, many such microvesicles are formed for a given activation of complement, accounting at least in part for the thrombophilia of the disease [28]. At any event, the thrombophilia appears to be dependent upon the activation of complement as interruption of the sequence by an antibody to C5 markedly diminishes the incidence of clinical thrombosis [29].

1.6 PNH and Aplastic Anemia

The relationship of PNH to aplastic anemia was first clarified by Lewis and Dacie in 1961 [30]. They noted the patients who had aplastic anemia before having PNH as well as the evidence of hypofunctional bone marrow in patients without such a history. Epidemiological studies showed that at least 75 % of PNH patients had either granulocytopenia and/or thrombocytopenia. Since these cells have a normal life span in the circulation, this implies that the cause of the cytopenia is diminished production. Finally, it was shown in several laboratories that the cell culture of bone marrow from all PNH patients (even those with apparently active marrow) yielded few colonies, much like the culture of marrow from aplastic anemia patients [31].

When the bone marrow of patients with aplastic anemia was examined for the presence of cells lacking GPI-linked proteins, such cells were detected in small but abnormal numbers in most patients [32]. Such cells are present in very small numbers in the marrow of many normal individuals [33]. How these very small populations increase in size so as to result in clinical symptoms is not clear.

It is clear that PNH can arise only in the marrow afflicted by aplastic anemia, the severity of which may range from subclinical to severe. Aplastic anemia is thought to arise from an immunological attack on hematopoietic stem cells (HSCs). The GPI-deficient HSCs characteristic of PNH may be able to resist this attack by some means as yet unknown. Further exponential increase in clone size occurs in some of these patients, leading to a controlled growth of the clone; the reason for this is entirely unknown but may be due to a second somatic mutation in the GPI-deficient line. The result is clinical PNH when the clone increases to 5–10% of the total marrow production.

Thus, PNH patients have two diseases: (1) hypoplastic/aplastic anemia caused by immunological attack of the hematopoietic stem cells and (2) PNH caused by a somatic mutation resulting in the deficiency of GPI-anchored proteins. Each disease must be considered and treated separately but often at the same time.

1.7 Specific Treatment

In Greek and much of subsequent medicine, treatment was of symptoms, not of disease. The same was true of the treatment of PNH for many years: blood transfusion, iron replacement, anticoagulation, etc. The first specific treatment based on understanding the disease was introduced in 2003 – eculizumab – a monoclonal antibody that totally inhibits the activation of the fifth component of complement, C5 [34]. The drug virtually completely stops the intravascular hemolysis and markedly inhibits thrombosis [27], thus treating the effects of the disease. It does not affect the underlying hypoplasia of the marrow affecting all patients, demonstrating that this is a disease separate from PNH. With this therapy, the quality of life is markedly improved, and life span is increased [35].

1.8 Summary

PNH offers an excellent example of the interaction of clinical observations and scientific investigation in delineating precisely a disease. Other examples exist but few are as clear-cut. It is through such careful definitions that specific treatment and further investigation are possible.

References

1. Gull WW (1866) A case of intermittent haematinuria, with remarks. Guys Hosp Rep 12:381–392
2. Strubing P (1882) Paroxysmale Hamoglobinurie. Dtsch Med Wochenschr 8:1–8
3. Hijmans van den Bergh AA (1911) Ictere hemolytique avec crises hemoglobinuriques. Fragiliute globulaire. Rev Med 31:63–69
4. Ross GD (1986) Introduction and history of complement research. In: Immunobiology of the complement system. Academic, Orlando, pp 1–19
5. Ham TH (1938) Chronic hemolytic anemia with paroxysmal nocturnal hemoglobinuria. A study of the mechanism of hemolysis in relation to acid-base equilibrium. N Engl J Med 217:915–917

6. Dacie JV, Israels MCG, Wilkinson JF (1938) Paroxysmal nocturnal haemoglobinuria of the Marchiafava type. Lancet 1:479–482
7. Jordan FLJ (1938) Etudes sur l'hemoglobinurie. Acta Med Scand 95:319–340
8. Pillemer L, Blum L, Lepow IH et al (1954) The properdin system and immunity. I. Demonstration and isolation of a new serum protein, properdin, and its role in immune phenomena. Science 120:279
9. Muller-Eberhard HJ, Gotze O (1972) Paroxysmal nocturnal hemoglobinuria. Hemolysis initiated by the C3 activator system. N Engl J Med 286:180–184
10. Rosse WF, Dacie JV (1966) Immune lysis of normal human and paroxysmal nocturnal hemoglobinuria red blood cells: I. The sensitivity of PNH red cells to lysis by complement and specific antibody. J Clin Invest 45:736–748
11. Rosse WF, Adams JP, Thorpe AM (1974) The population of cells in paroxysmal nocturnal haemaglobinuria of intermediate sensitivity to complement: Significance and mechanism of increased immune lysis. Br J Haematol 28:181–190
12. Logue GL, Rosse WF, Adams JP (1973) Mechanism of immune lysis of red blood cells in vitro. I. Paroxysmal nocturnal hemoglobinuria cells. J Clin Invest 42:1129–1137
13. Parker CJ, Baker PJ, Rosse WF (1982) Increased enzymatic activity of the alternative pathway convertase when bound to the erythrocytes of paroxysmal nocturnal hemoglobinuria. J Clin Invest 69:337–346
14. Nicholson-Weller A, March JP, Rosenfeld SL, Austen KF (1983) Affected erythrocytes of patients with paroxysmal nocturnal hemoglobinuria are deficient in the complement regulatory protein, decay accelerating factor. Proc Soc Natl Acad Sci USA 80:5430–5434
15. Rosse WF, Logue GL, Parker J, Crookston JH (1974) Mechanisms of immune lysis of the red cells in hereditary erythroblastic multinuclearity with a positive acidified serum lysis test and paroxysmal nocturnal hemoglobinuria. J Clin Invest 53:31–43
16. Holguin MH, Frederick LR, Bernshaw NJ, Wilcox LA, Parker CJ (1989) Isolation and characterization of a membrane protein from normal human erythrocytes that inhibits reactive lysis of erythrocytes of paroxysmal nocturnal hemoglobinuria. J Clin Invest 84:7–17
17. Holguin MH, Wilcox LA, Bernshaw NJ, Rosse WF, Parker CJ (1989) Relationship between the membrane inhibitor of reactive lysis and erythrocyte phenotypes of paroxysmal nocturnal hemoglobinuria. J Clin Invest 84:1387–1394
18. Hall S, Rosse WF (1996) The use of monoclonal antibodies and flow cytometry in the diagnosis of PNH. Blood 87:5332–5340
19. Kuntsling TR, Rosse WF (1969) Erythrocyte acetylcholinesterase in PNH. Blood 33:607–616
20. Lewis SM, Dacie JV (1965) Neutrophil (leukocyte) alkaline phosphatase in paroxysmal nocturnal haemoglobinuria. Br J Haematol 11:549–557
21. Low MG (1989) Glycosyl-phophatidylinositol: a versatile anchor for cell surface proteins. FASEB J 3:1600–1608
22. Davitz MA, Low MG, Nussenzweig V (1986) Release of decay-accelerating factor (DAF) from the cell membrane by phosphatidylinositol-specific phospholipase C (PIPLC). J Exp Med 163:1150–1161
23. Takeda J, Miyata T, Kawagoe K, Iida Y, Endo Y, Fugita T, Takahashi M, Kitani T, Kinoshita T (1993) Deficiency of the GPI anchor caused by a somatic mutation of the OIG-A gene in paroxysmal nocturnal hemoglobinuria. Cell 73:703–711
24. Aster RH, Enright SE (1969) A platelet and granulocyte membrane defect in paroxysmal nocturnal hemoglobinuria: Usefulness for the detection of platelet antibodies. J Clin Invest 48:1199–1210
25. Hill A, Kelly RJ, Hillmen P (2013) Thrombosis in paroxysmal nocturnal hemoglobinuria. Blood 121:4985–4995
26. Crosby WH, Dameshek W (1950) Paroxysmal nocturnal hemoglobinuria. The mechanisms of hemolysis and its relation to the coagulation mechanism. Blood 5:822–842

27. Sims PJ, Faioni EM, Wiedmer T, Shattil SJ (1988) Complement proteins C5b-9 cause release of membrane vesicles from platelet surface that are enriched in the membrane receptor for coagulation factor Va and express prothrombinase activity. J Biol Chem 263:18205–18212
28. Wiedmer T, Hall SE, Ortel TL, Kane WH, Rosse WF, Sims PJ (1993) Complement-induced vesiculation and exposure of membrane prothrombinase sites in platelets of paroxysmal nocturnal hemoglobinuria. Blood 82:1192–1196
29. Hillmen P, Muus P, Duhrsen U et al (2007) Effect of the complement inhibitor eculizumab o n thromboembolism in patients with paroxysmal nocturnal hemoglobinuria. Blood 110:4123–4128
30. Dacie JV, Lewis SM (1961) Paroxysmal nocturnal haemoglobinuria: variation in clinical severity and association with bone marrow hypoplasia. Br J Haematol 7:442–457
31. Maciejewski JP, Sloand EM, Sato T, Anderson S, Young NS (1997) Impaired hematopoiesis in paroxysmal nocturnal hemoglobinuria/aplastic anemia is not associated with a selective proliferative defect in the glycosylphosphatidylinositol-anchored protein-deficient clone. Blood 79:1173–1181
32. Pu JJ, Mukhina G, Wang H, Savage WJ, Brodsky RA (2011) Natural history of paroxysmal nocturnal hemoglobinuria clones in patients presenting as aplastic anemia. Eur J Haematol 87:37–45
33. Araten DJ, Nafa K, Pakdeesuwan K, Luzzatto L (1999) Clonal populations of hematopoietic cells with paroxysmal nocturnal hemoglobinuria genotype and phenotype are present in normal individuals. Proc Natl Acad Sci U S A 96:5209–5214
34. Hillmen P, Hall C, Marsh JC, Elebute M, Bombara MP, Petro BE, Cullen MJ, Richards SJ, Mojcik CF, Rother RP (2004) Effect of eculizumab on hemolysis and transfusion requirements in patients with paroxysmal nocturnal hemoglobinuria. N Engl J Med 350:552–559
35. Hillmen P, Muus P, Roth A, Elebute MO, Risitano AM, Schrezenmeier H, Szer J, Browne P, Maciejewski JP, Schubert J, Urbano-Ispizua A, de Castro C, Socie G, Brodsky RA (2013) Long-term safety and efficacy of sustained eculizumab treatment in patients with paroxysmal nocturnal haemoglobinuria. Br J Haemat 162:62–73

Part I
Basic Sciences in PNH

Chapter 2
Synthesis, Genetics, and Congenital Diseases of GPI-Anchored Proteins

Yusuke Maeda, Yoshiko Murakami, and Taroh Kinoshita

Abstract In this chapter, we present basic research covering paroxysmal nocturnal hemoglobinuria (PNH). PNH is characterized by impaired regulation of the complement system because of reduced surface expression of complement regulatory molecules, CD55 (DAF) and CD59. Both proteins are glycosylphosphatidylinositol-anchored proteins (GPI-APs) present in wide variety of cells exposed to complement. GPI-AP deficiency is caused by somatic mutation of *PIGA* in hematopoietic stem cells, the primary defect in PNH. Clinical manifestations, such as hemolytic anemia, also occur when other factors induce clonal expansion of the affected hematopoietic stem cells. Although a defect in any 20 or more genes essential for GPI biosynthesis and/or remodeling can cause PNH, only *PIGA*, encoding an enzyme catalyzing the first step in GPI biosynthesis, was known to be a gene responsible for PNH over the last two decades. This is because among the more than 20 genes, *PIGA* is the only gene located on the *X*-chromosome and a single mutation is sufficient to cause PIG-A dysfunction. PNH caused by compound defects of somatic and germ line mutations in the *PIGT* gene located on chromosome 20 was recently found. In addition to PNH, revolutionary development of next-generation sequencing (NGS) has enabled the identification of inherited GPI deficiencies with various clinical phenotypes, such as intellectual disability, developmental delay, seizures, and hypotonia. Currently, individuals with mutations in 12 genes along the GPI biosynthetic pathway have been identified. Further development of NGS will facilitate discovery of more inherited GPI deficiencies and possibly PNH. Therefore, characterizing the biosynthetic pathway of GPI is increasingly more important for understanding the pathology of GPI deficiencies.

Y. Maeda (✉) • Y. Murakami, M.D., Ph.D.
Department of Immunoregulation, Research Institute for Microbial Diseases, Osaka University, 3-1 Yamadaoka, Suita, Osaka 565-0871, Japan

Department of Immunoglycobiology, WPI Immunology Frontier Research Center, Osaka University, 3-1 Yamadaoka, Suita, Osaka 565-0871, Japan
e-mail: ymaeda@biken.osaka-u.ac.jp

T. Kinoshita
Research Institute for Microbial Diseases, Osaka University, 3-1 Yamadaoka, Suita 565-0871, Osaka, Japan

WPI Immunology Frontier Research Center, Osaka University, 3-1 Yamadaoka, Suita 565-0871, Osaka, Japan

Y. Kanakura et al. (eds.), *Paroxysmal Nocturnal Hemoglobinuria*,
DOI 10.1007/978-4-431-56003-6_2

Keywords Biosynthesis • Glycosylphosphatidylinositol • Congenital disease • PGAP

2.1 Introduction

Glycosylphosphatidylinositol-anchored proteins (GPI-APs) are cell-surface proteins that are anchored to the outer leaflet of plasma membranes by GPI, a glycolipid, covalently linked to the carboxyl (C)-terminus of proteins. Protein modification with GPI occurs in all eukaryotes and the basic structure of GPI is conserved among a wide range of organisms. The addition of GPI takes place in the endoplasmic reticulum (ER) as a posttranslational modification to the protein. Precursor GPI that has been assembled is en bloc added to the C-terminus of proteins that have been newly generated from precursor proteins by the removal of a GPI-additional signal peptide present at the C-terminus. This transamidation reaction is catalyzed by the GPI-transamidase complex, which forms an amide bond between the terminal ethanolamine of GPI and the C-terminal amino acid of a processed protein, termed the ω site. After the GPI is attached to proteins, the GPI moiety is subjected to further modifications, i.e., removal of an ethanolamine phosphate (EtNP) and an acyl chain in the ER and the addition of lateral sugar chains and lipid remodeling in the Golgi apparatus during transport, and eventually mature GPI-APs are expressed on the plasma membrane. One-hundred and thirty-four human proteins with a diverse range of functions, including enzymes, receptors, adhesion molecules, and miscellaneous proteins such as prion and complement regulators, are reported to be modified with GPI in the UniProt database (the reviewed proteins are listed with their entry numbers in Table 2.1) (http://www.uniprot.org/uniprot/?query=location:%22GPI-anchor%20[SL-9902]%22&fil=organism%3A%22Homo+sapiens+%28Human%29+[9606]%22). At least ten other proteins are reported to be GPI-anchored, making a total of ~150 human GPI-APs. GPI-APs have common features, because of the physical nature of GPI. GPI-APs are enriched in specialized microdomains, so-called lipid rafts, and can be released from the surface by the cleavage of the GPI. This chapter focuses mainly on the structure, biosynthesis pathway, and transport of mammalian GPI-APs.

2.2 Structure of GPI-APs

The basic structures of mature (cell-surface) GPI-APs are peptide-linked EtNP-6-Man-α1, 2-Man-α1, 6-(EtNP-2)-Man-α1, 4-GlcN-α1, 6-myoPI (Man, mannose; GlcN, glucosamine; PI, phosphatidylinositol). The three mannoses are herein termed the first, second, and third according to their biosynthetic orders, i.e., the mannose linked to GlcN represents the first since GPI is synthesized from PI (Fig. 2.1).

Table 2.1 List of human GPI-anchored proteins

(Reviewed by UniProt)				
Entry	**Protein names**	**Gene names**	**Length**	**Mass**
P21589	5′-Nucleotidase (5′-NT) (EC 3.1.3.5) (ecto-5′-nucleotidase) (CD antigen CD73)	NT5E NT5 NTE	574	63,368
P22303	Acetylcholinesterase (AChE) (EC 3.1.1.7)	ACHE	614	67,796
Q10588	ADP-ribosyl cyclase/cyclic ADP-ribose hydrolase 2 (EC 3.2.2.6) (ADP-ribosyl cyclase 2) (bone marrow stromal antigen 1) (BST-1) (cyclic ADP-ribose hydrolase 2) (cADPr hydrolase 2) (CD antigen CD157)	BST1	318	35,724
Q10589	Bone marrow stromal antigen 2 (BST-2) (HM1.24 antigen) (tetherin) (CD antigen CD317)	BST2	180	19,769
O95971	CD160 antigen (natural killer cell receptor BY55) (CD antigen CD160)	CD160 BY55	181	19,810
P55290	Cadherin-13 (heart cadherin) (H-cadherin) (P105) (truncated cadherin) (T-cad) (T-cadherin)	CDH13 CDHH	713	78,287
P22748	Carbonic anhydrase 4 (EC 4.2.1.1) (carbonate dehydratase IV) (Carbonic anhydrase IV) (CA-IV)	CA4	312	35,032
P14384	Carboxypeptidase M (CPM) (EC 3.4.17.12)	CPM	443	50,514
Q6YHK3	CD109 antigen (150 kDa TGF-beta-1-binding protein) (C3 and PZP-like alpha-2-macroglobulin domain-containing protein 7) (platelet-specific Gov antigen) (p180) (r150) (CD antigen CD109)	CD109 CPAMD7	1445	161,689
P08571	Monocyte differentiation antigen CD14 (myeloid cell-specific leucine-rich glycoprotein) (CD antigen CD14) [cleaved into: monocyte differentiation antigen CD14, urinary form; monocyte differentiation antigen CD14, membrane-bound form]	CD14	375	40,076

(continued)

Table 2.1 (continued)

(Reviewed by UniProt)				
Entry	**Protein names**	**Gene names**	**Length**	**Mass**
Q8N6Q3	CD177 antigen (human neutrophil alloantigen 2a) (HNA-2a) (NB1 glycoprotein) (NB1 GP) (polycythemia rubra vera protein 1) (PRV-1) (CD antigen CD177)	CD177 NB1 PRV1 UNQ595/PRO1181	437	46,363
P25063	Signal transducer CD24 (small cell lung carcinoma cluster 4 antigen) (CD antigen CD24)	CD24 CD24A	80	8097
P09326	CD48 antigen (B-lymphocyte activation marker BLAST-1) (BCM1 surface antigen) (leukocyte antigen MEM-102) (SLAM family member 2) (SLAMF2) (signaling lymphocytic activation molecule 2) (TCT.1) (CD antigen CD48)	CD48 BCM1 BLAST1	243	27,683
P31358	CAMPATH-1 antigen (CDw52) (Cambridge pathology 1 antigen) (epididymal secretory protein E5) (Human epididymis-specific protein 5) (He5) (CD antigen CD52)	CD52 CDW52 HE5	61	6614
P13987	CD59 glycoprotein (1 F5 antigen) (20 kDa homologous restriction factor) (HRF-20) (HRF20) (MAC-inhibitory protein) (MAC-IP) (MEM43 antigen) (membrane attack complex inhibition factor) (MACIF) (membrane inhibitor of reactive lysis) (MIRL) (protectin) (CD antigen CD59)	CD59 MIC11 MIN1 MIN2 MIN3 MSK21	128	14,177
P06731	Carcinoembryonic antigen-related cell adhesion molecule 5 (carcinoembryonic antigen) (CEA) (meconium antigen 100) (CD antigen CD66e)	CEACAM5 CEA	702	76,795
P40199	Carcinoembryonic antigen-related cell adhesion molecule 6 (nonspecific cross-reacting antigen) (normal cross-reacting antigen) (CD antigen CD66c)	CEACAM6 NCA	344	37,195
Q14002	Carcinoembryonic antigen-related cell adhesion molecule 7 (carcinoembryonic antigen CGM2)	CEACAM7 CGM2	265	29,379
P31997	Carcinoembryonic antigen-related cell adhesion molecule 8 (CD67 antigen) (carcinoembryonic antigen CGM6) (nonspecific cross-reacting antigen NCA-95) (CD antigen CD66b)	CEACAM8 CGM6	349	38,154

P0CG37	Cryptic protein (cryptic family protein 1)	CFC1	223	24,612
P26992	Ciliary neurotrophic factor receptor subunit alpha (CNTF receptor subunit alpha) (CNTFR-alpha)	CNTFR	372	40,633
Q12860	Contactin-1 (glycoprotein gp135) (neural cell-surface protein F3)	CNTN1	1018	113,320
Q02246	Contactin-2 (axonal glycoprotein TAG-1) (axonin-1) (transient axonal glycoprotein 1) (TAX-1)	CNTN2 AXT TAG1 TAX1	1040	113,393
Q9P232	Contactin-3 (brain-derived immunoglobulin superfamily protein 1) (BIG-1) (plasmacytoma-associated neuronal glycoprotein)	CNTN3 KIAA1496 PANG	1028	112,883
Q8IWV2	Contactin-4 (brain-derived immunoglobulin superfamily protein 2) (BIG-2)	CNTN4	1026	113,454
O94779	Contactin-5 (neural recognition molecule NB-2) (hNB-2)	CNTN5	1100	120,686
Q9UQ52	Contactin-6 (neural recognition molecule NB-3) (hNB-3)	CNTN6	1028	113,956
P08174	Complement decay-accelerating factor (CD antigen CD55)	CD55 CR DAF	381	41,400
P16444	Dipeptidase 1 (EC 3.4.13.19) (dehydropeptidase-I) (microsomal dipeptidase) (renal dipeptidase) (hRDP)	DPEP1 MDP RDP	411	45,674
Q9H4A9	Dipeptidase 2 (EC 3.4.13.19)	DPEP2 UNQ284/PRO323	486	53,306
Q9H4B8	Dipeptidase 3 (EC 3.4.13.19)	DPEP3 UNQ834/PRO1772	488	53,687
P20827	Ephrin-A1 (EPH-related receptor tyrosine kinase ligand 1) (LERK-1) (immediate early response protein B61) (tumor necrosis factor alpha-induced protein 4) (TNF alpha-induced protein 4) [cleaved into: ephrin-A1, secreted form]	EFNA1 EPLG1 LERK1 TNFAIP4	205	23,787
O43921	Ephrin-A2 (EPH-related receptor tyrosine kinase ligand 6) (LERK-6) (HEK7 ligand) (HEK7-L)	EFNA2 EPLG6 LERK6	213	23,878
P52797	Ephrin-A3 (EFL-2) (EHK1 ligand) (EHK1-L) (EPH-related receptor tyrosine kinase ligand 3) (LERK-3)	EFNA3 EFL2 EPLG3 LERK3	238	26,350

(continued)

Table 2.1 (continued)

(Reviewed by UniProt)				
Entry	**Protein names**	**Gene names**	**Length**	**Mass**
P52798	Ephrin-A4 (EPH-related receptor tyrosine kinase ligand 4) (LERK-4)	EFNA4 EPLG4 LERK4	201	22,386
P52803	Ephrin-A5 (AL-1) (EPH-related receptor tyrosine kinase ligand 7) (LERK-7)	EFNA5 EPLG7 LERK7	228	26,297
Q6UWR7	Ectonucleotide pyrophosphatase/phosphodiesterase family member 6 (E-NPP 6) (NPP-6) (EC 3.1.4.-) (EC 3.1.4.38) (choline-specific glycerophosphodiester phosphodiesterase) (glycerophosphocholine cholinephosphodiesterase) (GPC-Cpde)	ENPP6 UNQ1889/PRO4334	440	50,241
O75015	Low affinity immunoglobulin gamma Fc region receptor III-B (Fc-gamma RIII-beta) (Fc-gamma RIII) (Fc-gamma RIIIb) (FcRIII) (FcRIIIb) (FcR-10) (IgG Fc receptor III-1) (CD antigen CD16b)	FCGR3B CD16B FCG3 FCGR3 IGFR3	233	26,216
P15328	Folate receptor alpha (FR-alpha) (adult folate-binding protein) (FBP) (folate receptor 1) (folate receptor, adult) (KB cells FBP) (ovarian tumor-associated antigen MOv18)	FOLR1 FOLR	257	29,819
P14207	Folate receptor beta (FR-beta) (folate receptor 2) (folate receptor, fetal/placental) (placental folate-binding protein) (FBP)	FOLR2	255	29,280
P54826	Growth arrest-specific protein 1 (GAS-1)	GAS1	345	35,693
P56159	GDNF family receptor alpha-1 (GDNF receptor alpha-1) (GDNFR-alpha-1) (GFR-alpha-1) (RET ligand 1) (TGF-beta-related neurotrophic factor receptor 1)	GFRA1 GDNFRA RETL1 TRNR1	465	51,456
O00451	GDNF family receptor alpha-2 (GDNF receptor alpha-2) (GDNFR-alpha-2) (GFR-alpha-2) (GDNF receptor beta) (GDNFR-beta) (neurturin receptor alpha) (NRTNR-alpha) (NTNR-alpha) (RET ligand 2) (TGF-beta-related neurotrophic factor receptor 2)	GFRA2 GDNFRB RETL2 TRNR2	464	51,544
O60609	GDNF family receptor alpha-3 (GDNF receptor alpha-3) (GDNFR-alpha-3) (GFR-alpha-3)	GFRA3 UNQ339/PRO538/PRO3664	400	44,511

Q9GZZ7	GDNF family receptor alpha-4 (GDNF receptor alpha-4) (GDNFR-alpha-4) (GFR-alpha-4) (persephin receptor)	GFRA4	299	31,670
Q99445	Glycosylphosphatidylinositol-anchored molecule-like protein	GML LY6DL	158	17,730
P55259	Pancreatic secretory granule membrane major glycoprotein GP2 (pancreatic zymogen granule membrane protein GP-2) (ZAP75)	GP2	537	59,480
P35052	Glypican-1 [cleaved into: secreted glypican-1]	GPC1	558	61,680
Q8N158	Glypican-2 [cleaved into: secreted glypican-2]	GPC2	579	62,830
P51654	Glypican-3 (GTR2-2) (intestinal protein OCI-5) (MXR7) [cleaved into: secreted glypican-3]	GPC3 OCI5	580	65,563
O75487	Glypican-4 (K-glypican) [cleaved into: secreted glypican-4]	GPC4 UNQ474/PRO937	556	62,412
P78333	Glypican-5 [cleaved into: secreted glypican-5]	GPC5	572	63,707
Q9Y625	Glypican-6 [cleaved into: secreted glypican-6]	GPC6 UNQ369/PRO705	555	62,736
Q8IV16	Glycosylphosphatidylinositol-anchored high-density lipoprotein-binding protein 1 (GPI-HBP1) (GPI-anchored HDL-binding protein 1) (high-density lipoprotein-binding protein 1)	GPIHBP1 HBP1	184	19,806
Q12891	Hyaluronidase-2 (Hyal-2) (EC 3.2.1.35) (hyaluronoglucosaminidase-2) (lung carcinoma protein 2) (LuCa-2)	HYAL2 LUCA2	473	53,860
P38567	Hyaluronidase PH-20 (Hyal-PH20) (EC 3.2.1.35) (hyaluronoglucosaminidase PH-20) (sperm adhesion molecule 1) (sperm surface protein PH-20)	SPAM1 HYAL3 PH20	509	57,848
Q8WWA0	Intelectin-1 (ITLN-1) (endothelial lectin HL-1) (galactofuranose-binding lectin) (intestinal lactoferrin receptor) (omentin)	ITLN1 INTL ITLN LFR UNQ640/PRO1270	313	34,962
A6ND01	Sperm-egg fusion protein Juno (folate receptor 4) (folate receptor delta) (FR-delta) (IZUMO1 receptor protein JUNO)	IZUMO1R FOLR4 JUNO	250	28,672
P19256	Lymphocyte function-associated antigen 3 (Ag3) (surface glycoprotein LFA-3) (CD antigen CD58)	CD58 LFA3	250	28,147
P06858	Lipoprotein lipase (LPL) (EC 3.1.1.34)	LPL LIPD	475	53,162
Q8NI32	Ly6/PLAUR domain-containing protein 6B	LYPD6B	183	20,656

(continued)

Table 2.1 (continued)

(Reviewed by UniProt)				
Entry	**Protein names**	**Gene names**	**Length**	**Mass**
Q13449	Limbic system-associated membrane protein (LSAMP) (IgLON family member 3)	LSAMP IGLON3 LAMP	338	37,393
O95867	Lymphocyte antigen 6 complex locus protein G6c	LY6G6C C6orf24 G6C NG24 UNQ1947/PRO4430	125	13,821
O95868	Lymphocyte antigen 6 complex locus protein G6d (protein Ly6-D) (megakaryocyte-enhanced gene transcript 1 protein)	LY6G6D C6orf23 G6D MEGT1 NG25	133	13,691
Q14210	Lymphocyte antigen 6D (Ly-6D) (E48 antigen)	LY6D E48	128	13,286
Q16553	Lymphocyte antigen 6E (Ly-6E) (retinoic acid-induced gene E protein) (RIG-E) (stem cell antigen 2) (SCA-2) (Thymic shared antigen 1) (TSA-1)	LY6E 9804 RIGE SCA2 TSA1	131	13,507
O94772	Lymphocyte antigen 6H (Ly-6H)	LY6H	140	14,669
Q17RY6	Lymphocyte antigen 6 K (Ly-6 K)	LY6K CO16	165	18,673
Q9BZG9	Ly-6/neurotoxin-like protein 1 (secreted Ly-6/uPAR domain-containing protein 2) (secreted Ly-6/uPAR-related protein 2) (SLURP-2)	LYNX1 SLURP2	131	14,026
Q8N2G4	Ly6/PLAUR domain-containing protein 1 (putative HeLa tumor suppressor) (PHTS)	LYPD1 LYPDC1 PSEC0181 UNQ3079/PRO9917	141	15,240
Q6UXB3	Ly6/PLAUR domain-containing protein 2	LYPD2 LYPDC2 UNQ430/PRO788	125	13,115
O95274	Ly6/PLAUR domain-containing protein 3 (GPI-anchored metastasis-associated protein C4.4A homologue) (matrigel-induced gene C4 protein) (MIG-C4)	LYPD3 C4.4A UNQ491/PRO1007	346	35,971
Q6UWN0	Ly6/PLAUR domain-containing protein 4	LYPD4 UNQ2552/PRO6181	246	26,763
Q6UWN5	Ly6/PLAUR domain-containing protein 5	LYPD5 UNQ1908/PRO4356	251	26,936
Q6UX82	Ly6/PLAUR domain-containing protein 8	LYPD8 UNQ511/PRO1026	237	25,284
Q8NFP4	MAM domain-containing glycosylphosphatidylinositol anchor protein 1 (GPI and MAM protein) (GPIM) (glycosylphosphatidylinositol-MAM) (MAM domain-containing protein 3)	MDGA1 MAMDC3	955	105,790

Q7Z553	MAM domain-containing glycosylphosphatidylinositol anchor protein 2 (MAM domain-containing protein 1)	MDGA2 MAMDC1 UNQ8188/ PRO23197	956	107,436
Q9ULZ9	Matrix metalloproteinase-17 (MMP-17) (EC 3.4.24.-) (membrane-type matrix metalloproteinase 4) (MT-MMP 4) (MTMMP4) (membrane-type-4 matrix metalloproteinase) (MT4-MMP) (MT4MMP)	MMP17 MT4MMP	603	66,653
Q9NPA2	Matrix metalloproteinase-25 (MMP-25) (EC 3.4.24.-) (leukolysin) (membrane-type matrix metalloproteinase 6) (MT-MMP 6) (MTMMP6) (membrane-type-6 matrix metalloproteinase) (MT6-MMP) (MT6MMP)	MMP25 MMP20 MMPL1 MT6MMP	562	62,554
Q13421	Mesothelin (CAK1 antigen) (pre-pro-megakaryocyte-potentiating factor) [cleaved into: megakaryocyte-potentiating factor (MPF); mesothelin, cleaved form]	MSLN MPF	630	68,986
Q9BZM6	NKG2D ligand 1 (N2DL-1) (NKG2DL1) (ALCAN-beta) (retinoic acid early transcript 1I) (UL16-binding protein 1)	ULBP1 N2DL1 RAET1I	244	27,997
Q9BZM5	NKG2D ligand 2 (N2DL-2) (NKG2DL2) (ALCAN-alpha) (retinoic acid early transcript 1H) (UL16-binding protein 2)	ULBP2 N2DL2 RAET1H UNQ463/ PRO791	246	27,368
Q9BZM4	NKG2D ligand 3 (N2DL-3) (NKG2DL3) (ALCAN-gamma) (retinoic acid early transcript 1 N)	ULBP3 N2DL3 RAET1N	244	27,949
P52961	GPI-linked NAD(P)(+)--arginine ADP-ribosyltransferase 1 (EC 2.4.2.31) (ADP-ribosyltransferase C2 and C3 toxin-like 1) (ARTC1) (mono(ADP-ribosyl)transferase 1) (CD antigen CD296)	ART1	327	36,335
Q13508	Ecto-ADP-ribosyltransferase 3 (EC 2.4.2.31) (ADP-ribosyltransferase C2 and C3 toxin-like 3) (ARTC3) (mono(ADP-ribosyl)transferase 3) (NAD(P)(+)--arginine ADP-ribosyltransferase 3)	ART3 TMART	389	43,923
Q93070	Ecto-ADP-ribosyltransferase 4 (EC 2.4.2.31) (ADP-ribosyltransferase C2 and C3 toxin-like 4) (ARTC4) (Dombrock blood group carrier molecule) (mono(ADP-ribosyl) transferase 4) (NAD(P)(+)--arginine ADP-ribosyltransferase 4) (CD antigen CD297)	ART4 DO DOK1	314	35,878

(continued)

Table 2.1 (continued)

(Reviewed by UniProt)				
Entry	**Protein names**	**Gene names**	**Length**	**Mass**
P13591	Neural cell adhesion molecule 1 (N-CAM-1) (NCAM-1) (CD antigen CD56)	NCAM1 NCAM	858	94,574
Q7Z3B1	Neuronal growth regulator 1 (IgLON family member 4)	NEGR1 IGLON4 UNQ2433/PRO4993	354	38,719
Q496H8	Neuritin-like protein	NRN1L UNQ2446/PRO5725	165	17,786
Q9NPD7	Neuritin	NRN1 NRN	142	15,333
Q9Y2I2	Netrin-G1 (laminet-1)	NTNG1 KIAA0976 LMNT1 UNQ571/ PRO1133	539	60,541
Q96CW9	Netrin-G2 (laminet-2)	NTNG2 KIAA1857 LMNT2 UNQ9381/ PRO34206	530	59,799
Q9P121	Neurotrimin (hNT) (IgLON family member 2)	NTM IGLON2 NT UNQ297/PRO337	344	37,971
P23515	Oligodendrocyte-myelin glycoprotein	OMG OMGP	440	49,608
Q14982	Opioid-binding protein/cell adhesion molecule (OBCAM) (OPCML) (opioid-binding cell adhesion molecule) (IgLON family member 1)	OPCML IGLON1 OBCAM	345	38,008
Q7RTW8	Otoancorin	OTOA	1153	128,533
Q96GW7	Brevican core protein (brain-enriched hyaluronan-binding protein) (BEHAB) (chondroitin sulfate proteoglycan 7)	BCAN BEHAB CSPG7 UNQ2525/ PRO6018	911	99,118
Q6UQ28	Placenta-expressed transcript 1 protein	PLET1 C11orf34	207	23,385
P05187	Alkaline phosphatase, placental type (EC 3.1.3.1) (alkaline phosphatase Regan isozyme) (placental alkaline phosphatase 1) (PLAP-1)	ALPP PLAP	535	57,954
P09923	Intestinal-type alkaline phosphatase (IAP) (intestinal alkaline phosphatase) (EC 3.1.3.1)	ALPI	528	56,812
P10696	Alkaline phosphatase, placental-like (EC 3.1.3.1) (ALP-1) (alkaline phosphatase Nagao isozyme) (germ cell alkaline phosphatase) (GCAP) (placental alkaline phosphatase-like) (PLAP-like)	ALPPL2 ALPPL	532	57,377

P05186	Alkaline phosphatase, tissue-nonspecific isozyme (AP-TNAP) (TNSALP) (EC 3.1.3.1) (alkaline phosphatase liver/bone/kidney isozyme)	ALPL	524	57,305
P04156	Major prion protein (PrP) (ASCR) (PrP27-30) (PrP33-35C) (CD antigen CD230)	PRNP ALTPRP PRIP PRP	253	27,661
Q9UKY0	Prion-like protein doppel (PrPLP) (prion protein 2)	PRND DPL UNQ1830/PRO3443	176	20,293
Q7RTY9	Putative serine protease 41 (EC 3.4.21.-) (testis serine protease 1) (TESSP-1)	PRSS41 TESSP1	318	35,078
O43653	Prostate stem cell antigen	PSCA UNQ206/PRO232	123	12,912
Q86UN2	Reticulon-4 receptor-like 1 (nogo receptor-like 2) (nogo-66 receptor homologue 2) (nogo-66 receptor-related protein 3) (NgR3)	RTN4RL1 NGRH2 NGRL2	441	49,065
Q86UN3	Reticulon-4 receptor-like 2 (nogo receptor-like 3) (nogo-66 receptor homologue 1) (nogo-66 receptor-related protein 2) (NgR2)	RTN4RL2 NGRH1 NGRL3	420	46,106
O95980	Reversion-inducing cysteine-rich protein with Kazal motifs (hRECK) (suppressor of tumorigenicity 15 protein)	RECK ST15	971	106,457
Q6H3X3	Retinoic acid early transcript 1G protein (UL-16 binding protein 5) (ULBP5)	RAET1G	334	37,106
Q5VY80	Retinoic acid early transcript 1 L protein	RAET1L	246	27,509
Q96B86	Repulsive guidance molecule A (RGM domain family member A)	RGMA RGM	450	49,347
Q6NW40	RGM domain family member B (DRG11-responsive axonal guidance and outgrowth of neurite) (DRAGON)	RGMB	437	47,547
Q6ZVN8	Hemojuvelin (hemochromatosis type 2 protein) (RGM domain family member C)	HFE2 HJV RGMC	426	45,080
Q9BZR6	Reticulon-4 receptor (nogo receptor) (NgR) (nogo-66 receptor)	RTN4R NOGOR UNQ330/PRO526	473	50,708

(continued)

Table 2.1 (continued)

(Reviewed by UniProt)

Entry	Protein names	Gene names	Length	Mass
Q8TDM5	Sperm acrosome membrane-associated protein 4 (sperm acrosomal membrane-associated protein 14)	SPACA4 SAMP14 UNQ3046/PRO9862	124	13,004
O75326	Semaphorin-7A (CDw108) (JMH blood group antigen) (John-Milton-Hargen human blood group Ag) (semaphorin-K1) (sema K1) (semaphorin-L) (sema L) (CD antigen CD108)	SEMA7A CD108 SEMAL	666	74,824
Q5BIV9	Shadow of prion protein (protein shadoo)	SPRN SHO	151	14,522
P13385	Teratocarcinoma-derived growth factor 1 (cripto-1 growth factor) (CRGF) (epidermal growth factor-like cripto protein CR1)	TDGF1 CRIPTO	188	21,169
O75443	Alpha-tectorin	TECTA	2155	239,527
Q96PL2	Beta-tectorin	TECTB	329	36,956
Q9Y6M0	Testisin (EC 3.4.21.-) (Eosinophil serine protease 1) (ESP-1) (serine protease 21)	PRSS21 ESP1 TEST1 UNQ266/PRO303	314	34,884
P10646	Tissue factor pathway inhibitor (TFPI) (extrinsic pathway inhibitor) (EPI) (lipoprotein-associated coagulation inhibitor) (LACI)	TFPI LACI TFPI1	304	35,015
P04216	Thy-1 membrane glycoprotein (CDw90) (Thy-1 antigen) (CD antigen CD90)	THY1	161	17,935
O14798	Tumor necrosis factor receptor superfamily member 10C (antagonist decoy receptor for TRAIL/Apo-2 L) (decoy TRAIL receptor without death domain) (decoy receptor 1) (DcR1) (lymphocyte inhibitor of TRAIL) (TNF-related apoptosis-inducing ligand receptor 3) (TRAIL receptor 3) (TRAIL-R3) (TRAIL receptor without an intracellular domain) (CD antigen CD263)	TNFRSF10C DCR1 LIT TRAILR3 TRID UNQ321/PRO366	259	27,407
O43280	Trehalase (EC 3.2.1.28) (Alpha,alpha-trehalase) (Alpha,alpha-trehalose glucohydrolase)	TREH TREA	583	66,568
P08582	Melanotransferrin (melanoma-associated antigen p97) (CD antigen CD228)	MFI2 MAP97	738	80,215

Q9BY14	Testis-expressed sequence 101 protein (cell-surface receptor NYD-SP8) (scleroderma-associated autoantigen) (spermatogenesis-related gene protein)		TEX101 SGRG UNQ867/PRO1884	249	26,667
Q03405	Urokinase plasminogen activator surface receptor (U-PAR) (uPAR) (monocyte activation antigen Mo3) (CD antigen CD87)		PLAUR MO3 UPAR	335	36,978
P07911	Uromodulin (Tamm-Horsfall urinary glycoprotein) (THP) [cleaved into: uromodulin, secreted form]		UMOD	640	69,761
O95497	Pantetheinase (EC 3.5.1.92) (Pantetheine hydrolase) (Tiff66) (vascular noninflammatory molecule 1) (vanin-1)		VNN1	513	57,012
O95498	Vascular noninflammatory molecule 2 (vanin-2) (EC 3.5.1.92) (glycosylphosphatidyl inositol-anchored protein GPI-80) (protein FOAP-4)		VNN2	520	58,503
Q9NY84	Vascular noninflammatory molecule 3 (vanin-3) (EC 3.5.1.92)		VNN3	501	56,118
O43895	Xaa-Pro aminopeptidase 2 (EC 3.4.11.9) (aminoacylproline aminopeptidase) (membrane-bound aminopeptidase P) (membrane-bound APP) (membrane-bound AmP) (mAmP) (X-Pro aminopeptidase 2)		XPNPEP2	674	75,625
(Proteins not reviewed by UniProt but reported by publications (refer to PMID))					
Entry	**Protein names**	**PMID**	**Gene names**	**Length**	**Mass**
Q16651	Prostasin	16822939	PRSS8	343	36,431
Q7RTU9	Stereocilin	12445334	STRC	1775	192,967
Q8IVL8	Carboxypeptidase O	21921028	CPO	374	42,529
Q92485	Acid sphingomyelinase-like phosphodiesterase 3b (ASM-like phosphodiesterase 3b) (EC 3.1.4.-)	24001144	SMPDL3B, ASML3B	455	50,814
Q9GZU5	Nyctalopin	15905181	NYX, CLRP	481	52,000

(continued)

Table 2.1 (continued)

(Reviewed by UniProt)

Entry	Protein names		Gene names	Length	Mass
P54289	Voltage-dependent calcium channel subunit alpha-2/delta-1 (voltage-gated calcium channel subunit alpha-2/delta-1) [cleaved into: voltage-dependent calcium channel subunit alpha-2-1; voltage-dependent calcium channel subunit delta-1]	20080692	CACNA2D1, CACNL2A, CCHL2A, MHS3	1103	124,568
Q9NY47	Voltage-dependent calcium channel subunit alpha-2/delta-2 (voltage-gated calcium channel subunit alpha-2/delta-2) [cleaved into: voltage-dependent calcium channel subunit alpha-2-2; voltage-dependent calcium channel subunit delta-2]	20080692	CACNA2D2, KIAA0558	1150	129,817
Q8IZS8	Voltage-dependent calcium channel subunit alpha-2/delta-3 (voltage-gated calcium channel subunit alpha-2/delta-3) [cleaved into: voltage-dependent calcium channel subunit alpha-2-3; voltage-dependent calcium channel subunit delta-3]	20080692	CACNA2D3	1091	123,011
Q7Z3S7	Voltage-dependent calcium channel subunit alpha-2/delta-4 (voltage-gated calcium channel subunit alpha-2/delta-4) [cleaved into: voltage-dependent calcium channel subunit alpha-2-4; voltage-dependent calcium channel subunit delta-4]	20080692	CACNA2D4	1137	127,938
P00450	Ceruloplasmin	22178061	CP	1065	122,205

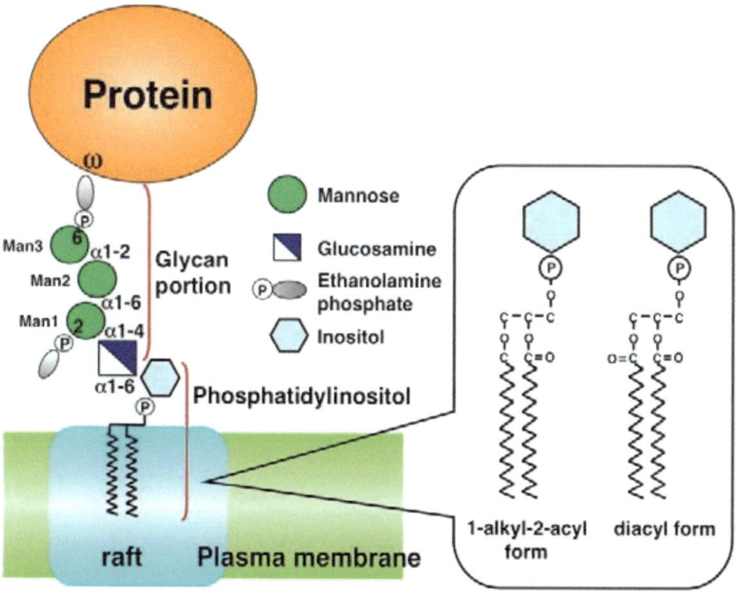

Fig. 2.1 The conserved backbone structure of the mammalian cell-surface GPI-APs. EtNP-Man-Man-(EtNP)Man-GlcN-PI is covalently linked to the C-terminal omega (ω) site of the processed precursor protein through an amide bond. In mammalian nucleated cells, 1-stearyl, 2-stearoyl PI is the predominant composition. Some GPI-APs have side branches such as GalNAc (on Man1) and a fourth Man (on Man3). In yeast, many GPI-APs use inositolphosphoceramide instead of PI. Numbers indicate the linkage positions

The first prominent structural characteristic of GPI is the presence of a non-*N*-acetylated glucosamine, which is the sole example of a glucosamine without *N*-acetylation in mammalian sugar chains. This unique structure, possibly together with inositol, may act as a target for proteins with lectin activities that have specific recognition involved in particular biological phenomena. The second prominent characteristic is within the lipid moiety. GPI is synthesized from PI whose major lipid composition is the diacyl form harboring an unsaturated acyl chain, typically arachidonic acid, at the *sn*-2 position. In contrast, the majority of mature cell-surface GPI-APs contain a saturated *sn*-2-linked acyl chain, typically stearic acid, in addition to a saturated fatty chain at the *sn*-1 position. A saturated acyl chain at the *sn*-2 position is produced by the replacement of an unsaturated chain with a saturated one, so-called fatty acid remodeling, which occurs in the Golgi apparatus. The fatty acid remodeling is especially significant, because the physical attributes afforded by saturated chains are critical for the enrichment of GPI-APs in lipid rafts. Thus, a defect in fatty acid remodeling impairs enrichment and dimerization of GPI-APs in lipid rafts in cells and an immunological response in mice models. In addition, in a significant population of GPI-APs, lipid chains at the *sn*-1 position are covalently linked to the glycerol moiety via an alkyl bond, which differs from the diacyl form of PI. The replacement of the diacyl form with the 1-alkyl-2-acyl form during GPI biosynthesis takes place in the ER, but the molecular machinery for the replacement and biological significance remains to be solved.

GPI may have some additional modifications with sugars, depending on proteins, cells, tissues, and mammalian species, which produce a diversity of biological functions. One of these additional sugar modifications is the addition of a fourth mannose to the third mannose via the α1,2 linkage catalyzed by PIG-Z. It has been reported that the fourth mannose modification is observed in brain tissue. Other side chain sugar modifications include the addition of *N*-acetyl galactosamine to the first mannose via a β1, 4 linkage, which may be followed by further addition of galactose via the β1, 3 linkage. The galactose may further be modified by sialic acid. The glycosyltransferases involved in these modifications have not been identified. In the fourth mannose and the *N*-acetyl galactosamine side chains, the mechanisms that regulate what GPI-APs and how much of them are modified and the biological significance of these modifications remain to be solved.

2.3 GPI Biosynthetic Pathway and the Genes Involved

The GPI biosynthetic pathway can be divided into two processes. The first process ranges from the biosynthesis of the GPI precursor from PI to its addition to proteins. This process takes place in the ER and the genes involved are generally named *PIGA* to *PIGZ*. The second process is the maturation of GPI-APs, which takes place after the first process and includes the removal of EtNP and the acyl chain in the ER, and fatty acid remodeling in the Golgi (Fig. 2.2 and Table 2.2).

Fig. 2.2 A scheme for the full GPI-APs biosynthetic pathway and structural modification. GPI is synthesized in the ER from free PI through more than 10 steps and 20 genes, most of them are named PIG genes. Steps 1 and 2 take place on the cytoplasmic side of the ER, and then the GPI intermediate flips and subsequent steps occur on the luminal side. GPI intermediates with a *red* PI portion (steps 1–4) indicate that they are the diacyl-form, whereas a considerable amount of intermediates in latter steps possess alkyl-acyl chains (symbolized in *black*) by an exchange of the lipid part (step 5). Synthesis of alkyl lipids in the peroxisome is required for the synthesis of the 1-alkyl-2-acyl form GPIs. A mannose donor is derived from dolichol-phosphate-mannose (DPM), which is synthesized by the DPM synthase complex composed of DPM1, DPM2, and DPM3. Mature GPI (H8) is transferred en bloc to the ω site of separately synthesized precursor proteins by a GPI-transamidase complex as a posttranslational modification. After proteins are linked with GPI, further structural modification and remodeling occurs on the glycan and lipid portions of the GPI, which involves PGAP (post-GPI-attachment to proteins) genes. p24 family members function as cargo receptors for GPI-APs to sort to and exit them from ER exit sites. GPI-APs are then transported to the cell surface through the Golgi, where additional structural remodeling, namely, fatty acid remodeling, occurs. This remodeling enables GPI-APs to be enriched in lipid rafts, which endows GPI-APs unique characteristics for their behavior and signaling. Genes symbolized in red indicate the presence of inherited GPI deficiencies caused by defects within the genes

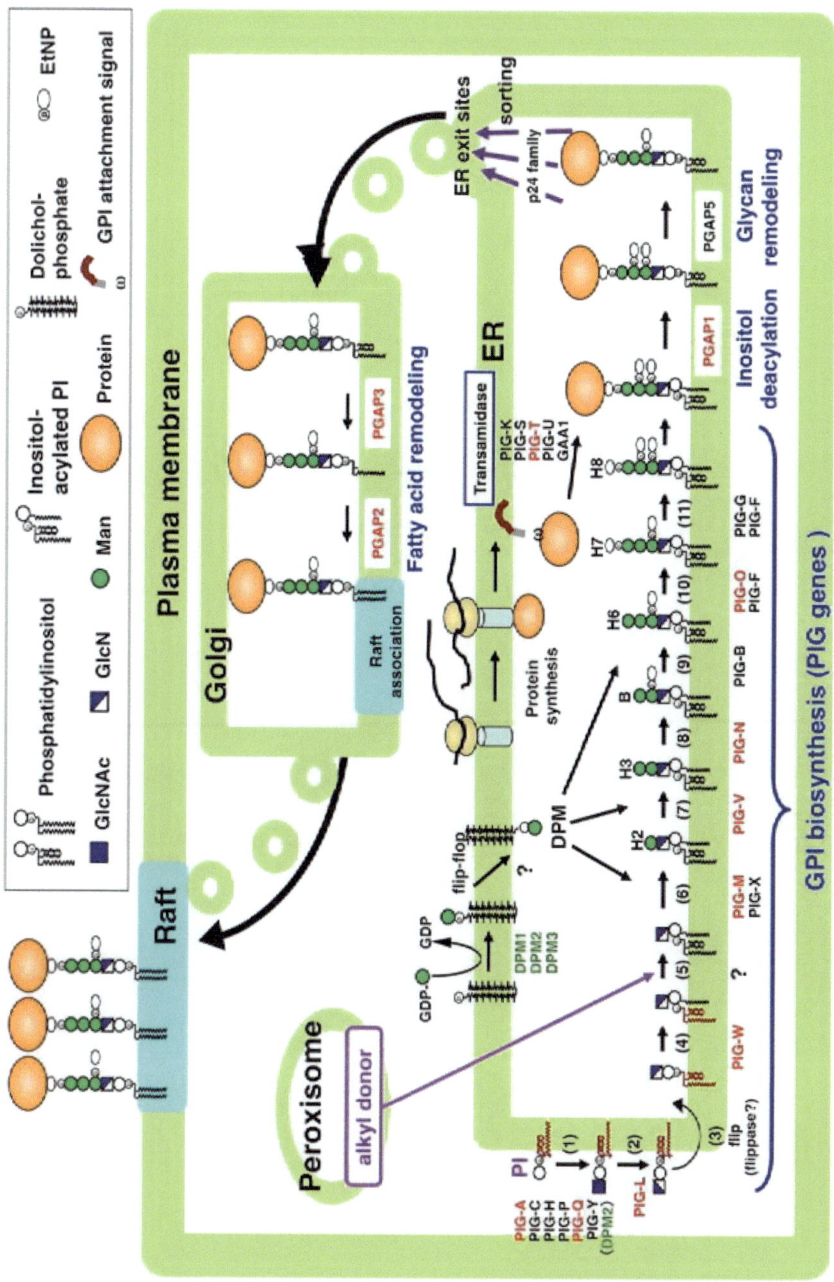
Phosphatidylinositol
GlcNAc
GlcN
Man
Inositol-acylated PI
Protein
Dolichol-phosphate
GPI attachment signal
EtNP
Plasma membrane
Raft
Golgi
Raft association
PGAP2
PGAP3
Fatty acid remodeling
ER exit sites
sorting
p24 family
Peroxisome
alkyl donor
ER
Transamidase
PIG-K
PIG-S
PIG-T
PIG-U
GAA1
Protein synthesis
flip-flop
GDP
DPM1
DPM2
DPM3
DPM
PI
PIG-A
PIG-C
PIG-H
PIG-P
PIG-Q
PIG-Y
(DPM2)
PIG-L
flip
(flippase?)
PIG-W
PIG-M
PIG-X
PIG-V
PIG-N
PIG-B
PIG-O
PIG-F
PIG-G
PIG-F
PGAP1
PGAP5
Inositol deacylation
Glycan remodeling
GPI biosynthesis (PIG genes)

Table 2.2 GPI biosynthetic pathway and the genes involved

Step		Donor substrate	Gene	Entry	Length	TM	Chromosome	Diseases	Yeast homologue
(I) Biosynthesis of precursor GPI									
1	Phosphatidylinositol N-acetylglucosaminyltransferase (GPI-GnT) (EC: 2.4.1.198)	UDP-GlcNAc	PIGA	P37287	484	1	Xp22.1	Paroxysmal nocturnal hemoglobinuria, ferro-cerebro-cutaneous syndrome, multiple congenital anomalies-hypotonia-seizures syndrome type 2, West syndrome	GPI3
			PIGC	Q92535	297	4	1q23-q25		GPI2
			PIGH	Q14442	188	0	14q24.1		GPI15
			PIGP	P57054	158	2	21q22.2		GPI19
			PIGQ	Q9BRB3	760	5	16p13.3	Early infantile epileptic encephalopathy	GPI1
			PIGY	Q3MUY2	71	2	4q22.1		ERI1
			DPM2	O94777	84	2	9q34.13	Congenital disorder of glycosylation 1U	–
2	N-acetylglucosaminyl-phosphatidylinositol de-N-acetylase (EC:3.5.1.89)		PIGL	Q9Y2B2	252	1	17p12-p11.2	Coloboma, congenital heart disease, ichthyosiform dermatosis, mental retardation and ear anomalies syndrome, HPMR	GPI12
3	Flippase?		Not identified						
4	Glucosaminyl-phosphatidylinositol acyltransferase	Palmitoyl-CoA	PIGW	Q7Z7B1	504	12	17q12	Hyperphosphatasia with mental retardation syndrome type 5	GWT1
5	Transform of diacyl-form to alkyl-acyl intermediate	PE?	Not identified						—

6	GPI mannosyltransferase 1 (EC:2.4.1.-) (GPI-MTI)	Dol-P-Man	PIGM	Q9H3S5	423	10	1q23.1	Inherited glycosylphosphatidylinositol deficiency	GPI14
			PIGX	Q8TBF5	258	1	3q29		PBN1
7	GPI mannosyltransferase 2 (EC:2.4.1.-) (GPI-MTII)	Dol-P-Man	PIGV	Q9NUD9	493	10	1p36.11	Hyperphosphatasia with mental retardation syndrome type 1	GPI18
			—						PGA1
8	GPI-ethanolamine phosphate transferase 1 (GPI-ETI)	PE	PIGN	O95427	931	15	18q21.33	Multiple congenital anomalies-hypotonia -seizures syndrome type 1	MCD4
9	GPI mannosyltransferase 3 (EC:2.4.1.-) (GPI-MTIII)	Dol-P-Man	PIGB	Q92521	554	9	15q21.3		GPI10
M4	GPI mannosyltransferase 4 (EC:2.4.1.-) (GPI-MTIV)	Dol-P-Man	PIGZ	Q86VD9	579	8	3q29		SMP3
10	GPI-ethanolamine phosphate transferase 3 (GPI-ETIII)	PE	PIGO	Q8TEQ8	1089	14	9p13.3	Hyperphosphatasia with mental retardation syndrome type 2	GPI13
			PIGF	Q07326	219	6	2p21-p16		GPI11
11	GPI-ethanolamine phosphate transferase 2 (GPI-ETII)	PE	PIGG	Q5H8A4	983	12	4p16.3		GPI7
			PIGF	Q07326	219	6	2p21-p16		GPI11
(II) Addition of GPI to precursor protein									
12	GPI-anchor transamidase (GPI-TA)		PIGK	Q92643	395	1	1p31.1		GPI8
			GPAA1	O43292	621	7	8q24.3		GAA1
			PIGS	Q96S52	555	2	17p13.2		GPI17
			PIGT	Q969N2	578	1	20q12-q13.12	Multiple congenital anomalies-hypotonia-seizures syndrome type 3	GPI16
			PIGU	Q9H490	435	9	20q11.22		GAB1

(continued)

Table 2.2 (continued)

Step		Donor substrate	Gene	Entry	Length	TM	Chromosome	Diseases	Yeast homologue
(III) Structural modification of GPI moiety									
1	GPI inositol-deacylase		PGAP1	Q75T13	922	7	2q33.1	Mental retardation, autosomal recessive	BST1
2	Ethanolamine phosphate phosphodiesterase (metallophosphoesterase 1)		PGAP5 (MPPE1)	Q53F39	396	2	18p11.21		CDC1 TED1
3a	GPI phospholipase A2		PGAP3	Q96FM1	320	7	17q12	Hyperphosphatasia with mental retardation syndrome type 4	PER1
3b	Lyso-GPI acyltransferase	Stearyl-CoA ?	PGAP2	Q9UHJ9	254	5	11p15.5	Hyperphosphatasia with mental retardation syndrome type 3	—
			Not identified						GUP1

(Note) Entry number of proteins (entry), number of amino acids (length), and number of transmembrane domains (TM) are obtained from UniProt database

2.3.1 (I) Biosynthesis of Precursor GPI

Precursor GPI is synthesized via more than ten steps on the ER membrane and transferred en bloc to processed proteins by the GPI-transamidase complex as a posttranslational modification. The biosynthetic steps include sequential addition of each component to PI, a flip of the intermediate from the cytosolic to luminal sides (step 3) and lipid remodeling to produce alkyl chain-containing GPI (step 5). Twenty-two genes involved in ten of the 12 steps have been identified, whereas genes for steps 3 and 5 are still unknown.

2.3.1.1 Step (1)

The first step is the transfer of *N*-acetylglucosamine (GlcNAc) to the 6 position of inositol in PI, which produces GlcNAc-PI. The reaction occurs on the cytosolic face of the ER membrane, and uridine diphosphate (UDP)-GlcNAc is used as the GlcNAc donor. Common species of PI are used as acceptors, because the PI moiety in GlcNAc-PI has a chain composition similar to cellular PI as shown by mass spectrometry, namely, both have stearic acid at the *sn*-1 position and an unsaturated acyl chain, such as arachidonic acid, at the *sn*-2 position [27, 40]. The enzyme that mediates this step PI-*N*-acetylglucosaminyltransferase (EC: 2.4.1.198), so-called GPI-GnT, is composed of seven proteins, PIG-A, PIG-C, PIG-H, PIG-P, PIG-Q, PIG-Y, and DPM2, and is one of the most complex glycosyltransferase enzymes [32, 35, 58, 64, 107, 109]. PIG-A, which belongs to the glycosyltransferase family (GT) 4 in CAZy classification, has a binding site for UDP-GlcNAc and a catalytic site. PIG-A, PIG-C, PIG-H, and PIG-P are all indispensable for GPI-GnT activity, and the loss of PIG-Q or PIG-Y causes a severe decrease in GPI-GnT activity, but their precise functions are still unclear. DPM2 is an essential component of the dolichol-phosphate mannose (DPM) synthase complex. Therefore, a defect in DPM2 causes a lack of the donor for all mannoses in GPI biosynthesis [50]. In addition, the loss of DPM2 decreases the GPI-GnT activity to one-third, indicating that synthesis of GPI and DPM may have a common regulation system [109].

2.3.1.2 Step (2)

The second step is de-*N*-acetylation of GlcNAc-PI, resulting in GlcN-PI. This reaction is catalyzed by PIG-L, an *N*-acetylglucosaminyl-phosphatidylinositol de-*N*-acetylase (EC: 3.5.1.89) [68, 110]. PIG-L belongs to an enzyme family that includes *N*-acetyl-1-D-*myo*-inositol-2-amino-2-deoxy-α-D-glucopyranoside (GlcNAc-inositol) deacetylase, which is involved in the biosynthesis of mycothiol, an unusual thiol compound found in *Actinobacteria* [71]. PIG-L has a transmembrane domain in the amino-terminal region, and the other part faces to the cytosol. Therefore, the reaction occurs on the cytosolic face of the ER membrane. PIG-L has consensus sequences, (P/A)-H-(P/A)-DD and HxxH, conserved among this family, which are critical for metal binding [19, 98]. PIG-L activity is enhanced by divalent metals, such as Zn^{2+} [110].

2.3.1.3 Step (3)

The third step is the flip of GlcN-PI from the cytosolic side to the ER luminal side. Since spontaneous flipping of GlcN-PI is considered to be slow, there is likely to be machinery that catalyzes this step. Nevertheless, any molecule involved in this process has not been identified, irrespective of extensive efforts to establish flip-defective mutant cells. This suggests that the flip is catalyzed by multiple functionally redundant proteins or that the protein involved has functions more than solely flipping GlcN-PI and the defect is lethal to cells.

2.3.1.4 Step (4)

The fourth step is the addition of an acyl chain from acyl-CoA, usually palmitoyl-CoA, to the C2 position of inositol, generating GlcN-(acyl)PI. From this step, the biosynthesis is executed on the luminal side. This reaction is catalyzed by PIG-W, the acyltransferase [65]. This acyl chain is removed in the ER immediately after transfer of GPI to proteins. Therefore, this acyl chain may be a hallmark of GPI intermediates that is recognized by key enzymes further downstream in the biosynthetic pathway. Importantly, a defect in PIG-W allows the reactions of a few further steps, but eventually impairs the addition of GPI to proteins and severely decreases the surface expression of GPI-APs [65].

2.3.1.5 Step (5)

It is well known that GPI is synthesized from the diacyl form of PI, but a sizable fraction of the cell-surface mature GPI-APs have the 1-alkyl-2-acyl glycerol form of GPI [40]. A mass spectrometric analysis revealed that the 1-alkyl-2-acyl glycerol form of the GPI intermediate was high in GlcN-(acyl)PI [27]. Thus, this lipid remodeling is positioned as step 5; however, nothing is known about the molecular mechanisms of lipid remodeling. It was shown that remodeling of the diacyl form to 1-alkyl-2-acyl requires the 1-alkyl-glycerone-phosphate synthesis pathway of the peroxisome [37, 38]. Thus, mutant CHO cells defective in either the first or second step in the peroxisome pathway generated only the diacyl form of GPI anchors. Although the exact mechanism is yet to be clarified, this GPI lipid remodeling appears to be a replacement of the entire lipid moiety, including the glycerol part, either diacyl glycerol or phosphatidic acid. 1-Alkyl-glycerone phosphate generated in the peroxisome may be converted to some phospholipid in the ER and thereby acts as a donor for GPI lipid remodeling. It should be noted that acyl chain compositions of GlcN-PI and the diacyl-form GlcN-(acyl)PI are significantly different, indicating that even diacyl GlcN-(acyl)PI is the product of lipid remodeling. We assume that the donor phospholipid consists of 1-alkyl-2-acyl and diacyl forms. Based on the composition of fatty chains, we have proposed that phosphatidylethanolamine (PE) is a good lipid donor candidate [37]. Since no gene involved in the step is known and genetic manipulation is currently not possible, the precise biological significance is unclear, but it was reported that defects of the enzymes catalyzing the alkyl phospholipid in the peroxisome enhance the surface expression of certain GPI-APs, such as uPAR/CD87, indicating that this lipid remodeling may regulate GPI biosynthesis and/or the localization of GPI-APs by altering the physical nature of the lipid moiety in GPI-APs [38].

2.3.1.6 Step (6)

The sixth step, addition of the first mannose from DPM to GlcN of GlcN-(acyl)PI via the α1, 4 linkage, is catalyzed by a complex of PIG-M and PIG-X [4, 51, 78]. Both PIG-M and PIG-X are essential for GPI biosynthesis. PIG-M is a GPI mannosyltransferase 1 (GPI-MTI) that belongs to the GT50 family in CAZy classification. All GPI-MTs (I–IV) are also classified into a GT-C superfamily of integral membrane glycosyltransferases with a modified DxD motif in the first luminal loop [47]. The superfamily includes *N*-glycosylation-related mannosyltransferase (ALG3, ALG9, and ALG12), glycosyltransferases (ALG6, ALG8, and ALG10), and protein *O*-mannosyltransferases (POMT1 and POMT2) [78]. They all use the dolichol-linked sugar as a donor in the ER lumen. It is not known whether the conserved modified DxD motif, such as D/E-D/E and D/ExD/E, binds a divalent cation, similarly to nucleotide-diphosphosugar-dependent transferases of the GT-A superfamily whose conserved DxD motif binds a divalent cation. The replacement of D to A in the conserved DxD motif in PIG-M abolishes enzyme activity [51]. PIG-X stabilizes PIG-M, but the precise function of PIG-M is unclear [4].

2.3.1.7 Step (7)

Step 7 is the addition of the second mannose from donor DPM to Man of Man-GlcN-(acyl)PI, the product of step 6, via the α1, 6 linkage, generating Man-Man-GlcN-(acyl)PI. PIG-V, GPI mannosyltransferase 2 (GPI-MTII), catalyzes this step and belongs to the GT76 family in CAZy classification and the GT-C superfamily [36]. There is a WD motif close to the C-terminus of the first luminal loop, and the motif is conserved among various species. Mutation of the WD motif abolishes enzyme activity [36]. It has been demonstrated that PIG-V is a limiting enzyme among the three GPI mannosyltransferases (GPI-GTI-III) [21].

2.3.1.8 Step (8)

The eighth step is the addition of EtNP from PE to the C2 position of the first mannose of Man-Man-GlcN-(acyl)PI as a side branch. This reaction is catalyzed by PIG-N, GPI-EtNP transferase 1 (GPI-ETI) [25]. Three GPI-EtNP transferases,

GPI-ETI, II, and III (see below), form a family and have a type I phosphodiesterase domain in their N-terminal halves. YW3548/BE49385A, a terpenoid lactone that is obtained from *Codinea simplex*, inhibits PIG-N activity [25, 88]. Although the EtNP is a side branch, this modification is conserved among mammalian cells and is critical for GPI biosynthesis, and the loss of PIG-N leads to a reduction in surface expression of GPI-APs lacking this side branch. The basis for the reduced levels may be either a decrease in the generation of GPI-APs because of inefficient recognition by enzymes further down the biosynthetic pathway, especially the GPI-transamidase complex, or higher turnover of the side-branch-less GPI-APs, or both [100].

2.3.1.9 Step (9)

The third mannose from donor DPM is transferred to the second mannose of Man-(EtNP)Man-GlcN-(acyl)PI, the product of step 8, via the α1, 2 linkage, generating Man-Man-(EtNP)Man-GlcN-(acyl)PI. PIG-B is a GPI mannosyltransferase 3 (GPI-MTIII), which belongs to the GT22 family in CAZy classification and the GT-C superfamily, and is essential for this step [91].

2.3.1.10 Step (10)

This step is an addition of EtNP from donor PE to the C6 position of the third mannose of Man-Man-(EtNP)Man-GlcN-(acyl)PI, which is catalyzed by the PIG-O/PIG-F complex, GPI-EtNP transferase 3 (GPI-ETIII) [24, 31]. Because this EtNP links GPI covalently to the processed C-terminus of proteins, the modification is essential for the biosynthesis of GPI-APs. PIG-O belongs to the GPI-EtNP transferase family and is a catalytic subunit of the enzyme complex. PIG-F forms a complex either with PIG-O or PIG-G, a GPI-ETII (see below), and stabilizes the catalytic subunits. Since PIG-F binds to PIG-O and PIG-G through distinct molecular domains, PIG-O, PIG-G, and PIG-F may form a trimer to complete their modifications more efficiently, although a different possibility was proposed, in which PIG-O and PIG-G compete for binding to PIG-F [85, 87]. Truncated PIG-F that retains the ability to bind PIG-O and PIG-G cannot complement the defective phenotype of PIG-F mutants, suggesting that PIG-F has functions other than stabilizing enzyme complexes [87].

2.3.1.11 Step (11)

The final step to complete GPI biosynthesis is the addition of EtNP from donor PE to the C6 position of the second mannose of EtNP-Man-Man-(EtNP)Man-GlcN-(acyl)PI, resulting in EtNP-Man-(EtNP)Man-(EtNP)Man-GlcN-(acyl)PI, a mature

GPI. This reaction is catalyzed by the PIG-G/PIG-F complex, a GPI-EtNP transferase 2 (GPI-ETII) [85]. An RNAi-mediated knockdown of PIG-G was found to cause accumulation of the intermediate product synthesized in step10, indicating that step 11 follows step 10. Nevertheless, the surface expression levels of GPI-APs did not change, most likely due to the alternative use of the product synthesized in step 10 to produce GPI-APs. The EtNP attached in this step is removed after linkage of the GPI with proteins (see 3.3.3.2 Step 2)

2.3.2 (II) Addition of GPI to Precursor Proteins

Finally, the mature GPI is transferred to precursor proteins by a GPI-transamidase complex. The C-terminal portion of the precursor protein, so-called GPI-attachment signal peptide, is removed, and the resultant new carboxyl amino acid whose position is the ω site is covalently linked with an amino group of EtNP at the third mannose of the mature GPI. The GPI-attachment signal peptide does not have a conserved consensus sequence but has the following characteristics: (1) small side chain amino acids are located at the ω and ω + 2 sites; (2) a stretch of 5 – 10 hydrophilic amino acids start from the ω + 3 site; and (3) this is followed by a stretch of 10 – 20 hydrophobic amino acids ending at the C-terminus [30, 96]. The precursor protein also has an amino-terminal signal peptide for ER translocation. It is believed that ER translocation occurs co-translationally in a signal recognition particle (SRP)-dependent manner. However, it was reported recently for yeast GPI-APs that some, but not all, precursor GPI-APs are entirely translated in the cytosol before entering the ER lumen. The translated precursor proteins are recognized by GET3 (guided entry of tail-anchored proteins 3) along with Apj1 and Jjj3, both are Hsp40 family members, and targeted to translocon machinery in the ER [5]. The GPI-attachment signal is cleaved by GPI transamidase after transversing into the ER lumen. It remains to be solved whether TRC40, a mammalian homologue of Get3, plays a similar role on GPI-APs. The GPI-transamidase complex is composed of five proteins, PIG-K, GPAA1, PIG-S, PIG-T, and PIG-U, and all of these proteins are indispensable for GPI-transamidase activity [7, 18, 22, 26, 75, 76]. PIG-K is a C13 cysteine protease with a predicted structure resembling those of gingipain R and caspases. PIG-K cleaves the GPI-attachment signal peptide of the precursor protein and forms an intermediate with the protein via a thioester bond between the catalytic cysteine residue and a carboxyl group of ω site amino acid [57]. GPAA1 binds GPI at the carboxyl transmembrane region and was recently reported to be a M28 family metallo-peptide-synthetase that catalyzes the peptide bond formation between EtNP at the third mannose and the ω site amino acid [12, 99]. PIG-T covalently binds PIG-K through a disulfide bond and the destruction of the disulfide bond impairs GPI-transamidase activity; although, the precise functions of PIG-T as well as PIG-S and PIG-U are not known [77].

2.3.3 (III) Structural Modifications of the GPI Moiety of GPI-APs

GPI-APs synthesized in the ER by the addition of GPI to precursor proteins are transported to the cell surface through the Golgi apparatus. During transport, the GPI moiety is further modified in several steps. These modifications are executed by post-GPI-attachment to proteins (PGAP) proteins as described below. Removal of the acyl chain attached to inositol by PGAP1 (step 1) and removal of EtNP attached to the second mannose by PGAP5 (step 2) occur in the ER, whereas fatty acid remodeling catalyzed by PGAP3 and PGAP2 occurs in the Golgi apparatus. Unique characteristics in structural remodeling occurring in the ER are that the moieties to be removed by PGAP1 and PGAP5 have been added to GPI intermediates during GPI biosynthesis; therefore, the significance of these moieties should be evaluated.

2.3.3.1 Step (1)

An acyl chain, typically palmitic acid, is added to the C2 position of inositol by PIG-W during GPI biosynthesis, as mentioned above. This acyl chain is removed soon after GPI is attached to precursor proteins by PGAP1 [94]. PGAP1 is an ER-resident multi-spanning membrane protein that has a lipase motif GxSxG on the luminal side. Bacillus PI-specific phospholipase C (PI-PLC) is very useful to examine whether a certain surface protein is anchored by GPI, because most GPI-APs are cleaved by PI-PLC and detached from the cell surface, which results in a clear decrease in surface expression of GPI-APs when examined by flow cytometry. As an exception, GPI-APs harboring an extra lipid chain at the inositol are resistant to PI-PLC, because the hydroxyl group at the C2 position is used to produce cyclic phosphoinositol in the process of PI-PLC cleavage [103]. Moreover, GPI-APs expressed on the surface of red blood cells, which harbor an extra inositol acyl chain due to the lack of deacylase activity, are resistant to PI-PLC [82]. It seems that the GPI anchor with three fatty chains is more advantageous than those with two chains in preventing spontaneous release of GPI-APs from the surface of very long-living red blood cells.

In cultured cells, a defect in PGAP1 causes accumulation of GPI-APs in the ER due to inefficient exit from the ER [17, 94]. The slowed ER exit is caused by impaired binding of GPI-APs to the p24 family cargo receptor complex, which is also observed in PGAP5-defective cells (see below) [9, 17, 93]. The defect in PGAP1 also prevents fatty acid remodeling in the Golgi by inhibiting PGAP3 activity (see Step 3 in this section) [49]. Therefore, GPI-APs with unusual GPI structures are expressed on the cell surface, but importantly the surface expression levels of various GPI-APs are comparable to those in normal cells [94]. Nevertheless, studies with *Pgap1* knockout mice demonstrated the critical significance of the deacylation of inositol. These mice had developmental defects such as otocephaly or holoprosencephaly accompanying impaired formation of the face and jaw, and most mice die immediately after birth, most likely due to the failure of milk uptake [56, 97, 112]. The *Pgap1* knockout males who survived the critical neonatal period demonstrated infertility caused by their sperm being incapable of climbing up the oviduct [97]. The inherited *PGAP1* deficiency in humans was recently reported [66]. The affected individuals show intellectual disability as a main symptom in addition to developmental abnormalities, yet somewhat different from those observed in mice. The basis for the defects is considered to be different from the bases in other inherited GPI deficiencies, which cause a decrease in the surface expression of GPI-APs. The precise mechanisms of abnormalities caused by *PGAP1* deficiency remain unclear, but one possible explanation is that the regulated cleavages and releases of GPI-APs from the cell surface by GPI-cleaving enzymes, such as GPI-specific phospholipase D (GPI-PLD) [106], angiotensin-converting enzyme (ACE) [14, 41], and glycerophosphodiester phosphodiesterase (GDE) family [79], are inhibited in a similar manner to PI-PLC. Alternatively, the altered physical nature of GPI caused by the presence of an extra acyl chain and an *sn*2-linked unsaturated chain due to impaired fatty lipid remodeling in the Golgi may affect the behavior of and signal transduction by GPI-APs, similar to PGAP3 deficiency (see Step3).

2.3.3.2 Step (2)

This step is the removal of EtNP attached to the second mannose of GPI and is catalyzed by PGAP5 [15]. PGAP5 has a phosphodiesterase motif and requires manganese ion for activity. PGAP5 also has an ER-retention signal KxKxx and recycles between the ER and Golgi, but the removal of EtNP is considered to take place in the ER, because this process is required for the efficient binding to the p24 cargo receptor and therefore efficient exit from the ER [15]. This is supported by the finding that a defect in PGAP5 causes a delay in transport from the ER. PGAP5 seems to function after PGAP1, because PGAP1 is an ER-resident protein, whereas PGAP5 is recycled. If surface GPI-APs in PGAP1-defective cells maintain EtNP on the second mannose, it would provide definitive evidence to show that PGAP5 functions after PGAP1. The EtNP is added to the second mannose by GPI-ETII in the last step of GPI biosynthesis just before its transfer to precursor protein and is removed in the ER after production of GPI-APs. Interestingly, in cultured cells no defective phenotypes in surface expression and transport of GPI-APs are observed when PIG-G, a catalytic subunit of GPI-ETII, is defective. This is not surprising because the structure of the GPI in GPI-APs is normal in PIG-G defective cells. Therefore, the significance of EtNP added to the second mannose remains unresolved.

Yeast has two structural homologues of PGAP5, Ted1p and Cdc1p. Manzano-Lopez, et al. reported that Ted1p is required for removal of EtNP linked to the second mannose and, therefore, is the functional homologue of PGAP5 [52]. EtNP linked to the first mannose remains in mammalian GPI-APs, whereas it is removed in yeast during GPI-AP maturation. Vazquez, et al. demonstrated that Cdc1p is involved in removal of EtNP from the first mannose, suggesting that Cdc1p is also a phosphodiesterase [102].

2.3.3.3 Step (3)

The *sn*-2-linked fatty acid of the GPI moiety in GPI-APs transported to the Golgi apparatus is remodeled in this step. As described above, the lipid part of GlcN-(acyl)PI is remodeled in the ER and after this remodeling, GPI has an unsaturated lipid chain, such as arachidonic acid (C20:4) and docosapentaenoic acid (C22:5) at the *sn*-2 position of the glycerol backbone [27, 40]. Conversely, GPI expressed on the cell surface has a saturated lipid chain, mainly stearic acid (C18:0), at the *sn*-2 position [49, 55]. This replacement termed "GPI-fatty acid remodeling" is carried out in the Golgi [49]. This step involves at least two proteins working consecutively, PGAP3 and PGAP2 [49, 95]. First, an unsaturated fatty acid is removed by PGAP3. PGAP3 is considered to be a phospholipase A2, because PGAP3 belongs to a superfamily of transmembrane hydrolases including an alkaline ceramidase. Additionally, mutagenesis of putative catalytic amino acids conserved among this superfamily members impaired PGAP3 activity, although there is no direct experimental evidence [16, 81]. Defect of PGAP1 activity inhibits the cleavage catalyzed by PGAP3, leading to surface expression of un-remodeled GPI-APs with an extra acyl chain at inositol [49]. The defect of PGAP3 also causes the surface expression of un-remodeled GPI-APs, accompanying a decrease in the surface expression levels to various extents ranging from almost normal to one-third of the normal level. The variation in the observed levels may depend on proteins, cell types, and animal species [62, 83, 105]. Although the precise mechanisms responsible for the decrease remains to be solved, fatty acid remodeling may render membrane-association of GPI-APs more stable either by enhancing the interaction of GPI with cholesterol and sphingolipids or by inducing GPI-dependent dimer/oligomer formation [89]. GPI facilitates the packing of GPI-APs into specialized microdomains, so-called lipid rafts, through the straight saturated lipid chains [86]. Defective GPI-fatty acid remodeling alters the physical nature and weakens the association of GPI-APs with lipid rafts due to the unsaturated lipid chains [33, 49, 83]. It may also enhance the sensitivity to lipases/GPIase, which leads to abnormal secretion and decrease of surface expression [41]. There are reports regarding *Pgap3*-knockout mice and inherited diseases defective in *PGAP3* [28, 62, 105]. *Pgap3*-knockout mice show growth retardation and minor abnormalities such as kinked tail and short heads, and a significant number of aged *Pgap3*-knockout mice develop autoimmune-like symptoms [105]. PGAP3-deficient patients exhibit hyperphosphatasia, which is caused by secretion of GPI-anchored alkaline phosphatases, growth retardation, intellectual disability, and seizure, indicating the biological significance of GPI-fatty acid remodeling [28].

The second part of this step is the addition of a saturated fatty acid, mostly stearic acid to the hydrolyzed *sn*-2 position [49]. The acyl donor is most likely acyl-CoA because acyl-CoA is used in similar GPI-fatty acid remodeling in yeast [10]. PGAP2 is essential for this step [95]. PGAP2 is a transmembrane protein and has no similarity to known acyltransferases. At present, it is unclear whether PGAP2 is an enzyme or a regulator. If PGAP2 functions as a regulator, then other unknown enzymes must be involved. If PGAP2 function is impaired, GPI-APs bearing the lyso-form GPI are transported to the cell surface and are promptly cleaved by unknown enzymes with phospholipase D activity on the cell surface or after spontaneous release from the membrane because of the weakened membrane-anchoring capacity of lyso-GPI. Thus, surface GPI-APs are significantly decreased (usually below one-tenth of the wild-type levels) in PGAP2-deficient cells.

2.4 PIGA and Its Somatic Mutation in PNH

2.4.1 PIGA *Gene*

PIGA was identified by expression cloning using a GPI-deficient cell line JY5 as a recipient of a cDNA library [58]. JY5 cells were derived from human B-lymphoblastoid JY cells as a GPI-AP-deficient mutant and were later shown to be deficient in the first step in GPI biosynthesis and belong to complementation group "class A" of GPI-deficient mutant cells. After stable transfection of a HeLa cell cDNA library, JY5 cells with restored cell-surface expression of CD59 were collected by a flow cytometer, and this enrichment process was repeated three times before recovery of transfected plasmids. Cloned cDNAs were individually transfected to JY5 cells to assess the ability to restore CD59 expression. In this way, *PIGA* cDNA was cloned.

PIGA encodes the PIG-A protein, a catalytic subunit of GPI-N-acetylglucosamine (GlcNAc) transferase (GPI-GnT) that mediates the first reaction of GPI biosynthesis. The *PIGA* gene consists of six exons located in the short arm of the X-chromosome (Fig. 2.3) [29, 92]. It was initially reported that *PIGA* resides at Xp22.1 [92], but was later reported to reside at Xp22.2. *PIGA* is the only X-linked gene among the approximately 30 genes involved in biosynthesis, attachment to proteins, structural remodeling of GPI, and transport of GPI-APs (Table 2.2).

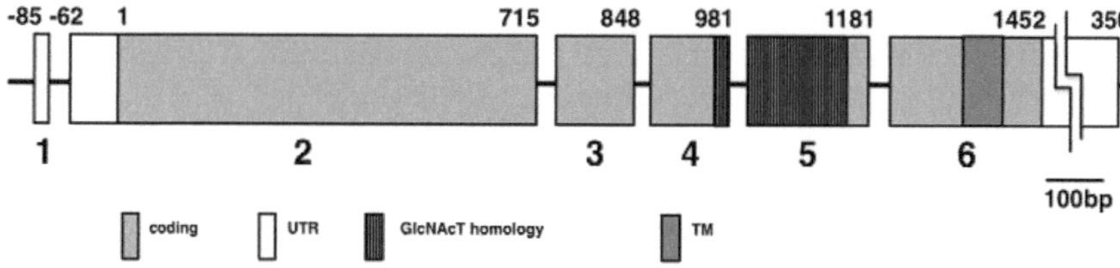

Fig. 2.3 Schematics of *PIGA* gene. *PIGA* consists of 6 exons. Coding regions (*shaded*) spans exons 2–6. 5′ untranslated region (UTR) spans exons 1 and 2. *Black* striped areas, region homologous to GlcNAc transferase; *gray* area, transmembrane domain (TM). Nucleotide numbers of mRNA with A in the initiation codon as 1 are shown above exons. Bars between exons indicate introns, and flanking exons 1 and 6 indicate intragenic regions

2.4.2 PIG-A Protein

PIG-A is an ER-resident, single-pass transmembrane protein consisting of 484 amino acids. PIG-A consists of an N-terminal large cytoplasmic region, a transmembrane domain, and a short C-terminal luminal domain [108]. The cytoplasmic domain contains a binding site for UDP-GlcNAc and has sequence homology to glycosyltransferases belonging to the glycosyltransferase family 4 [42]. PIG-A and six other proteins, PIG-C, PIG-H, PIG-P, PIG-Q, PIG-Y, and DPM2, form a complex [107, 109]. The complex solubilized from cell lysates by 1 % digitonin and purified by affinity beads had GPI-GnT activity in vitro when incubated with bovine PI and UDP-GlcNAc [107]. GPI-GnT is the most complex glycosyltransferase known.

2.4.3 Outcome of PIGA Defect

Proteins that undergo GPI anchoring are translated as preproproteins bearing an N-terminal signal peptide for translocation across the ER membrane and a C-terminal signal peptide that directs GPI attachment [30, 96]. After translocation into the ER lumen, the N-terminal signal peptide is cleaved, generating a proprotein, which is thought to be transiently associated with the ER membrane via a hydrophobic part of the C-terminal signal peptide. GPI transamidase recognizes the C-terminal GPI-attachment signal peptide, cleaves it, and replaces the peptide with preassembled GPI, generating an immature, ER-form, GPI-anchored protein. Complete loss of *PIGA* function by mutation causes complete loss of GPI-GnT activity and a lack of the GPI precursor. In the absence of any GPI intermediate, GPI transamidase does not cleave or cleaves only very inefficiently the C-terminal signal peptide, and the proprotein accumulates and is eventually degraded presumably by ER-associated degradation (ERAD) [63]. This results in complete deficiency of the cell-surface GPI-APs. If a *PIGA* mutation causes a partial loss of PIG-A activity, an amount of the GPI precursor decreases, and a fraction of the proproteins that normally receive GPI attachment may decrease. Those proproteins that do not receive GPI are subjected to ERAD, resulting in a partial deficiency of the cell-surface expression of GPI-APs. Different proproteins have different C-terminal GPI-attachment signal sequences. The efficiencies of recognition by GPI transamidase are thought to be different among various signal sequences. Under partial loss of GPI, various proproteins compete with each other for the limited amounts of GPI. Proteins with weaker C-terminal signal sequences may be less likely to be GPI-anchored and, thus, more likely to be degraded by ERAD and lost from the cell surface.

All cell-surface GPI-APs, including two complement regulatory proteins DAF and CD59, are completely deficient in type III PNH cells, in which PIG-A activity is null. GPI-APs are partially deficient on type II PNH cells, in which PIG-A activity is partially lost [13]. On type II erythrocytes, CD59 is sometimes nearly completely lost, whereas DAF is only weakly reduced, suggesting that the C-terminal signal sequence of DAF is stronger than that of CD59.

2.4.4 Somatic Mutations of *PIGA* in PNH

Somatic mutation of *PIGA* was first found in a CD59- and DAF-deficient B-lymphoblastoid cell line established from a patient with PNH [92]. This mutation was a single-base deletion in a splice donor site in intron 3, causing deletion of the exon 3 in mRNA. This mutation was not found in a CD59- and DAF-positive B-lymphoblastoid cell line from the same patient, indicating a somatic origin of the mutation. The patient was female and the mutation was found in one of the two X chromosomes. Only the abnormally spliced *PIGA* mRNA was found in the affected cells; therefore, the mutation existed in the active X-chromosome. The same mutation was found in granulocytes and lymphocytes from the same patient, suggesting that the somatic mutation occurred in the hematopoietic stem cell that gave rise to both affected granulocytes and lymphocytes [92].

Analyses of *PIGA* in B-lymphoblastoid cell lines and/or granulocytes from approximately 20 patients with PNH demonstrated *PIGA* somatic mutations in each patient [8, 59]. Therefore, it was established that GPI deficiency in PNH is caused by somatic mutations in the *PIGA* gene.

As described above, only *PIGA* is X-linked and all other genes involved in GPI-anchored biosynthesis and protein attachment are autosomal. For X-linked *PIGA*, one hit of loss-of-function mutation to the active allele in females or to one allele in males causes GPI-deficiency, whereas for autosomal genes, such as *PIGB* and *PIGC*, hits to two alleles are required to generate a GPI-deficient cell. The frequency of two somatic mutations of the same gene in a cell is so low that there is no such case found to date, and all patients with PNH analyzed in these studies were due to *PIGA* mutations.

As of 2000, data on 174 somatic *PIGA* mutations had been accumulated and their spectrum summarized [67]. *PIGA* somatic mutations were predominantly small mutations, and only three were deletions of the entire or a large part of *PIGA*. Most of the mutations were unique to respective patients, and only 16 of them were found in more than one patient. They were widely distributed in all coding exons and splice sites. There is no obvious mutation hot spot in *PIGA* [48]. Approximately one-third of the somatic mutations were base substitutions, including nonsense mutations, splice site mutations, and missense mutations causing amino acid changes. Another one-third was single-base deletions, causing primarily frame shifts or less frequently splice abnormalities. The rest of the mutations include single-base insertions, deletions or insertions of several bases, and combinations of small deletions and insertions [67]. A similar spectrum of *PIGA* somatic mutations was found by recent whole exome sequencing of PNH cells, although somewhat higher frequency of large deletions was found [84].

At least 25–30% of the patients with PNH had more than two independent *PIGA* mutants. There is a report of a patient bearing four PNH clones [13, 73]. A recent whole exome sequence study demonstrated six somatic mutations in a patient [84]. In many cases with multiple clones, one is predominant and the others are minor. Therefore, finding oligo clones is not rare.

2.4.5 Clinical Manifestation of PIGA Somatic Mutations

At least 150 different proteins are anchored at the cell surface via GPI (Table 2.1). Complete or severe partial loss of PIG-A function results in complete or partial lack of many, if not all, GPI-APs from the cell surface. In fact, multiple GPI-APs such as CD16, DAF, and CD59 are reduced or lost from blood granulocytes bearing *PIGA* mutations. GPI-AP deficiency affects only a fraction of hematopoietic cells because *PIGA* somatic mutations occur in hematopoietic stem cells. One would expect that a wide range of clinical symptoms would result because of *PIGA* mutations; however, it is remarkable that complement-mediated intravascular hemolysis is by far the most prominent symptom [80]. Host cells are protected from membrane-destructive action of complement by cell-surface complement regulatory proteins. In particular, DAF and CD59, GPI-anchored complement regulators, are critical for red blood cell protection. Patients with PNH have clonally expanded affected red blood cells characterized by an absence of DAF and CD59. Those affected red blood cells are highly sensitive to complement-mediated membrane damage, causing hemolytic attack after or during infection or other events that systemically activate complement. Venous thrombosis is another common clinical symptom, which is also triggered by complement activation [80].

2.4.6 PIGA Somatic Mutations in Healthy Individuals and Patients with Idiopathic Aplastic Anemia (AA)

It should be noted that *PIGA* somatic mutations are not unique to PNH. The majority of healthy individuals have small numbers of CD59-deficient granulocytes in their peripheral blood (about 0.002 % of the granulocytes were CD59 negative) [3]. *PIGA* somatic mutations similar to those found in PNH were found in the CD59-negative granulocytes concentrated by a cell sorter. In one case, the same mutation was found again 65 days later but disappeared 174 days later, suggesting that the mutation existed in myeloid progenitor cells. Nakao and his group demonstrated the presence of hematopoietic stem cells with a *PIGA* somatic mutation in bone marrow from a healthy donor by analyzing a case of bone marrow transplantation to a patient with AA, in whom donor-derived GPI-AP-negative granulocytes appeared after transplantation [60].

Many of the patients with idiopathic AA have significantly higher numbers of CD59-/DAF-negative granulocytes. It was reported that greater than 0.03 % of granulocytes from 88 % of patients with untreated AA were CD59/DAF negative [104]. These CD59-/DAF-negative granulocytes were usually of clonal origin (bearing one kind of mutation), suggesting that the mutant granulocytes have clonally expanded to some extent.

2.5 PIGT and Its Mutations in PNH (PIGT-PNH)

If one allele of a particular autosomal PIG gene is congenitally inactive because of a mutation, the situation of that PIG gene in that particular individual is like *PIGA*, i.e., one hit of loss-of-function somatic mutation in hematopoietic stem cells causes a GPI-AP-deficient stem cell clone. A case of PNH occurring in such a way was found recently [43]. Analysis of *PIGA* in blood cells from a female patient with PNH did not find a somatic mutation, and accordingly ultra-deep sequencing of all exons of all known genes involved in GPI-anchored synthesis was carried out. Germ line and somatic mutations were identified in the *PIGT* gene, which is located on chromosome 20. The germ line mutation, confirmed by its presence in blood cells and buccal epithelial cells, was a single-base substitution in the splice acceptor site of intron 10. The somatic mutation, confirmed by the presence in granulocytes and the absence in T-lymphocytes, was an 8.2-Mb deletion, including the entire *PIGT* gene. The two mutations resided in different alleles, indicating that *PIGT* activity in the mutant cells should be very low, if not negative, and consistent with GPI-AP deficiency.

PIG-T is a component of GPI transamidase that attaches preassembled GPI to proteins [75]. GPI transamidase consists of five subunits, PIG-K, GPAA1, PIG-S, PIG-T, and PIG-U. Within the complex, PIG-T acts to stabilize the complex and is covalently linked by a disulfide bond to PIG-K, a cysteine protease-like subunit, which cleaves the C-terminal GPI-attachment signal peptide [77]. In *PIGT*-defective cells, in which GPI-transamidase activity is reduced, the C-terminal GPI-attachment signal peptide is not cleaved, resulting in the degradation of proproteins in the ER [63]. GPI is assembled but is not transferred to proteins and accumulates [75]. The accumulation of preassembled GPI is a unique condition of *PIGT*-defective cells, which does not occur in *PIGA*-defective cells.

The patient with *PIGT*-PNH had urticaria before the onset of PNH and developed ulcerative colitis after the onset of PNH and initiation of eculizumab therapy [43]. Whether the *PIGT* mutation and its consequences, such as accumulation of GPI, are causally related to these immune-related symptoms not usually seen in *PIGA*-PNH is currently not clear.

2.6 CD59 Deficiency

A male Japanese patient with CD59 deficiency showing intravascular hemolysis similar to PNH was reported in 1990 [111]. CD59 on his erythrocytes was absent, whereas the DAF level was normal, indicating that CD59 is critical for protection of erythrocytes from complement. CD59 was deficient not only in blood cells but also in skin fibroblasts. His parents were cousins and both had a partial decrease in CD59 levels. The patient had a homozygous mutation in CD59 and his parents were heterozygous for the mutation [61].

The second case of CD59 deficiency was found in a familial chronic hemolysis in infants of Northern-African Jewish origin in four unrelated families [70]. The affected individuals had a homozygous mutation in the CD59 gene different from the mutation found in the Japanese patient.

The third case of CD59 deficiency was found in Germany, and this patient had yet another homozygous mutation in the *CD59* gene [23]. Although only complement-mediated intravascular hemolysis was reported for the Japanese patient, relapsing immune-mediated polyneuropathy was seen in the second set of patients [70], and progressive neurological impairment was observed in the third patient [23], in addition to PNH-like intravascular hemolysis. This set of results indicates that complement activation can occur on the surface of neuronal cells and that their protection is dependent upon CD59.

2.7 Inherited GPI Deficiency (IGD)

Male *Piga* knockout mice were lethal in the early stage of embryogenesis [74]. Heterozygous *Piga* knockout female mice, in which tissues become mosaic in expression of Pig-a protein due to X-chromosomal localization of the *Piga* gene, developed to near term but were not born, showing abnormal development of the head [74]. Therefore, GPI biosynthesis is essential for embryonic development, and systemic complete deficiency in GPI biosynthesis would not be compatible with birth. In PNH, where most of the *PIGA* mutations caused complete GPI deficiency, the mutations occur after birth and affect only hematopoietic cells, leading to manifestation as an acquired hemolytic disorder. In contrast, individuals with GPI deficiency caused by mutations in germ line PIG and PGAP genes have been recently found. In these individuals, mutations are of hypomorphic nature and consequently GPI deficiency is partial. Currently, individuals with mutations in 12 genes involved in GPI biosynthesis and remodeling have been reported [2, 11, 20, 28, 34, 44–46, 53, 54, 66, 72]. Expression of GPI-AP on blood cells from patients is decreased only in granulocytes and that on red blood cells is almost normal, so IGD patients do not exhibit hemolytic attack. The major symptoms of IGDs include intellectual disability, epilepsy, coarse facial features, and multiple organ anomalies. These symptoms vary in severity depending upon the degree of the defect and/or position in the pathway of the affected gene.

2.7.1 Inherited PIGA Deficiency

The first cases of inherited *PIGA* deficiency were reported by Johnston and colleagues in 2012 [34]. There have been five reports, which include seven families of *PIGA* deficiency [6, 39, 90, 101]. Johnston analyzed a family with an X-linked lethal disorder involving cleft palate, neonatal seizures, contractures, central nervous system (CNS) structural malformations (a thin corpus callosum, white-matter immaturity, no septum pellucidum, a dilated left lateral ventricle, and a small cerebellum), and other anomalies. By an X-chromosome exome sequencing screen of an affected boy, they identified a single nonsense *PIGA* mutation, c.1234C > T, which predicts p.Arg412*. Transfection of a mutant p.Arg412* PIG-A construct into *PIGA*-null cells showed partial restoration of GPI-APs, suggesting that this mutant *PIGA* has residual function. Another affected boy had the same mutation. This mutation was derived from their mother. Although the mother was expected to be a mosaic for PIG-A expression, GPI-AP levels of her blood cells determined by FACS analysis were normal and she had no clinical abnormalities. It is most likely that GPI-AP-deficient cells generated by inactivation of the X-chromosome bearing the intact *PIGA* allele may be eliminated during development.

We found five individuals from four families of *PIGA* deficiency among 172 patients with early onset epileptic encephalopathy, including early myoclonic encephalopathy, Ohtahara syndrome, and West syndrome, in Japan [39]. Severe forms involved myoclonus and asymmetrical suppression bursts on electroencephalogram (EEG), organ anomalies with a dysmorphic face, and delayed myelination with restricted diffusion patterns in specific areas of brain stem. One patient showed severe hydronephrosis caused by the vesicoureteral reflux and hepatoblastoma with facial dysmorphism, which resembled Schinzel-Giedion syndrome. The less severe form presented with intellectual disability and treatable seizures without facial dysmorphism.

Suwoboda and colleagues reported three male patients from a single family of *PIGA* deficiency (a single amino acid deletion, p.Leu110del) [90]. Affected boys were born without anomalies and were neurologically normal prior to onset of seizures at around 6 months of age. One died at 7 years, the other died at 16 years and one remains alive. All boys had ichthyosis or seborrheic dermatitis to varying degrees, progressive neurologic abnormalities, oral abnormalities including microdontia, widely spaced and pointed teeth, and gingival overgrowth. They also developed progressive hepatosplenomegaly and systemic iron overload. The authors suggested that those disorders should be designated as the Ferro-Cerebro-Cutaneous syndrome. Those symptoms may be due to reduced expression of a GPI-AP, hemojuvelin, which regulates iron levels. Van der Crabben and colleagues reported a Caucasian boy with a missense mutation (c.278C > T, p.Pro93Leu) in the *PIGA* gene [101]. The patient had accelerated linear growth, obesity, central hypotonia, severe refractory epilepsy, cardiac anomalies (Atrial septal defect), and mild facial dysmorphic features. He had no teeth and showed deepened plantar creases. He showed mildly elevated alkaline phosphatase levels and CNS anomalies consisting of progressive cerebral atrophy, insufficient myelination, and cortical MRI signal abnormalities. Belet and colleagues reported a large Belgian family diagnosed with X-linked infantile spasm syndrome in five affected males suffering from profound retardation, axial hypotonia, epileptic seizures, and hypsarrhythmia [6]. Sequence analysis resulted in a frameshift that generates a stop codon after amino acid 28 (p.Y26Lfs*3) in the *PIGA* gene. In these patients, the second methionine at position 37 may be used for the translation of a 36 residue shorter PIG-A, which had partial activity.

Expression of various GPI-APs is reduced to various levels according to the degree of decreased activities of the mutant PIG-A proteins. Additionally, patients' symptoms are more variable because of their genetic background. Thus, inherited GPI deficiencies show a broad spectrum of symptoms.

2.7.2 IGD Other Than PIGA Deficiency

The first cases of inherited GPI deficiency were identified by homozygosity mapping analysis of two familial cases with venous thrombosis and seizures that were inherited in an autosomal recessive manner in two independent consanguineous families [2]. Three young affected individuals had exactly the same homozygous base substitution in the promoter region of the *PIGM* gene that disrupted an Sp1 binding site, resulting in decreased transcription of *PIGM*. PIG-M is an α4-mannosyltransferase involved in transfer of the second mannose. Reduction in *PIGM* transcription caused a partial decrease in this essential mannosyltransferase and resulted in a partial decrease in the cell-surface expression of GPI-APs. These individuals did not have abnormality in organogenesis, suggesting that *PIGM* expression during embryogenesis was sufficiently high and the decrease in transcription affected GPI-AP levels after completion of embryogenesis. Cell-surface levels of GPI-APs, such as CD59 and DAF, were only slightly reduced in blood granulocytes, but were not affected in red blood cells, and the individuals showed no signs of hemolysis. Two had hepatic vein thrombosis, which is often seen in patients with PNH, suggesting some common basis of the prominent symptoms associated with GPI deficiency.

The decreased transcription of *PIGM* due to disruption of an Sp1 site was partially restored by incubation of B-lymphoblastoid cells from the affected individuals with sodium butyrate at 10 mM for 3 days [1]. The surface expression of GPI-APs was also partially restored. Because one of the individuals had intractable seizures, she was administered sodium butyrate, and after a few months of treatment, a significant increase in the surface expression of GPI-APs on granulocytes was observed, and this treatment ameliorated her conditions immensely with the patient being able to walk and eat by herself.

The second case and most of the later cases of inherited GPI deficiency were identified by whole exome sequencing of individuals with rare inherited diseases [45]. Mutations in *PIGV* and *PIGO* genes were found in individuals with a rare autosomal recessive disease termed Mabry syndrome or hyperphosphatasia with mental retardation syndrome (HPMRS), characterized by elevated serum alkaline phosphatase levels usually associated with intellectual disability, developmental delay, seizures and characteristic facial dysmorphism, and sometimes brain tissue atrophy, brachytelephalangy, Hirschsprung's megacolon, anal stenosis, and other anomalies. Partial decreases in the level of one or a few GPI-APs were found in blood granulocytes [44, 45]. Among them, CD16 is the most sensitive GPI-AP marker to diagnose GPI deficiency. CD59 and DAF on red blood cells are not affected, consistent with a lack of hemolysis among these individuals. Elevated serum alkaline phosphatase is due to a release of tissue-nonspecific alkaline phosphatase (TNAP) from cells. In *PIGV*- and *PIGO*-defective cells, the amounts of complete GPI decrease due to a reduction in GPI biosynthesis, and a fraction of TNAP precursors do not receive GPI. Under such conditions with *PIGV* or *PIGO* deficiency, GPI transamidase cleaves the C-terminal GPI-attachment signal peptide and generates a substrate-enzyme intermediate linked by a thioester bond. The intermediate is attacked by water instead of GPI, and the soluble TNAP thus generated is then secreted [63]. TNAP precursors that are not attacked by GPI transamidase are subjected to ER-associated degradation. The fraction of TNAP precursor secreted or degraded appears to be dependent on which step in the biosynthetic pathway is defective. In individuals with *PIGA* mutations, hyperphosphatasia is not seen or occurs only mildly [34, 39, 101]. Hyperphosphatasia has also not been reported for patients with PNH. It appears that ER-associated degradation dominates in *PIGA* defective cells, in which no GPI intermediate accumulates. In contrast, GPI intermediates are accumulated in *PIGV* and *PIGO* defective cells. It seems that GPI transamidase more actively attacks proprotein and generates soluble TNAP when some GPI intermediates accumulate than when no GPI intermediate accumulates. It is noteworthy that in two cases of inherited *PIGT* deficiency, hypophosphatasia, rather than hyperphosphatasia, was reported [46, 69], consistent with GPI-transamidase-mediated removal of the GPI-attachment signal peptide and generation of soluble TNAP. In *PIGT*-deficient individuals bone abnormality due to hypophosphatasia was reported.

References

1. Almeida AM, Murakami Y, Baker A, Maeda Y, Roberts IA, Kinoshita T, Layton DM, Karadimitris A (2007) Targeted therapy for inherited GPI deficiency. N Engl J Med 356(16):1641–1647
2. Almeida AM, Murakami Y, Layton DM, Hillmen P, Sellick GS, Maeda Y, Richards S, Patterson S, Kotsianidis I, Mollica L, Crawford DH, Baker A, Ferguson M, Roberts I, Houlston R, Kinoshita T, Karadimitris A (2006) Hypomorphic promoter mutation in PIGM causes inherited glycosylphosphatidylinositol deficiency. Nat Med 12(7):846–851

3. Araten DJ, Nafa K, Pakdeesuwan K, Luzzatto L (1999) Clonal populations of hematopoietic cells with paroxysmal nocturnal hemoglobinuria genotype and phenotype are present in normal individuals. Proc Natl Acad Sci U S A 96:5209–5214
4. Ashida H, Hong Y, Murakami Y, Shishioh N, Sugimoto N, Kim YU, Maeda Y, Kinoshita T (2005) Mammalian PIG-X and yeast Pbn1p are the essential components of glycosylphosphatidylinositol-mannosyltransferase I. Mol Biol Cell 16(3):1439–1448
5. Ast T, Cohen G, Schuldiner M (2013) A network of cytosolic factors targets SRP-independent proteins to the endoplasmic reticulum. Cell 152(5):1134–1145. doi:10.1016/j.cell.2013.02.003
6. Belet S, Fieremans N, Yuan X, Van Esch H, Verbeeck J, Ye Z, Cheng L, Brodsky BR, Hu H, Kalscheuer VM, Brodsky RA, Froyen G (2013) Early frameshift mutation in PIGA identified in a large XLID family without neonatal lethality. Hum Mutat 35(3):350–355. doi:10.1002/humu.22498
7. Benghezal M, Benachour A, Rusconi S, Aebi M, Conzelmann A (1996) Yeast Gpi8p is essential for GPI anchor attachment onto proteins. EMBO J 15:6575–6583
8. Bessler M, Mason PJ, Hillmen P, Luzzatto L (1994) Mutations in the PIG-A gene causing partial deficiency of GPI-linked surface proteins (PNH II) in patients with paroxysmal nocturnal haemoglobinuria. Br J Haematol 87:863–866
9. Bonnon C, Wendeler MW, Paccaud JP, Hauri HP (2010) Selective export of human GPI-anchored proteins from the endoplasmic reticulum. J Cell Sci 123(Pt 10):1705–1715. doi:10.1242/jcs.062950
10. Bosson R, Jaquenoud M, Conzelmann A (2006) GUP1 of Saccharomyces cerevisiae encodes an O-acyltransferase involved in remodeling of the GPI anchor. Mol Biol Cell 17(6):2636–2645
11. Chiyonobu T, Inoue N, Morimoto M, Kinoshita T, Murakami Y (2014) Glycosylphosphatidylinositol (GPI) anchor deficiency caused by mutations in PIGW is associated with West syndrome and hyperphosphatasia with mental retardation syndrome. J Med Genet 51(3):203–207. doi:10.1136/jmedgenet-2013-102156
12. Eisenhaber B, Eisenhaber S, Kwang TY, Gruber G, Eisenhaber F (2014) Transamidase subunit GAA1/GPAA1 is a M28 family metallo-peptide-synthetase that catalyzes the peptide bond formation between the substrate protein's omega-site and the GPI lipid anchor's phosphoethanolamine. Cell Cycle 13(12):1912–1917
13. Endo M, Ware R, Vreeke T, Singh S, Howard T, Tomita A, Holguin M, Parker C (1996) Molecular basis of the heterogeneity of expression of glycosyl phosphatidylinositol anchored proteins in paroxysmal nocturnal hemoglobinuria. Blood 87:2546–2557
14. Fujihara Y, Tokuhiro K, Muro Y, Kondoh G, Araki Y, Ikawa M, Okabe M (2013) Expression of TEX101, regulated by ACE, is essential for the production of fertile mouse spermatozoa. Proc Natl Acad Sci U S A 110(20):8111–8116. doi:10.1073/pnas.1222166110
15. Fujita M, Maeda Y, Ra M, Yamaguchi Y, Taguchi R, Kinoshita T (2009) GPI glycan remodeling by PGAP5 regulates transport of GPI-anchored proteins from the ER to the Golgi. Cell 139(2):352–365. doi:10.1016/j.cell.2009.08.040
16. Fujita M, Umemura M, Yoko-o T, Jigami Y (2006) PER1 is required for GPI-phospholipase A2 activity and involved in lipid remodeling of GPI-anchored proteins. Mol Biol Cell 17(12):5253–5264. doi:10.1091/mbc.E06-08-0715
17. Fujita M, Watanabe R, Jaensch N, Romanova-Michaelides M, Satoh T, Kato M, Riezman H, Yamaguchi Y, Maeda Y, Kinoshita T (2011) Sorting of GPI-anchored proteins into ER exit sites by p24 proteins is dependent on remodeled GPI. J Cell Biol 194(1):61–75. doi:10.1083/jcb.201012074
18. Hamburger D, Egerton M, Riezman H (1995) Yeast Gaa1p is required for attachment of a completed GPI anchor onto proteins. J Cell Biol 129:629–639
19. Handa N, Terada T, Kamewari Y, Hamana H, Tame JR, Park SY, Kinoshita K, Ota M, Nakamura H, Kuramitsu S, Shirouzu M, Yokoyama S (2003) Crystal structure of the conserved protein TT1542 from Thermus thermophilus HB8. Protein Sci A Publ Protein Soc 12(8):1621–1632. doi:10.1110/gad.03104003

20. Hansen L, Tawamie H, Murakami Y, Mang Y, ur Rehman S, Buchert R, Schaffer S, Muhammad S, Bak M, Nothen MM, Bennett EP, Maeda Y, Aigner M, Reis A, Kinoshita T, Tommerup N, Baig SM, Abou Jamra R (2013) Hypomorphic mutations in PGAP2, encoding a GPI-anchor-remodeling protein, cause autosomal-recessive intellectual disability. Am J Hum Genet 92(4):575–583. doi:10.1016/j.ajhg.2013.03.008
21. Hirata T, Fujita M, Kanzawa N, Murakami Y, Maeda Y, Kinoshita T (2013) Glycosylphosphatidylinositol mannosyltransferase II is the rate-limiting enzyme in glycosylphosphatidylinositol biosynthesis under limited dolichol-phosphate mannose availability. J Biochem 154(3):257–264. doi:10.1093/jb/mvt045
22. Hiroi Y, Komuro I, Chen R, Hosoda T, Mizuno T, Kudoh S, Georgescu SP, Medof ME, Yazaki Y (1998) Molecular cloning of human homolog of yeast *GAA1* which is required for attachment of glycosylphosphatidylinositols to proteins. FEBS Lett 421:252–258
23. Hochsmann B, Dohna-Schwake C, Kyrieleis HA, Pannicke U, Schrezenmeier H (2014) Targeted therapy with eculizumab for inherited CD59 deficiency. N Engl J Med 370(1):90–92. doi:10.1056/NEJMc1308104
24. Hong Y, Maeda Y, Watanabe R, Inoue N, Ohishi K, Kinoshita T (2000) Requirement of PIG-F and PIG-O for transferring phosphoethanolamine to the third mannose in glycosylphosphatidylinositol. J Biol Chem 275:20911–20919
25. Hong Y, Maeda Y, Watanabe R, Ohishi K, Mishkind M, Riezman H, Kinoshita T (1999) Pig-n, a mammalian homologue of yeast Mcd4p, is involved in transferring phosphoethanolamine to the first mannose of the glycosylphosphatidylinositol. J Biol Chem 274:35099–35106
26. Hong Y, Ohishi K, Kang JY, Tanaka S, Inoue N, Nishimura J, Maeda Y, Kinoshita T (2003) Human PIG-U and yeast Cdc91p are the fifth subunit of GPI transamidase that attaches GPI-anchors to proteins. Mol Biol Cell 14:1780–1789
27. Houjou T, Hayakawa J, Watanabe R, Tashima Y, Maeda Y, Kinoshita T, Taguchi R (2007) Changes in molecular species profiles of glycosylphosphatidylinositol-anchor precursors in early stages of biosynthesis. J Lipid Res 48:1599–1606
28. Howard MF, Murakami Y, Pagnamenta AT, Daumer-Haas C, Fischer B, Hecht J, Keays DA, Knight SJ, Kolsch U, Kruger U, Leiz S, Maeda Y, Mitchell D, Mundlos S, Phillips JA 3rd, Robinson PN, Kini U, Taylor JC, Horn D, Kinoshita T, Krawitz PM (2014) Mutations in PGAP3 impair GPI-anchor maturation, causing a subtype of hyperphosphatasia with mental retardation. Am J Hum Genet 94(2):278–287. doi:10.1016/j.ajhg.2013.12.012
29. Iida Y, Takeda J, Miyata T, Inoue N, Nishimura J, Kitani T, Maeda K, Kinoshita T (1994) Characterization of genomic PIG-A gene:a gene for GPI-anchor biosynthesis and paroxysmal nocturnal hemoglobinuria. Blood 83:3126–3131
30. Ikezawa H (2002) Glycosylphosphatidylinositol (GPI)-anchored proteins. Biol Pharm Bull 25(4):409–417
31. Inoue N, Kinoshita T, Orii T, Takeda J (1993) Cloning of a human gene, PIG-F, a component of glycosylphosphatidylinositol anchor biosynthesis, by a novel expression cloning strategy. J Biol Chem 268:6882–6885
32. Inoue N, Watanabe R, Takeda J, Kinoshita T (1996) PIG-C, one of the three human genes involved in the first step of glycosylphosphatidylinositol biosynthesis is a homologue of Saccharomyces cerevisiae GPI2. Biochem Biophys Res Commun 226:193–199
33. Jaensch N, Correa IR Jr, Watanabe R (2014) Stable cell surface expression of GPI-anchored proteins, but not intracellular transport, depends on their fatty acid structure. Traffic 15(12):1305–1329. doi:10.1111/tra.12224
34. Johnston JJ, Gropman AL, Sapp JC, Teer JK, Martin JM, Liu CF, Yuan X, Ye Z, Cheng L, Brodsky RA, Biesecker LG (2012) The phenotype of a germline mutation in PIGA: the gene somatically mutated in paroxysmal nocturnal hemoglobinuria. Am J Hum Genet 90(2):295–300. doi:10.1016/j.ajhg.2011.11.031
35. Kamitani T, Chang HM, Rollins C, Waneck GL, Yeh ET (1993) Correction of the class H defect in glycosylphosphatidylinositol anchor biosynthesis in Ltk- cells by a human cDNA clone. J Biol Chem 268(28):20733–20736

36. Kang JY, Hong Y, Ashida H, Shishioh N, Murakami Y, Morita YS, Maeda Y, Kinoshita T (2005) PIG-V involved in transferring the second mannose in glycosylphosphatidylinositol. J Biol Chem 280(10):9489–9497. doi:10.1074/jbc.M413867200
37. Kanzawa N, Maeda Y, Ogiso H, Murakami Y, Taguchi R, Kinoshita T (2009) Peroxisome dependency of alkyl-containing GPI-anchor biosynthesis in the endoplasmic reticulum. Proc Natl Acad Sci U S A 106(42):17711–17716. doi:10.1073/pnas.0904762106
38. Kanzawa N, Shimozawa N, Wanders RJ, Ikeda K, Murakami Y, Waterham HR, Mukai S, Fujita M, Maeda Y, Taguchi R, Fujiki Y, Kinoshita T (2012) Defective lipid remodeling of GPI anchors in peroxisomal disorders, Zellweger syndrome, and rhizomelic chondrodysplasia punctata. J Lipid Res 53(4):653–663. doi:10.1194/jlr.M021204
39. Kato M, Saitsu H, Murakami Y, Kikuchi K, Watanabe S, Iai M, Miya K, Matsuura R, Takayama R, Ohba C, Nakashima M, Tsurusaki Y, Miyake N, Hamano S, Osaka H, Hayasaka K, Kinoshita T, Matsumoto N (2014) PIGA mutations cause early-onset epileptic encephalopathies and distinctive features. Neurology 82(18):1587–1596. doi:10.1212/WNL.0000000000000389
40. Kerwin JL, Tuininga AR, Ericsson LH (1994) Identification of molecular species of glycerophospholipids and sphingomyelin using electrospray mass spectrometry. J Lipid Res 35(6):1102–1114
41. Kondoh G, Tojo H, Nakatani Y, Komazawa N, Murata C, Yamagata K, Maeda Y, Kinoshita T, Okabe M, Taguchi R, Takeda J (2005) Angiotensin-converting enzyme is a GPI-anchored protein releasing factor crucial for fertilization. Nat Med 11(2):160–166
42. Kostova Z, Rancour DM, Menon AK, Orlean P (2000) Photoaffinity labelling with P^3-(4-azidoanilido)uridine 5′-triphosphate identifies Gpi3p as the UDP-GlcNAc-binding subunit of the enzyme that catalyses formation of GlcNAc-phosphatidylinositol, the first glycolipid intermediate in glycosylphosphatidylinositol synthesis. Biochem J 350:815–822
43. Krawitz PM, Hochsmann B, Murakami Y, Teubner B, Kruger U, Klopocki E, Neitzel H, Hoellein A, Schneider C, Parkhomchuk D, Hecht J, Robinson PN, Mundlos S, Kinoshita T, Schrezenmeier H (2013) A case of paroxysmal nocturnal hemoglobinuria caused by a germline mutation and a somatic mutation in PIGT. Blood 122(7):1312–1315. doi:10.1182/blood-2013-01-481499
44. Krawitz PM, Murakami Y, Hecht J, Kruger U, Holder SE, Mortier GR, Delle Chiaie B, De Baere E, Thompson MD, Roscioli T, Kielbasa S, Kinoshita T, Mundlos S, Robinson PN, Horn D (2012) Mutations in PIGO, a member of the GPI-anchor-synthesis pathway, cause hyperphosphatasia with mental retardation. Am J Hum Genet 91(1):146–151. doi:10.1016/j.ajhg.2012.05.004
45. Krawitz PM, Schweiger MR, Rodelsperger C, Marcelis C, Kolsch U, Meisel C, Stephani F, Kinoshita T, Murakami Y, Bauer S, Isau M, Fischer A, Dahl A, Kerick M, Hecht J, Kohler S, Jager M, Grunhagen J, de Condor BJ, Doelken S, Brunner HG, Meinecke P, Passarge E, Thompson MD, Cole DE, Horn D, Roscioli T, Mundlos S, Robinson PN (2010) Identity-by-descent filtering of exome sequence data identifies PIGV mutations in hyperphosphatasia mental retardation syndrome. Nat Genet 42(10):827–829. doi:10.1038/ng.653
46. Kvarnung M, Nilsson D, Lindstrand A, Korenke GC, Chiang SC, Blennow E, Bergmann M, Stodberg T, Makitie O, Anderlid BM, Bryceson YT, Nordenskjold M, Nordgren A (2013) A novel intellectual disability syndrome caused by GPI anchor deficiency due to homozygous mutations in PIGT. J Med Genet 50(8):521–528. doi:10.1136/jmedgenet-2013-101654
47. Liu J, Mushegian A (2003) Three monophyletic superfamilies account for the majority of the known glycosyltransferases. Protein Sci A Publ Protein Soc 12(7):1418–1431. doi:10.1110/ps.0302103
48. Luzzatto L, Nafa K (2000) Genetics of PNH. In: Young NS, Moss J (eds) Paroxysmal nocturnal hemoglobinuria and the glycosylphosphatidylinositol-linked proteins. Academic, San Diego, pp 21–47
49. Maeda Y, Tashima Y, Houjou T, Fujita M, Yoko-o T, Jigami Y, Taguchi R, Kinoshita T (2007) Fatty acid remodeling of GPI-anchored proteins is required for their raft association. Mol Biol Cell 18(4):1497–1506

50. Maeda Y, Tomita S, Watanabe R, Ohishi K, Kinoshita T (1998) DPM2 regulates biosynthesis of dolichol phosphate-mannose in mammalian cells: correct subcellular localization and stabilization of DPM1, and binding of dolichol phosphate. EMBO J 17:4920–4929
51. Maeda Y, Watanabe R, Harris CL, Hong Y, Ohishi K, Kinoshita K, Kinoshita T (2001) PIG-M transfers the first mannose to glycosylphosphatidylinositol on the lumenal side of the ER. EMBO J 20:250–261
52. Manzano-Lopez J, Perez-Linero AM, Aguilera-Romero A, Martin ME, Okano T, Silva DV, Seeberger PH, Riezman H, Funato K, Goder V, Wellinger RE, Muniz M (2015) COPII coat composition is actively regulated by luminal cargo maturation. Curr Biol 25(2):152–162. doi:10.1016/j.cub.2014.11.039
53. Martin HC, Kim GE, Pagnamenta AT, Murakami Y, Carvill GL, Meyer E, Copley RR, Rimmer A, Barcia G, Fleming MR, Kronengold J, Brown MR, Hudspith KA, Broxholme J, Kanapin A, Cazier JB, Kinoshita T, Nabbout R, Consortium WGS, Bentley D, McVean G, Heavin S, Zaiwalla Z, McShane T, Mefford HC, Shears D, Stewart H, Kurian MA, Scheffer IE, Blair E, Donnelly P, Kaczmarek LK, Taylor JC (2014) Clinical whole-genome sequencing in severe early-onset epilepsy reveals new genes and improves molecular diagnosis. Hum Mol Genet 23(12):3200–3211. doi:10.1093/hmg/ddu030
54. Maydan G, Noyman I, Har-Zahav A, Neriah ZB, Pasmanik-Chor M, Yeheskel A, Albin-Kaplanski A, Maya I, Magal N, Birk E, Simon AJ, Halevy A, Rechavi G, Shohat M, Straussberg R, Basel-Vanagaite L (2011) Multiple congenital anomalies-hypotonia-seizures syndrome is caused by a mutation in PIGN. J Med Genet 48(6):383–389. doi:10.1136/jmg.2010.087114
55. McConville MJ, Ferguson MA (1993) The structure, biosynthesis and function of glycosylated phosphatidylinositols in the parasitic protozoa and higher eukaryotes. Biochem J 294(Pt 2):305–324
56. McKean DM, Niswander L (2012) Defects in GPI biosynthesis perturb Cripto signaling during forebrain development in two new mouse models of holoprosencephaly. Biol open 1(9):874–883. doi:10.1242/bio.20121982
57. Meyer U, Benghezal M, Imhof I, Conzelmann A (2000) Active site determination of Gpi8p, a caspase-related enzyme required for glycosylphosphatidylinositol anchor addition to proteins. Biochemistry 39:3461–3471
58. Miyata T, Takeda J, Iida Y, Yamada N, Inoue N, Takahashi M, Maeda K, Kitani T, Kinoshita T (1993) Cloning of PIG-A, a component in the early step of GPI-anchor biosynthesis. Science 259:1318–1320
59. Miyata T, Yamada N, Iida Y, Nishimura J, Takeda J, Kitani T, Kinoshita T (1994) Abnormalities of PIG-A transcripts in granulocytes from patients with paroxysmal nocturnal hemoglobinuria. N Engl J Med 330:249–255
60. Mochizuki K, Sugimori C, Qi Z, Lu X, Takami A, Ishiyama K, Kondo Y, Yamazaki H, Okumura H, Nakao S (2008) Expansion of donor-derived hematopoietic stem cells with PIGA mutation associated with late graft failure after allogeneic stem cell transplantation. Blood 112(5):2160–2162. doi:10.1182/blood-2008-02-141325
61. Motoyama N, Okada N, Yamashina M, Okada H (1992) Paroxysmal nocturnal hemoglobinuria due to hereditary nucleotide deletion in the HRF20 (CD59) gene. Eur J Immunol 22:2669–2673
62. Murakami H, Wang Y, Hasuwa H, Maeda Y, Kinoshita T, Murakami Y (2012) Enhanced response of T lymphocytes from Pgap3 knockout mouse: Insight into roles of fatty acid remodeling of GPI anchored proteins. Biochem Biophys Res Commun 417(4):1235–1241. doi:10.1016/j.bbrc.2011.12.116
63. Murakami Y, Kanzawa N, Saito K, Krawitz PM, Mundlos S, Robinson PN, Karadimitris A, Maeda Y, Kinoshita T (2012) Mechanism for release of alkaline phosphatase caused by glycosylphosphatidylinositol deficiency in patients with hyperphosphatasia mental retardation syndrome. J Biol Chem 287(9):6318–6325. doi:10.1074/jbc.M111.331090
64. Murakami Y, Siripanyaphinyo U, Hong Y, Tashima Y, Maeda Y, Kinoshita T (2005) The initial enzyme for glycosylphosphatidylinositol biosynthesis requires PIG-Y, a seventh component. Mol Biol Cell 16(11):5236–5246

65. Murakami Y, Siripanyapinyo U, Hong Y, Kang JY, Ishihara S, Nakakuma H, Maeda Y, Kinoshita T (2003) PIG-W is critical for inositol acylation but not for flipping of glycosylphosphatidylinositol-anchor. Mol Biol Cell 14(10):4285–4295
66. Murakami Y, Tawamie H, Maeda Y, Buttner C, Buchert R, Radwan F, Schaffer S, Sticht H, Aigner M, Reis A, Kinoshita T, Jamra RA (2014) Null mutation in PGAP1 impairing Gpi-anchor maturation in patients with intellectual disability and encephalopathy. PLoS Genet 10(5):e1004320. doi:10.1371/journal.pgen.1004320
67. Nafa K, Bessler M, Castro-Malaspina H, Jhanwar S, Luzzatto L (1998) The spectrum of somatic mutations in the PIG-A gene in paroxysmal nocturnal hemoglobinuria includes large deletions and small duplications. Blood Cell Mol Dis 24:370–384
68. Nakamura N, Inoue N, Watanabe R, Takahashi M, Takeda J, Stevens VL, Kinoshita T (1997) Expression cloning of PIG-L, a candidate N-acetylglucosaminyl-phosphatidylinositol deacetylase. J Biol Chem 272:15834–15840
69. Nakashima M, Kashii H, Murakami Y, Kato M, Tsurusaki Y, Miyake N, Kubota M, Kinoshita T, Saitsu H, Matsumoto N (2014) Novel compound heterozygous PIGT mutations caused multiple congenital anomalies-hypotonia-seizures syndrome 3. Neurogenetics 15(3):193–200. doi:10.1007/s10048-014-0408-y
70. Nevo Y, Ben-Zeev B, Tabib A, Straussberg R, Anikster Y, Shorer Z, Fattal-Valevski A, Ta-Shma A, Aharoni S, Rabie M, Zenvirt S, Goldshmidt H, Fellig Y, Shaag A, Mevorach D, Elpeleg O (2013) CD59 deficiency is associated with chronic hemolysis and childhood relapsing immune-mediated polyneuropathy. Blood 121(1):129–135. doi:10.1182/blood-2012-07-441857
71. Newton GL, Av-Gay Y, Fahey RC (2000) N-Acetyl-1-D-myo-inosityl-2-amino-2-deoxy-alpha-D-glucopyranoside deacetylase (MshB) is a key enzyme in mycothiol biosynthesis. J Bacteriol 182(24):6958–6963
72. Ng BG, Hackmann K, Jones MA, Eroshkin AM, He P, Wiliams R, Bhide S, Cantagrel V, Gleeson JG, Paller AS, Schnur RE, Tinschert S, Zunich J, Hegde MR, Freeze HH (2012) Mutations in the glycosylphosphatidylinositol gene PIGL cause CHIME syndrome. Am J Hum Genet 90(4):685–688. doi:10.1016/j.ajhg.2012.02.010
73. Nishimura J, Inoue N, Wada H, Ueda E, Pramoonjago P, Hirota T, Machii T, Kageyama T, Kanamaru A, Takeda J, Kinoshita T, Kitani T (1997) A patient with paroxysmal nocturnal hemoglobinuria bearing four independent PIG-A mutant clones. Blood 89:3470–3476
74. Nozaki M, Ohishi K, Yamada N, Kinoshita T, Nagy A, Takeda J (1999) Developmental abnormalities of glycosylphosphatidylinositol-anchor-deficient embryos revealed by Cre/loxP system. Lab Invest 79:293–299
75. Ohishi K, Inoue N, Kinoshita T (2001) PIG-S and PIG-T, essential for GPI anchor attachment to proteins, form a complex with GAA1 and GPI8. EMBO J 20:4088–4098
76. Ohishi K, Inoue N, Maeda Y, Takeda J, Riezman H, Kinoshita T (2000) Gaa1p and gpi8p are components of a glycosylphosphatidylinositol (GPI) transamidase that mediates attachment of GPI to proteins. Mol Biol Cell 11:1523–1533
77. Ohishi K, Nagamune K, Maeda Y, Kinoshita T (2003) Two subunits of glycosylphosphatidylinositol transamidase, GPI8 and PIG-T, form a functionally important intermolecular disulfide bridge. J Biol Chem 278(16):13959–13967
78. Oriol R, Martinez-Duncker I, Chantret I, Mollicone R, Codogno P (2002) Common origin and evolution of glycosyltransferases using Dol-P-monosaccharides as donor substrate. Mol Biol Evol 19:1451–1463
79. Park S, Lee C, Sabharwal P, Zhang M, Meyers CL, Sockanathan S (2013) GDE2 promotes neurogenesis by glycosylphosphatidylinositol-anchor cleavage of RECK. Science 339(6117):324–328. doi:10.1126/science.1231921
80. Parker C, Omine M, Richards S, Nishimura J, Bessler M, Ware R, Hillmen P, Luzzatto L, Young N, Kinoshita T, Rosse W, Socie G, International PNHIG (2005) Diagnosis and management of paroxysmal nocturnal hemoglobinuria. Blood 106(12):3699–3709. doi:10.1182/blood-2005-04-1717

81. Pei J, Millay DP, Olson EN, Grishin NV (2011) CREST–a large and diverse superfamily of putative transmembrane hydrolases. Biol Direct 6:37. doi:10.1186/1745-6150-6-37
82. Roberts WL, Myher JJ, Kuksis A, Low MG, Rosenberry TL (1988) Lipid analysis of the glycoinositol phospholipid membrane anchor of human erythrocyte acetylcholinesterase. Palmitoylation of inositol results in resistance to phosphatidylinositol-specific phospholipase C. J Biol Chem 263:18766–18775
83. Seong J, Wang Y, Kinoshita T, Maeda Y (2013) Implications of lipid moiety in oligomerization and immunoreactivities of GPI-anchored proteins. J Lipid Res 54(4):1077–1091. doi:10.1194/jlr.M034421
84. Shen W, Clemente MJ, Hosono N, Yoshida K, Przychodzen B, Yoshizato T, Shiraishi Y, Miyano S, Ogawa S, Maciejewski JP, Makishima H (2014) Deep sequencing reveals stepwise mutation acquisition in paroxysmal nocturnal hemoglobinuria. J Clin Invest 124(10):4529–4538. doi:10.1172/JCI74747
85. Shishioh N, Hong Y, Ohishi K, Ashida H, Maeda Y, Kinoshita T (2005) GPI7 is the second partner of PIG-F and involved in modification of glycosylphosphatidylinositol. J Biol Chem 280(10):9728–9734
86. Simons K, Ikonen E (1997) Functional rafts in cell membranes. Nature 387:569–572
87. Stokes MJ, Murakami Y, Maeda Y, Kinoshita T, Morita YS (2014) New insights into the functions of PIGF, a protein involved in the ethanolamine phosphate transfer steps of glycosylphosphatidylinositol biosynthesis. Biochem J 463(2):249–256. doi:10.1042/BJ20140541
88. Sutterlin C, Horvath A, Gerold P, Schwarz RT, Wang Y, Dreyfuss M, Riezman H (1997) Identification of a species-specific inhibitor of glycosylphosphatidylinositol synthesis. EMBO J 16:6374–6383
89. Suzuki KG, Kasai RS, Hirosawa KM, Nemoto YL, Ishibashi M, Miwa Y, Fujiwara TK, Kusumi A (2012) Transient GPI-anchored protein homodimers are units for raft organization and function. Nat Chem Biol 8(9):774–783. doi:10.1038/nchembio.1028
90. Swoboda KJ, Margraf RL, Carey JC, Zhou H, Newcomb TM, Coonrod E, Durtschi J, Mallempati K, Kumanovics A, Katz BE, Voelkerding KV, Opitz JM (2014) A novel germline PIGA mutation in Ferro-Cerebro-Cutaneous syndrome: a neurodegenerative X-linked epileptic encephalopathy with systemic iron-overload. Am J Med Genet A 164(1):17–28. doi:10.1002/ajmg.a.36189
91. Takahashi M, Inoue N, Ohishi K, Maeda Y, Nakamura N, Endo Y, Fujita T, Takeda J, Kinoshita T (1996) PIG-B, a membrane protein of the endoplasmic reticulum with a large lumenal domain, is involved in transferring the third mannose of the GPI anchor. EMBO J 15(16):4254–4261
92. Takeda J, Miyata T, Kawagoe K, Iida Y, Endo Y, Fujita T, Takahashi M, Kitani T, Kinoshita T (1993) Deficiency of the GPI anchor caused by a somatic mutation of the PIG-A gene in paroxysmal nocturnal hemoglobinuria. Cell 73:703–711
93. Takida S, Maeda Y, Kinoshita T (2008) Mammalian GPI-anchored proteins require p24 proteins for their efficient transport from the ER to the plasma membrane. Biochem J 409(2):555–562. doi:10.1042/BJ20070234
94. Tanaka S, Maeda Y, Tashima Y, Kinoshita T (2004) Inositol deacylation of glycosylphosphatidylinositol-anchored proteins is mediated by mammalian PGAP1 and yeast Bst1p. J Biol Chem 279:14256–14263
95. Tashima Y, Taguchi R, Murata C, Ashida H, Kinoshita T, Maeda Y (2006) PGAP2 is essential for correct processing and stable expression of GPI-anchored proteins. Mol Biol Cell 17(3):1410–1420
96. Udenfriend S, Kodukula K (1995) How glycosylphosphatidylinositol-anchored membrane proteins are made. Annu Rev Biochem 64:563–591
97. Ueda Y, Yamaguchi R, Ikawa M, Okabe M, Morii E, Maeda Y, Kinoshita T (2007) PGAP1 knock-out mice show otocephaly and male infertility. J Biol Chem 282(42):30373–30380. doi:10.1074/jbc.M705601200
98. Urbaniak MD, Crossman A, Chang T, Smith TK, van Aalten DM, Ferguson MA (2005) The N-acetyl-D-glucosaminylphosphatidylinositol De-N-acetylase of glycosylphosphatidylinosi-

tol biosynthesis is a zinc metalloenzyme. J Biol Chem 280(24):22831–22838. doi:10.1074/jbc.M502402200

99. Vainauskas S, Menon AK (2004) A conserved proline in the last transmembrane segment of Gaa1 is required for glycosylphosphatidylinositol (GPI) recognition by GPI transamidase. J Biol Chem 279(8):6540–6545. doi:10.1074/jbc.M312191200
100. Vainauskas S, Menon AK (2006) Ethanolamine phosphate linked to the first mannose residue of glycosylphosphatidylinositol (GPI) lipids is a major feature of the GPI structure that is recognized by human GPI transamidase. J Biol Chem 281(50):38358–38364. doi:10.1074/jbc.M608896200
101. van der Crabben SN, Harakalova M, Brilstra EH, van Berkestijn FM, Hofstede FC, van Vught AJ, Cuppen E, Kloosterman W, Ploos van Amstel HK, van Haaften G, van Haelst MM (2014) Expanding the spectrum of phenotypes associated with germline PIGA mutations: a child with developmental delay, accelerated linear growth, facial dysmorphisms, elevated alkaline phosphatase, and progressive CNS abnormalities. Am J Med Genet A 164(1):29–35. doi:10.1002/ajmg.a.36184
102. Vazquez HM, Vionnet C, Roubaty C, Conzelmann A (2014) Cdc1 removes the ethanolamine phosphate of the first mannose of GPI anchors and thereby facilitates the integration of GPI proteins into the yeast cell wall. Mol Biol Cell 25(21):3375–3388. doi:10.1091/mbc.E14-06-1033
103. Volwerk JJ, Shashidhar MS, Kuppe A, Griffith OH (1990) Phosphatidylinositol-specific phospholipase C from Bacillus cereus combines intrinsic phosphotransferase and cyclic phosphodiesterase activities: a 31P NMR study. Biochemistry 29(35):8056–8062
104. Wang H, Chuhjo T, Yamazaki H, Shiobara S, Teramura M, Mizoguchi H, Nakao S (2001) Relative increase of granulocytes with a paroxysmal nocturnal haemoglobinuria phenotype in aplastic anaemia patients: the high prevalence at diagnosis. Eur J Haematol 66:200–205
105. Wang Y, Murakami Y, Yasui T, Wakana S, Kikutani H, Kinoshita T, Maeda Y (2013) Significance of glycosylphosphatidylinositol-anchored protein enrichment in lipid rafts for the control of autoimmunity. J Biol Chem 288(35):25490–25499. doi:10.1074/jbc.M113.492611
106. Watanabe K, Bianco C, Strizzi L, Hamada S, Mancino M, Bailly V, Mo W, Wen D, Miatkowski K, Gonzales M, Sanicola M, Seno M, Salomon DS (2007) Growth factor induction of Cripto-1 shedding by glycosylphosphatidylinositol-phospholipase D and enhancement of endothelial cell migration. J Biol Chem 282(43):31643–31655. doi:10.1074/jbc.M702713200
107. Watanabe R, Inoue N, Westfall B, Taron CH, Orlean P, Takeda J, Kinoshita T (1998) The first step of glycosylphosphatidylinositol biosynthesis is mediated by a complex of PIG-A, PIG-H, PIG-C and GPI1. EMBO J 17:877–885
108. Watanabe R, Kinoshita T, Masaki R, Yamamoto A, Takeda J, Inoue N (1996) PIG-A and PIG-H, which participate in glycosylphosphatidylinositol anchor biosynthesis, form a protein complex in the endoplasmic reticulum. J Biol Chem 271:26868–26875
109. Watanabe R, Murakami Y, Marmor MD, Inoue N, Maeda Y, Hino J, Kangawa K, Julius M, Kinoshita T (2000) Initial enzyme for glycosylphosphatidylinositol biosynthesis requires PIG-P and is regulated by DPM2. EMBO J 19:4402–4411
110. Watanabe R, Ohishi K, Maeda Y, Nakamura N, Kinoshita T (1999) Mammalian PIG-L and its yeast homologue Gpi12p are N-acetylglucosaminylphosphatidylinositol de-N-acetylases essential in glycosylphosphatidylinositol biosynthesis. Biochem J 339:185–192
111. Yamashina M, Ueda E, Kinoshita T, Takami T, Ojima A, Ono H, Tanaka H, Kondo N, Orii T, Okada N et al (1990) Inherited complete deficiency of 20-kilodalton homologous restriction factor (CD59) as a cause of paroxysmal nocturnal hemoglobinuria. N Engl J Med 323(17):1184–1189. doi:10.1056/NEJM199010253231707
112. Zoltewicz JS, Ashique AM, Choe Y, Lee G, Taylor S, Phamluong K, Solloway M, Peterson AS (2009) Wnt signaling is regulated by endoplasmic reticulum retention. PLoS One 4(7):e6191. doi:10.1371/journal.pone.0006191

Chapter 3
Animal Models of Paroxysmal Nocturnal Hemoglobinuria

Yoshiko Murakami and Taroh Kinoshita

Abstract Paroxysmal nocturnal hemoglobinuria (PNH) is caused by the somatic mutation of the *PIGA* gene of one or several hematopoietic stem cells, but how these stem cells acquire dominance to full expansion is not clearly elucidated. We and other groups have generated and studied several animal models to clarify this unknown. The first-generation models were simple *Piga* knockout mice that were shown to be lethal. The second-generation models were conditional *Piga* knockout mice using the *Cre/loxP* system, which indicated that a *Piga* mutation alone does not account for the dominance of the mutant stem cells and that other factors are involved in pathogenesis of PNH. From the observation of PNH clones in aplastic anemia patients, we hypothesize that immunological selection and additional abnormality, leading to benign tumorlike proliferation, would be necessary for clonal expansion of GPI-negative cells in addition to the *PIGA* mutation. Immunological selection was experimentally proven by our model mice in combination with bone marrow chimera. From the analysis of the PNH patients with a chromosome 12 abnormality, we identified the candidate gene, *HMGA2*, for the benign tumorlike proliferation. HMGA2-expressing hematopoietic stem cells showed increased proliferation in mice. Although the expression of HMGA2 in pluripotent stem cells requires testing, HMGA2 expression was found to increase in peripheral blood cells for 75 % of PNH patients examined.

Keywords HMGA2 • Cre/loxP system • X-inactivation • Autoreactive T cell • Bone marrow chimera

---

Y. Murakami, M.D., Ph.D. (✉)
Department of Immunoregulation, Research Institute for Microbial Diseases, Osaka University, 3-1 Yamadaoka, Suita, Osaka 565-0871, Japan

Department of Immunoglycobiology, WPI Immunology Frontier Research Center, Osaka University, 3-1 Yamadaoka, Suita, Osaka 565-0871, Japan
e-mail: yoshiko@biken.osaka-u.ac.jp

T. Kinoshita
Research Institute for Microbial Diseases, Osaka University, 3-1 Yamadaoka, Suita 565-0871, Osaka, Japan

WPI Immunology Frontier Research Center, Osaka University, 3-1 Yamadaoka, Suita 565-0871, Osaka, Japan

Y. Kanakura et al. (eds.), *Paroxysmal Nocturnal Hemoglobinuria*, DOI 10.1007/978-4-431-56003-6_3

3.1 Introduction

PNH is generally caused by somatic mutation of the X-linked *PIGA* gene in one or some hematopoietic stem cells. Recently, an atypical case of PNH caused by the combination of germline and somatic mutations of the autosomal *PIGT* gene was found. The affected stem cells were deficient in the biosynthesis of glycosylphosphatidylinositol (GPI) because of the mutations and cell surface expression of GPI-anchored proteins (GPI-APs), such as CD59 and DAF, were lost or very low. Because of the reduced levels of complement regulators, namely, CD59 and DAF, affected erythrocytes are highly sensitive to autologous complement. For clinical manifestation of PNH, the dominance of hematopoiesis by a GPI-negative clone is required. Deficiency of GPI caused by a *PIGA* mutation would be necessary for clonal expansion, but several lines of evidence suggest that this mutation alone is insufficient. Araten and colleagues reported that PNH clones were present in normal individuals, but they never expanded [2]. It is well known that aplastic anemia (AA) is often associated with PNH, and there are many AA cases in which PNH clones become noticeable. It has been reported that the existence of PNH clones in patients with AA is a good indicator of the effectiveness of immunosuppressive therapy [27]. Thus, from the observation of PNH clones in AA patients, it appears that GPI-negative clones are less sensitive to cytotoxic cells, which has been experimentally proven by animal models described in this chapter. Selective killing of normal stem cells results in survival and expansion of GPI-negative clones. However, most PNH clones in AA do not fully expand to develop PNH, which indicates that some additional genetic abnormalities are necessary for full expansion of GPI-negative clones during vigorous amplification within a bone marrow suppressive environment. Ectopic expression of *HMGA2* is a possible cause of a benign tumorlike character [11, 19]. Thus, three steps, a somatic mutation of the *PIGA* gene, immunological selection, and additional abnormalities leading to benign tumorlike proliferation, are necessary for clonal expansion of GPI-negative clones.

3.2 First-Generation *Piga* KO Mouse

To investigate whether a *PIGA* mutation alone is sufficient or whether other factors are also required for the clonal dominance of GPI-deficient cells seen in PNH, Kawagoe et al. generated chimeric mice using GPI-deficient embryonic stem (ES) cells [13]. For this, they first cloned *Piga*, the murine homologue of *PIGA*, confirmed that it was functionally and structurally similar to *PIGA*, and mapped it to XF3/4, a region syntenic to human Xp22.2 where *PIGA* is localized (*PIGA* localization was first reported to be Xp22.1 and is now known to be Xp22.2). Because of the X-chromosomal location of *Piga* and male origin of ES cells, the *Piga*-disrupted ES cells are defective in the biosynthesis of GPI and the surface expression of GPI-anchored proteins (GPI-APs). The researchers then generated chimeric mice using the *Piga*-disrupted ES cells and obtained mice only with less than 5 % chimerism. Mice with high chimerism were likely to be lethal. Six chimeric mice, which had a GPI-negative population in multiple hematopoietic lineages, were used to investigate whether a GPI-negative population increased with time. The percentage of GPI-negative cells in each peripheral blood cell lineage at different time points was determined by flow cytometric analysis. Among the six mice, five did not show any increase in a GPI-negative population for several months to 1 year, whereas one mouse showed a significant increase, indicating that GPI-deficient hematopoietic cells do not have the ability of immediate expansion. The result also suggested that one mouse may have acquired some additional factor for expansion [13].

Rosti et al. reported similar experiments showing that *Piga* inactivation does not confer a proliferative advantage to the hematopoietic stem cell [24].

These mice models have several drawbacks. First, the GPI-deficient and sufficient hematopoietic cell populations derived from different strains were compared in these chimeric mice because ES cells were derived from 129 strains, whereas recipient mice were of the ICR or C57Bl/6 strain. Second, these chimeric mice had GPI-negative cells not only in hematopoietic cells but also cells from other organs. They are not precise models of PNH, in which only the hematopoietic cells have a GPI-deficient population. Third, most mice died during the perinatal period and sufficient numbers of mice could not be obtained for analysis. For these reasons, second-generation mouse PNH models were prepared.

3.3 Second-Generation *Piga* Knockout: The Cre/loxP System

Both our group and Monica Bessler's group generated the *Pigafloxed* mice, in which two loxP sites flank either exon 6 [28] or a part of exon 2 [15, 31]. Taking advantage of the *Pigaflox* mice, we generated bone marrow chimeric mice, in which GPI-anchor negative cells are present only in the hematopoietic system [20]. For this, we first crossed *Piga*$^{flox/-}$ male mice with female transgenic mice bearing human cytomegalovirus promoter-driven *Cre* (*hCMV-Cre*) and obtained female offspring mice bearing the *Cre* transgene. Due to the systemic expression of Cre, their cells were heterozygous for the *Piga*-deleted allele body–widely and the mice became mosaic for GPI-AP expression at the cell level, because of X-chromosome inactivation. The mice were lethal before delivery but were alive up to 13–14 days post coitum and a significant fraction of the hematopoietic stem cells in fetal liver were GPI-anchor negative at that stage. We transplanted lethally irradiated mice with fetal liver cells from these female mice (Fig. 3.1). In the transplanted mice, cells of all hematopoietic lineages contained GPI-AP-negative cells. The proportions of GPI-AP-negative cells in various blood cell lineages were stable over a period of 42 weeks, indicating that the *Piga* mutation alone does not account for the dominance of the mutant stem cells and that other phenotypic changes either in bone marrow environments or in mutant stem cells are involved in pathogenesis of PNH [20].

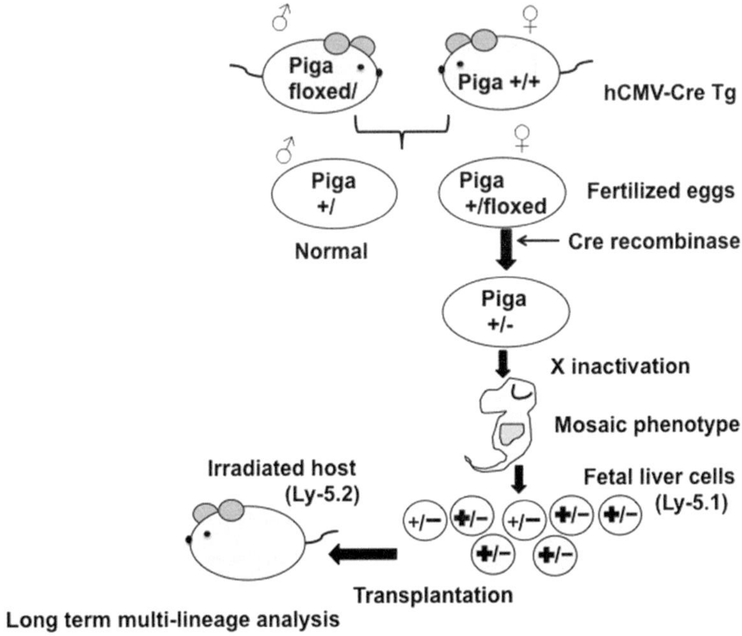

Fig. 3.1 Generation of PNH model mice. *Pigafloxed* male mice were crossed with heterozygous or homozygous *hCMV*-driven *Cre* transgenic female mice. *Piga*-targeted female embryos were heterozygous for the *Piga* defect and became mosaic for *Piga*-deficient and *Piga*-sufficient cells, because of random X-chromosome inactivation. Fetal liver cells of 14 days post coitum, which contained GPI-negative (*white*) and GPI-positive (*gray*) cells, were transplanted to the lethally irradiated C57BL/6 mice. To distinguish donor-derived cells from host-derived cells, mice with the Ly5.1 allele were used as donors and those with Ly5.2 were used as hosts. Peripheral blood cells from transplanted mice were analyzed by FACS

Bessler's group crossed hemizygous *Pigafloxed* male mice with homozygous adenovirus promoter-driven *EIIa-Cre* female mice [15, 31]. As expression of *EIIa-Cre* was transient in the relatively undifferentiated stages of oocytes and preimplantation embryos, the female offspring mice receiving the *Pigafloxed* allele showed varied efficiency of Cre-mediated *Piga* recombination owing to slight differences in the timing of Cre expression. When *Piga*-deleted cells were limited, mice were born alive. This situation was different from our experiments where *hCMV* promoter-driven Cre protein expression was present in all tissues. Additionally, these partially recombined female mice became mosaic because of X-inactivation. Analysis of highly recombined female mice showed that in the heart, lung, kidney, brain, and liver, mainly wild-type *Piga* was active, suggesting that these tissues require GPI-APs. In contrast, spleen, thymus, and red blood cells had almost equal numbers of cells expressing the wild type or the deleted allele, implying that GPI-APs are not essential for the derivation of these tissues. The observed percentage of GPI-negative populations in peripheral blood cells from mice with lower recombination extent for 12 months and the GPI-negative population did not show significant increase.

Although this model still contained GPI-negative cells in non-hematopoietic cells, it clearly showed that a *Piga* gene defect is not sufficient to cause expansion of GPI-AP-negative cells, as seen in PNH.

Both groups showed that GPI-negative red blood cells from *Piga*-defective mice were more sensitive to complement containing human serum than wild-type cells [20, 31].

Bessler's group generated human *c-fes* promoter-driven *Cre* transgenic mice (*Fes-Cre*) [14]. Human *c-fes* encodes a 92-kDa non-receptor protein tyrosine kinase (FES) that is preferentially expressed in hematopoietic progenitor cells in bone marrow and during myeloid differentiation. FES is also expressed in endothelial cells of blood vessels. Male mice in which hematopoietic cells were all GPI negative by crossing with *Pigafloxed* mice were generated. These mice had long-term bone marrow repopulating cells that lacked GPI-APs, as shown by bone marrow reconstitution experiments. *GATA-1* promoter-driven *Cre* transgenic mice (*GATA-1 Cre*) were also generated, and the researchers succeeded in making mice that have almost 100 % of the red blood cells deficient in GPI-AP by crossing with *Pigafloxed* mice and testing complement sensitivity [12].

We also found that *Tie2* promoter-driven *Cre* (*Tie2-Cre*) transgenic mice [16] crossed with *Piga*floxed mice had GPI-negative cells in hematopoietic cells, and the population did not increase during a 1-year observation (unpublished data).

3.4 PNH Model Mice Showing Clonal Expansion

As mentioned above, it was proven unequivocally that a *Piga* mutation alone does not account for the dominance of the mutant stem cells and that other phenotypic changes are involved in the pathogenesis of PNH. Bone marrow failure is one of the three major clinical symptoms of PNH. PNH is often preceded by aplastic anemia. The mechanism of bone marrow failure in PNH is thought to be common with idiopathic aplastic anemia, i.e., autoimmune-mediated reduction in hematopoiesis. One hypothetical mechanism for the clonal expansion of GPI-negative cells in PNH is that the mutant cells escape attacks by autoreactive cytotoxic cells that are thought to be responsible for aplastic anemia [25, 34]. We investigated this hypothesis using our model mice of PNH. For this, we took advantage of a pancytopenia model in which transplanted alloreactive CD4(+) T cells derived from bm12 mice suppress hematopoiesis in C57BL/6 mice. We transplanted lethally irradiated C57BL/6 mice with female C57BL/6 fetal liver cells bearing one disrupted allele of *Piga* with or without alloreactive CD4(+) T cells from bm12 mice. After several months, the contribution of GPI-negative cells in peripheral blood cells was clearly higher when bm12 CD4(+) T cells were cotransplanted, suggesting that GPI-positive hematopoietic cells were preferentially suppressed. It seems very likely that certain GPI-APs on target cells are important for recognition by alloreactive CD4(+) T cells. We also showed in an in vitro study that if a putative autoantigen recognized by cytotoxic cells is a GPI-AP, GPI-negative cells are less sensitive to cytotoxic cells. These results provide the first experimental evidence with mice for the hypothesis that GPI-negative cells expand by escaping immunologic attack [21].

3.5 *High-Mobility Group AT-Hook 2 (HMGA2)*-Transgenic Mice and PNH

We reported two patients with PNH whose GPI-negative cells had a concurrent, acquired rearrangement of chromosome 12. In both cases, der(12) had a break within the 3′ untranslated region (UTR) of *HMGA2* that caused ectopic expression of HMGA2 in bone marrow [11]. *HMGA2* is an architectural transcription factor gene deregulated in many benign mesenchymal tumors. The 3′ UTR of *HMGA2* contains seven binding sites for *let-7* miRNA, which regulates expression of this gene. Thus, truncation of the 3′ UTR leads to deregulated expression of HMGA2 [18]. These observations suggest that aberrant HMGA2 expression, in concert with mutant *PIGA*, accounts for clonal hematopoiesis in these two patients and the concept of PNH as a benign tumor of the bone marrow (BM) was proposed.

Consistent with this observation are the reports that ectopic activation of *HMGA2* in BM cells causes clonal expansion. In a successful case of gene therapy for β-thalassemia, bone marrow cells was inserted with the lentiviral vector bearing β-globin gene into intron 3 of *HMGA2*. This caused activation of the *HMGA2* gene and led to expansion of the clone, resulting in a contribution of approximately 10 % of the erythroblasts [5]. Expansion of clonal BM cells with insertion of the viral vector into *HMGA2* was also documented in a few other examples of gene therapy [33].

The HMGA2 protein is a member of the HMGA family of non-histone chromatin-binding proteins, which also includes HMGA1a, HMGA1b, and HMGA1c [26]. Exons 1 to 3 of the *HMGA2* gene encode DNA-binding AT-hook motifs. These motifs facilitate the preferential binding of the protein to AT-rich sequences in B-form DNA and induce conformational changes to promote the recruitment of transcription factors. Exon 4 acts as a linker and exon 5 encodes the acidic C-terminal domain of the protein and the 3′ UTR of the mRNA [23]. The HMGA2 protein is important in various biologic processes, including cell proliferation, cell-cycle progression [9], apoptosis, and senescence and plays a crucial role in self-renewal and control of differentiation of various stem cells [22].

Hmga2 null mice showed reduction of body size and are called "pigmy mice" and are resistant to diet-induced obesity because of a reduction in the total number of cells in the fat pads [1, 36]. In contrast, transgenic mice expressing a truncated form of *HMGA2 (T-HMGA2)* showed enhanced adipogenesis, a high prevalence of lipomas and significant weight gain in young mice [3]. Adipocyte-specific promoter-driven *T-HMGA2*-tg mice showed fibroadenomas of the breast, salivary gland hyperplasia, or endometrial hyperplasia [35]. Transgenic mice expressing the full-length *HMGA2* transcript under the control of the CMV promoter showed high

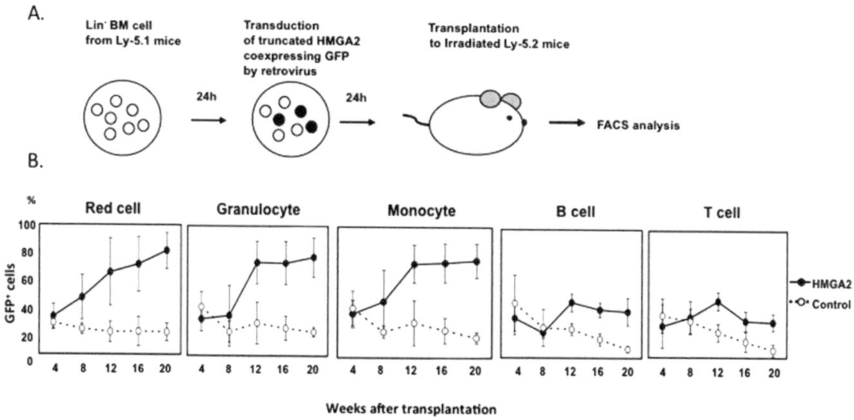

Fig. 3.2 Expansion of HMGA2-expressing cells in all hematopoietic lineages of bone marrow (BM) reconstituted mice. A. Lineage marker-negative BM cells from Ly-5.1 mice were transduced with a retrovirus vector bearing a truncated human HMGA2 and GFP, or GFP only as a control, and were transplanted to lethally irradiated Ly-5.2 mice. Peripheral blood cells from transplanted cells were analyzed by FACS. B. Mean percentages of GFP-expressing Ly-5.1 cells in each lineage of peripheral blood cells from BM-reconstituted mice (Reproduced from Murakami et al. [19])

frequency of pituitary adenomas, sporadic breast carcinomas, and lung and large cell lymphomas [7].

We have generated CAG-driven *HMGA2*-transgenic mice to analyze their hematopoietic phenotype. These mice expressed a truncated form of HMGA2 (containing the first three exons). We transplanted BM cells derived from *HMGA2*-transgenic mice (Ly-5.2) together with those from wild-type mice (Ly-5.1) to observe the proliferative phenotype of HMGA2-expressing hematopoietic stem cells. However, no increase of the population of HMGA2-expressing cells against wild-type cells was observed. Additionally we crossed *Tie2-Cre* mice [16] expressing a truncated form of HMGA2 with *Pigafloxed* mice to test the proliferative phenotype of GPI-negative cells with a HMGA2-expressing background, but the GPI-negative population did not increase (our unpublished result). We speculate that the expression level of HMGA2 in the hematopoietic stem cells is insufficient in these mice because the fatty phenotype of these mice became less apparent after several generations.

Then, we generated another system to test whether high expression of HMGA2 in bone marrow stem cells causes clonal expansion. The retrovirus expressing a truncated form of HMGA2 (containing the first three exons) and GFP was transduced to lineage marker-negative BM cells from mice (Ly-5.1), and those BM cells were intravenously injected into lethally irradiated recipient mice (Ly-5.2). After transplantation, the mice that were transplanted with *HMGA2*-transduced BM cells showed expansion of GFP-positive cells in all lineages (Fig. 3.2). Additionally, we investigated HMGA2 expression in PNH patients without chromosomal abnormalities. The expression of short *HMGA2* mRNA with a latent exon was significantly high in peripheral blood cells from 18 of the 24 patients (Fig. 3.3). Although the

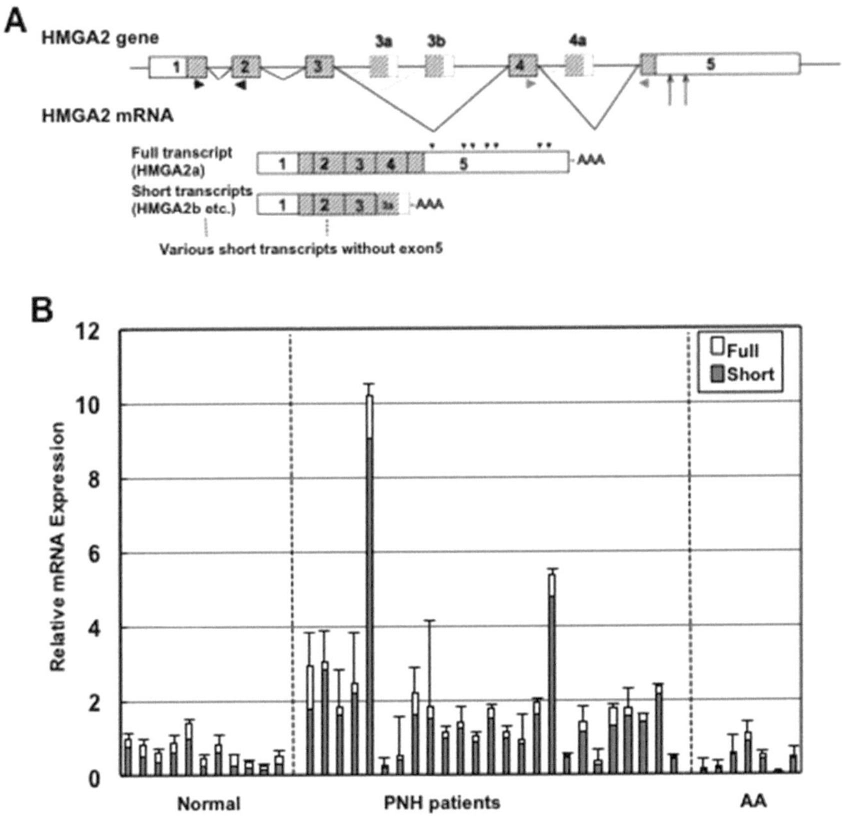

Fig. 3.3 Schematics of *the HMGA2* gene and various *HMGA2* mRNAs and their levels in blood cells of PNH patients. A. Structure of the *HMGA2* gene and its full transcript (*HMGA2a*) and short variants (*HMGA2b*). Black arrowheads, the primer pair for amplification of the total transcripts; gray arrowheads, the primer pair for amplification of the full-length transcript; long arrows, break points in two PNH patients with chromosome 12 rearrangements; and small arrow heads, binding sites of *let-7*. B. Relative *HMGA2* mRNA expression in the peripheral blood cells from patients with PNH in comparison with normal volunteers (Normal) and patients with aplastic anemia or with aplastic anemia and a small PNH clone (AA). White bars, full-length transcript; gray bars, short transcripts; *, the patient with a chromosome 12 rearrangement. Relative mRNA expression, a ratio of normalized *HMGA2* mRNA levels in each sample to that in one normal volunteer are indicated by **. Data are the mean + SD from triplicate measurements (Reproduced from Murakami et al. [19])

expression of HMGA2 in pluripotent stem cells of PNH patients requires testing, these results support the concept that deregulated expression of HMGA2 causes expansion of PNH cells [19].

Ikeda and colleagues succeeded to show the proliferative phenotype of hematopoietic cells expressing HMGA2 [10]. PGK-driven *Hmga2* transgenic mice were generated that contained the full coding region of the *Hmga2* cDNA, but lacked most of the 3′ UTR. These mice showed proliferative hematopoiesis with increased numbers in all lineages of peripheral blood cells, hypercellular BM, splenomegaly with extramedullary erythropoiesis, and erythropoietin-independent erythroid colony formation. The BM cells of the mice had a growth advantage over wild-type cells in competitive repopulation and serial transplantation experiments.

The molecular targets of HMGA2 are not clearly known but appear to include cyclin A [29], E2F1 transcription factor [8], the AP1 complex [32], and NF-κB [23]. As for the transcriptional regulation of *HMGA2*, TGF-β signaling was reported to regulate its expression [30], and growth factors, such as PDGF and EGF-1, were reported to strongly induce *HMGA2* expression in pre-adipocyte cells via the phosphatidylinositol 3-kinase and mitogen-activated protein kinase pathways [4]. Recently, there is a report showing that *Hmga2* is a direct target of RUNX1 [17]. They performed RUNX1 chromatin immunoprecipitation with high-throughput sequencing (Chip-seq) and identified *Hmga2* as a direct target of RUNX. RUNX1 is a master transcription factor in hematopoiesis and mediates the specification and homeostasis of hematopoietic stem and progenitor cells (HSCs). Hmga2 was strongly upregulated in RUNX1-deficient HSCs, which exhibited expansion of HSPCs and myeloid progenitors, which is canceled by knocking out both factors. It was concluded that *Hmga2* is a transcriptional target of RUNX1 and a critical regulator of myeloid progenitor expansion.

Lin28b has been known to regulate let-7 expression, which regulates HMGA2 expression. A recent report showed that overexpression of Lin28 in adult HSCs elevates their self-renewal activity in transplanted irradiated hosts through upregulation of *Hmga2* [6]. Lin28b acts as a master regulator of developmentally timed changes in HSC programs with *Hmga2* serving as its specific downstream modulator of HSC self-renewal potential. Based on this evidence, it is clear that *HMGA2* has an important role in expansion of hematopoietic progenitors especially in myeloid progenitors, which fits with the observation that dominance of GPI-negative cells can be seen more strongly in myeloid lineage in PNH patients. Our observation that the expression of short *HMGA2* with a latent exon was significantly high in peripheral blood cells for 75 % of PNH patients (Fig. 3.3) may suggest that some additional abnormality enhances HMGA2 expression leading to clonal expansion in these patients [19]. However, a significant population of PNH patients did not show high expression of HMGA2, suggesting that there are yet other mechanisms that lead to clonal expansion.

References

1. Anand A, Chada K (2000) In vivo modulation of Hmgic reduces obesity. Nat Genet 24(4):377–380. doi:10.1038/74207
2. Araten DJ, Nafa K, Pakdeesuwan K, Luzzatto L (1999) Clonal populations of hematopoietic cells with paroxysmal nocturnal hemoglobinuria genotype and phenotype are present in normal individuals. Proc Natl Acad Sci USA 96:5209–5214
3. Arlotta P, Tai AK, Manfioletti G, Clifford C, Jay G, Ono SJ (2000) Transgenic mice expressing a truncated form of the high mobility group I-C protein develop adiposity and an abnormally high prevalence of lipomas. J Biol Chem 275(19):14394–14400

4. Ayoubi TA, Jansen E, Meulemans SM, Van de Ven WJ (1999) Regulation of HMGIC expression: an architectural transcription factor involved in growth control and development. Oncogene 18(36):5076–5087
5. Cavazzana-Calvo M, Payen E, Negre O, Wang G, Hehir K, Fusil F, Down J, Denaro M, Brady T, Westerman K, Cavallesco R, Gillet-Legrand B, Caccavelli L, Sgarra R, Maouche-Chretien L, Bernaudin F, Girot R, Dorazio R, Mulder GJ, Polack A, Bank A, Soulier J, Larghero J, Kabbara N, Dalle B, Gourmel B, Socie G, Chretien S, Cartier N, Aubourg P, Fischer A, Cornetta K, Galacteros F, Beuzard Y, Gluckman E, Bushman F, Hacein-Bey-Abina S, Leboulch P (2010) Transfusion independence and HMGA2 activation after gene therapy of human beta-thalassaemia. Nature 467(7313):318–322
6. Copley MR, Babovic S, Benz C, Knapp DJ, Beer PA, Kent DG, Wohrer S, Treloar DQ, Day C, Rowe K, Mader H, Kuchenbauer F, Humphries RK, Eaves CJ (2013) The Lin28b-let-7-Hmga2 axis determines the higher self-renewal potential of fetal haematopoietic stem cells. Nat Cell Biol 15(8):916–925. doi:10.1038/ncb2783
7. Fedele M, Battista S, Kenyon L, Baldassarre G, Fidanza V, Klein-Szanto AJ, Parlow AF, Visone R, Pierantoni GM, Outwater E, Santoro M, Croce CM, Fusco A (2002) Overexpression of the HMGA2 gene in transgenic mice leads to the onset of pituitary adenomas. Oncogene 21(20):3190–3198
8. Fedele M, Visone R, De Martino I, Troncone G, Palmieri D, Battista S, Ciarmiello A, Pallante P, Arra C, Melillo RM, Helin K, Croce CM, Fusco A (2006) HMGA2 induces pituitary tumorigenesis by enhancing E2F1 activity. Cancer Cell 9(6):459–471
9. Fusco A, Fedele M (2007) Roles of HMGA proteins in cancer. Nat Rev Cancer 7(12):899–910. doi:10.1038/nrc2271
10. Ikeda K, Mason PJ, Bessler M (2011) 3′ UTR-truncated Hmga2 cDNA causes MPN-like hematopoiesis by conferring a clonal growth advantage at the level of HSC in mice. Blood 117(22):5860–5869
11. Inoue N, Izui-Sarumaru T, Murakami Y, Endo Y, Nishimura J, Kurokawa K, Kuwayama M, Shime H, Machii T, Kanakura Y, Meyers G, Wittwer C, Chen Z, Babcock W, Frei-Lahr D, Parker CJ, Kinoshita T (2006) Molecular basis of clonal expansion of hematopoiesis in 2 patients with paroxysmal nocturnal hemoglobinuria (PNH). Blood 108(13):4232–4236. doi:10.1182/blood-2006-05-025148
12. Jasinski M, Keller P, Fujiwara Y, Orkin SH, Bessler M (2001) GATA1-Cre mediates Piga gene inactivation in the erythroid/megakaryocytic lineage and leads to circulating red cells with a partial deficiency in glycosyl phosphatidylinositol-linked proteins (paroxysmal nocturnal hemoglobinuria type II cells). Blood 98(7):2248–2255
13. Kawagoe K, Kitamura D, Okabe M, Taniuchi I, Ikawa M, Watanabe T, Kinoshita T, Takeda J (1996) GPI-anchor deficient mice: implications for clonal dominance of mutant cells in paroxysmal nocturnal hemoglobinuria. Blood 87:3600–3606
14. Keller P, Payne JL, Tremml G, Greer PA, Gaboli M, Pandolfi PP, Bessler M (2001) FES-Cre targets phosphatidylinositol glycan class A (PIGA) inactivation to hematopoietic stem cells in the bone marrow. J Exp Med 194:581–589
15. Keller P, Tremml G, Rosti V, Bessler M (1999) X inactivation and somatic cell selection rescue female mice carrying a Piga-null mutation. Proc Natl Acad Sci U S A 96:7479–7483
16. Kisanuki YY, Hammer RE, Miyazaki J, Williams SC, Richardson JA, Yanagisawa M (2001) Tie2-Cre transgenic mice: a new model for endothelial cell-lineage analysis in vivo. Dev Biol 230(2):230–242
17. Lam K, Muselman A, Du R, Harada Y, Scholl AG, Yan M, Matsuura S, Weng S, Harada H, Zhang DE (2014) Hmga2 is a direct target gene of RUNX1 and regulates expansion of myeloid progenitors in mice. Blood 124(14):2203–2212. doi:10.1182/blood-2014-02-554543
18. Mayr C, Hemann MT, Bartel DP (2007) Disrupting the pairing between let-7 and Hmga2 enhances oncogenic transformation. Science 315(5818):1576–1579
19. Murakami Y, Inoue N, Shichishima T, Ohta R, Noji H, Maeda Y, Nishimura J, Kanakura Y, Kinoshita T (2012) Deregulated expression of HMGA2 is implicated in clonal expansion of PIGA deficient cells in paroxysmal nocturnal haemoglobinuria. Br J Haematol 156(3):383–387. doi:10.1111/j.1365-2141.2011.08914.x

20. Murakami Y, Kinoshita T, Maeda Y, Nakano T, Kosaka H, Takeda J (1999) Different roles of glycosylphosphatidylinositol in various hematopoietic cells as revealed by model mice of paroxysmal nocturnal hemoglobinuria. Blood 94:2963–2970
21. Murakami Y, Kosaka H, Maeda Y, Nishimura J, Inoue N, Ohishi K, Okabe M, Takeda J, Kinoshita T (2002) Inefficient response of T lymphocytes to GPI-anchor-negative cells: implications for paroxysmal nocturnal hemoglobinuria. Blood 100:4116–4122
22. Nishino J, Kim I, Chada K, Morrison SJ (2008) Hmga2 promotes neural stem cell self-renewal in young but not old mice by reducing p16Ink4a and p19Arf Expression. Cell 135(2):227–239
23. Noro B, Licheri B, Sgarra R, Rustighi A, Tessari MA, Chau KY, Ono SJ, Giancotti V, Manfioletti G (2003) Molecular dissection of the architectural transcription factor HMGA2. Biochemistry 42(15):4569–4577
24. Rosti V, Tremmi G, Soares V, Pandolfi PP, Luzzatto L, Bessler M (1997) Murine embryonic stem cells without pig-a gene activity are competent for hematopoiesis with the PNH phenotype but not for clonal expansion. J Clin Invest 100:1028–1036
25. Rotoli B, Luzzatto L (1989) Paroxysmal nocturnal haemoglobinuria. Baillieres Clin Haematol 2:113–138
26. Sgarra R, Rustighi A, Tessari MA, Di Bernardo J, Altamura S, Fusco A, Manfioletti G, Giancotti V (2004) Nuclear phosphoproteins HMGA and their relationship with chromatin structure and cancer. FEBS Lett 574(1–3):1–8. doi:10.1016/j.febslet.2004.08.013
27. Sugimori C, Chuhjo T, Feng X, Yamazaki H, Takami A, Teramura M, Mizoguchi H, Omine M, Nakao S (2006) Minor population of CD55-CD59- blood cells predicts response to immunosuppressive therapy and prognosis in patients with aplastic anemia. Blood 107(4):1308–1314. doi:10.1182/blood-2005-06-2485
28. Tarutani M, Itami S, Okabe M, Ikawa M, Tezuka T, Yoshikawa K, Kinoshita T, Takeda J (1997) Tissue specific knock-out of the mouse Pig-a gene reveals important roles for GPI-anchored proteins in skin development. Proc Natl Acad Sci U S A 94:7400–7405
29. Tessari MA, Gostissa M, Altamura S, Sgarra R, Rustighi A, Salvagno C, Caretti G, Imbriano C, Mantovani R, Del Sal G, Giancotti V, Manfioletti G (2003) Transcriptional activation of the cyclin A gene by the architectural transcription factor HMGA2. Mol Cell Biol 23(24):9104–9116
30. Thuault S, Valcourt U, Petersen M, Manfioletti G, Heldin CH, Moustakas A (2006) Transforming growth factor-beta employs HMGA2 to elicit epithelial-mesenchymal transition. J Cell Biol 174(2):175–183
31. Tremml G, Dominguez C, Rosti V, Zhang Z, Pandolfi PP, Keller P, Bessler M (1999) Increased sensitivity to complement and a decreased red cell life span in mice mosaic for a non-functional Piga gene. Blood 94:2945–2954
32. Vallone D, Battista S, Pierantoni GM, Fedele M, Casalino L, Santoro M, Viglietto G, Fusco A, Verde P (1997) Neoplastic transformation of rat thyroid cells requires the junB and fra-1 gene induction which is dependent on the HMGI-C gene product. Embo J 16(17):5310–5321
33. Wang GP, Berry CC, Malani N, Leboulch P, Fischer A, Hacein-Bey-Abina S, Cavazzana-Calvo M, Bushman FD (2010) Dynamics of gene-modified progenitor cells analyzed by tracking retroviral integration sites in a human SCID-X1 gene therapy trial. Blood 115(22):4356–4366. doi:10.1182/blood-2009-12-257352
34. Young NS (1992) The problem of clonality in aplastic anemia: Dr Dameshek's riddle, restated. Blood 79:1385–1392
35. Zaidi MR, Okada Y, Chada KK (2006) Misexpression of full-length HMGA2 induces benign mesenchymal tumors in mice. Cancer Res 66(15):7453–7459. doi:10.1158/0008-5472.CAN-06-0931
36. Zhou X, Benson KF, Ashar HR, Chada K (1995) Mutation responsible for the mouse pygmy phenotype in the developmentally regulated factor HMGI-C. Nature 376(6543):771–774. doi:10.1038/376771a0

Chapter 4
Complement and PNH

Charles J. Parker

Abstract The intravascular hemolysis that is the defining clinical feature of PNH is complement-mediated. PNH erythrocytes undergo spontaneous lysis in vivo because they lack decay-accelerating factor (DAF, CD55) and membrane inhibitor of reactive lysis (MIRL, CD59), glycosylphosphatidylinositol-anchored proteins, that regulate complement at two different steps in the cascade. DAF controls the formation and stability of the alternative pathway C3 and C5 convertases, whereas CD59 inhibits the terminal pathway by blocking the formation of the cytolytic membrane attack complex. Investigation into the mechanisms underlying the hemolysis of PNH has produced a remarkable number of important discoveries about the workings of the human complement system, including confirmation of the existence of the alternative pathway, characterization of the function of DAF, and discovery of CD59. Insightful analysis of complement sensitivity assays identified the phenotypic mosaicism characteristic of the PNH, revealed the clonal nature of the disease, and demonstrated its origin in the hematopoietic stem cell. Ultimately, research into the basis of the complement-mediated hemolysis of PNH led to development of symptomatically effective therapy for the disease.

Keywords Complement • PNH • Alternative pathway of complement • Hemolysis

4.1 Introduction

The defining clinical feature of PNH, chronic intravascular hemolysis, is a consequence of the combined deficiency of two proteins, CD55 (also known as decay-accelerating factor (DAF)) and CD59 (also known as membrane inhibitor of reactive lysis (MIRL)). The function of these two proteins is to protect the erythrocyte from complement-mediated destruction. As a result of the absence (or marked deficiency) of both DAF and CD59, PNH erythrocytes undergo spontaneous intravascular hemolysis. The hemolysis of PNH is mediated by the alternative pathway of

C.J. Parker, M.D. (✉)
Division of Hematology and Hematologic Malignancies, University of Utah School of Medicine, 30 N 1900 E RM 5C402, Salt Lake City, UT 84132-2101, USA
e-mail: Charles.Parker@hsc.utah.edu

Y. Kanakura et al. (eds.), *Paroxysmal Nocturnal Hemoglobinuria*,
DOI 10.1007/978-4-431-56003-6_4

complement (APC), and processes such as infection, trauma, or surgery that generate an inflammatory response, and thereby stimulate APC activation, account for the exacerbations of hemolysis that give the disease an episodic nature.

Almost from the discovery by Jules Bordet in 1895 of the system that "complemented" the activity of the antibody-dependent humoral immune system, participation of complement in the hemolysis of PNH has been investigated. Researchers working in the early part of the twentieth century, however, concluded that the hemolysis of PNH was not complement-mediated. Although the lytic activity in plasma that mediated the hemolysis of PNH erythrocytes in vitro could be inactivated by heating (a hallmark of complement-mediated processes), the activity could not be restored by the addition, to the heat-inactivated serum, of a small amount of unheated serum (another feature that, at the time, was thought to be a fundamental property of complement-mediated processes). Interest in the role of complement in PNH hemolysis was revived by the work of Thomas Hale Ham. His seminal studies, published in the late 1930s, built on the results of earlier experiments by others that showed that PNH erythrocytes underwent hemolysis in serum that was mildly acidified [45]. After rigorously dissecting the abnormal hemolysis of PNH erythrocytes, he concluded (along with his coauthor, John Dingle) that "The serum factor essential for hemolysis was closely associated with, if not indistinguishable from complement or alexin (the name used by Bordet for what came to be know as complement) of human serum" [45]. Ham and Dingle had to equivocate about the role of complement in the lysis of PNH erythrocytes in acidified serum because their experiments demonstrated that the process was antibody independent. While their findings challenged the existing dogma that complement activation was an antibody-dependent process, the rigorous design of their experiments and the compelling nature of their results made it difficult to dismiss their conclusions as artifactual. Other investigators confirmed and extended the observations of Ham and Dingle, and while evidence continued to build in favor of complement as the mechanism that mediated PNH hemolysis, it was not until the discovery of the antibody-independent "properdin pathway" (now known as the APC) by Louis Pillemer in 1954 that Ham's observations were explained [94]. In addition to their impact on the understanding of the pathophysiology of PNH, Ham's studies lead to implementation of the first clinical diagnostic test for PNH, the acidified serum test (or as it came to be known informally, Ham's Test). This simple but highly specific assay stood for 50 years as the standard diagnostic test for PNH until it was supplanted by flow cytometric analysis in the early 1990s.

4.2 The Complement System

The Classical Pathway and the Lectin Pathway There are three pathways that initiate activation of the complement system, the classical pathway, the lectin pathway, and the APC. All three of these initiation pathways activate the terminal pathway that mediates formation of the cytolytic membrane attack complex (MAC). Although the hemolysis of PNH erythrocytes is a consequence of lack of the capacity to con-

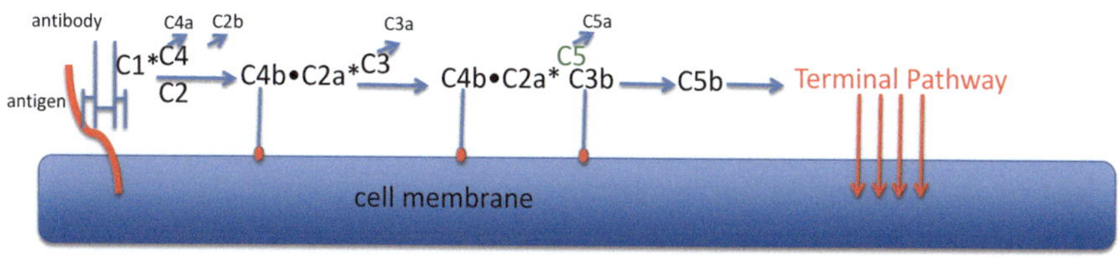

Fig. 4.1 *The classical pathway of complement.* The classical pathway is activated when C1 binds to a site in the Fc region of IgG or IgM antibodies that are antigen bound. C1 is composed of three subunits. C1q is the binding subunit, while C1r and C1s have enzymatic activity. The structural integrity of C1 is calcium dependent. Activation of C4 and C2 by C1s generates the classical pathway C3 convertase. C2a is the enzymatic subunit of the C3 and C5 convertases. Activation of C4 and C3 induces a conformational change that exposes an internal thioester that can form a covalent bond with the immunoglobulin molecule or with a protein or glycoprotein on the cell surface. Activation of C5 by the C2a component of the C5 convertase initiates formation of the terminal pathway of complement that generates the cytolytic MAC. Complement activation products C4a, C3a, and C5a are anaphylatoxins. * indicates enzymatic activity; • indicates magnesium-dependent binding

trol APC activation, an overview of the classical pathway is included in this review to provide readers with a perspective on the differences between the two pathways. The lectin pathway is similar to the classical pathway. It has no direct role in the pathophysiology of PNH, however, and therefore is mentioned only briefly in relationship to its similarity to the classical pathway.

The complement system discovered by Bordet is now known as the classical pathway (Fig. 4.1). The classical pathway is activated when IgG or IgM antibodies bind to antigen, exposing binding sites for C1, the first component of complement [18]. C1 is composed of three subunits, C1q, C1r, and C1s, in a stoichiometry of 1:2:2, respectively. C1q is a distinctive molecule with six globular heads extending from a collagen-like stem (under electron microscopy, the side view of the molecule looks remarkably similar to a bouquet of tulips). Each of the six globular heads of C1q has a binding site that is specific for the Fc region of the immunoglobulin molecule (Fig. 4.1). Both C1r and C1s are serine proteases that exist in their native state as zymogens (inactive proenzymes). C1 enzymatic activity is expressed following autoactivation of the two C1r zymogens that is initiated by a conformational change that occurs in C1q upon binding to immunoglobulin. The two C1s zymogens are converted to active enzymes by the proteolytic action of the activated C1r molecules. The natural substrates for the enzymatic component of C1 ($C1s_2$) are C2 and C4. Enzymatic cleavage of C4 into C4a and C4b fragments by $C1s_2$ exposes an internal thioester bond in the C4b moiety through which, via acyl transfer, the molecule binds covalently by forming an ester or imidoester bond with the antigen-bound immunoglobulin molecule or with a nearby membrane protein or glycoprotein (e.g., glycophorin A on human erythrocytes) [56, 61]. The covalent attachment of C4b serves as the nidus for formation of the C3 convertase of the classical pathway by providing a binding site for C2, another zymogen belonging to the family of serine proteases [58]. Upon enzymatic cleavage by $C1s_2$, activated C2 (C2a) remains bound to C4b and functions as the enzymatic subunit of the classical pathway C3 convertase (Fig. 4.1). The classical pathway C5 convertase is formed when C2a cleaves C3. As with C4, enzymatic cleavage of C3 exposes an internal thioester bond that results in covalent binding of activated C3 (C3b) to immunoglobulin or to a nearby cell surface protein or glycoprotein [16, 39, 62]. Covalently bound C3b serves as the binding site for C5 and positions it for cleavage by C2a (Fig. 4.1). Unlike C4b and C3b, activated C5b does not contain an internal thioester bond and thus does not bind covalently to the cell membrane [61]. Rather C5b serves as the nidus for the formation of the terminal pathway of complement, leading to generation of the MAC that inserts into the lipid bilayer, disrupting the integrity of the cell membrane and consequently inducing complement-mediated cytolysis.

The activity of the classical pathway is inhibited by both plasma- and membrane-associated proteins. C1 inhibitor, a plasma protein belonging to the serpin family of protease inhibitors, binds to activated C1r and C1s, dissociating these enzymes from the C1 molecular complex, leaving the C1q component bound to immunoglobulin [18]. The plasma constituent, C4b-binding protein regulates the formation and stability of the classical pathway C3 convertase by inhibiting binding of C2 to C4b and by accelerating the decay of the C4bC2a complex [41, 118, 138]. C4b-binding protein also serves as a cofactor for the enzymatic degradation of C4b by the serine protease, factor I. The activity of the classical pathway C3 convertase is also regulated by two erythrocyte membrane proteins, DAF and complement receptor type 1 (CR1, CD35). CR1 regulates the convertase activity in much the same way as C4b-binding protein (i.e., it binds to C4b preventing formation of the complex, accelerating the decay of the C4b2b complex, and serving as a factor I cofactor) [55, 69, 107]. In contrast, DAF lacks factor I cofactor activity, and it does not appear to block convertase formation. Rather (as its name suggests), DAF restricts convertase activity by accelerating the decay of the C4b2b complex [76]. Membrane cofactor protein (MCP, CD46) is another cellular protein that inhibits complement activation [5]. As does CR1, MCP (CD46) serves as a cofactor for the factor I-mediated cleavage of C4b (and C3b). MCP (CD46), however, is not an inhibitor of immune hemolysis because it is not expressed on erythrocytes.

The Lectin Pathway This ancient pathway that is a component of the innate immune system differs from the classical pathway only at the beginning of the initiation process [137]. Whereas activation of the classical pathway is initiated by binding of C1q to antibody, the lectin pathway is activated when mannose-binding lectin recognizes mannose, glucose, or other molecularly similar carbohydrate-based ligands on the surface of microorganisms. Structurally, mannose-binding lectin closely resembles C1q. In the lectin pathway, mannose-associated serine protease-1 and mannose-associated serine protease-2 serve a function comparable to that of C1r and C1s of the classical pathway, respectively, cleaving C2 and C4 to generate the C3 convertase. The structure of mannose-associated serine protease-1 and mannose-associated serine protease-2 is also analogous to that of C1r and C1s, and these proteins appear to have arisen as a consequence of gene duplication. Formation of the C5 convertase and activation of the terminal pathway proceed in the same fashion as described above for the classical pathway. C1 inhibitor controls the activation of the lectin pathway in a manner that parallels the mechanism by which it controls activation of the classical pathway. In the case of the lectin pathway, C1 inhibitor binds to mannose-associated serine protease-1 and mannose-associated serine protease-2, thereby dissociating the enzymatic subunits from the mannose-binding lectin complex.

The APC The classical pathway is a component of the system of acquired immunity that evolved to support (complement) antibody-mediated destruction of invading microorganisms in the immune host. Under normal physiologic conditions, host cells do not require protection against the classical pathway because antibodies against self-antigens are eliminated in the process of immune homeostasis. In contrast, the APC is a component of the innate immune system that evolved to protect the nonimmune host from microbial pathogens. Thus, the APC lacks the antibody-determined specificity of the classical pathway. Rather, the APC is activated by certain microorganisms because the biochemical properties of the potential pathogen promote the formation and stability of the APC C3 convertase [32, 33]. On such APC activators, the binding of the catalytic subunit, factor B, of the APC C3 convertase is favored over binding of the convertase inhibitory plasma protein, factor H. Human erythrocytes are exposed to the same plasma factors as invading organisms, and yet normal red cells are completely resistant to injury mediated by the APC. The resistance is mediated by a combination of mechanisms including the biochemical properties of the cell that favors binding of factor H over binding of factor B to cell-bound C3b and by expression of cell surface proteins that inhibit the formation and stability of the C3 convertase of the APC. That normal erythrocytes never undergo immune destruction mediated by the APC is a testament to the effectiveness of these inhibitors. On the other hand, the hemolysis of PNH is a consequence of deficiency of two of these regulatory proteins, DAF and CD59, confirming the essential role that cell surface inhibitors play in protecting erythrocytes from APC-mediated cytolysis in vivo.

In plasma, the APC is in a state of continuous, low-grade activation. Thus, the system is primed for attack at all times (as would be expected for a physiologically relevant component of innate immunity). Activation of the APC is initiated when the internal thioester bond of C3 undergoes spontaneous hydrolysis to form C3(H_2O) [84] (Fig. 4.2). Nascent C3(H_2O) undergoes a conformational change that transiently exposes a magnesium-dependent binding site for factor B [84] (Fig. 4.2). The catalytic subunit (Bb) of the APC C3 convertase [C3(H_2O)Bb] is generated when factor B that is bound to C3(H_2O) is cleaved by factor D into Ba and Bb fragments. Factor D, a trace plasma protein, is a serine protease that is activated from its zymogen form by MASP-3 of the lectin pathway. Factor B is both structurally and functionally homologous to C2 of the classical pathway. Like C2, factor B is a serine protease that exists in its native state as a zymogen with enzymatic cleavage being required for activation. Further, activated C2 (C2a) and factor B (Bb) have the same natural substrates (i.e., C3 and C5). Although factor B and C2 share only modest amino acid sequence homology (37 %), the genes that encode these two proteins

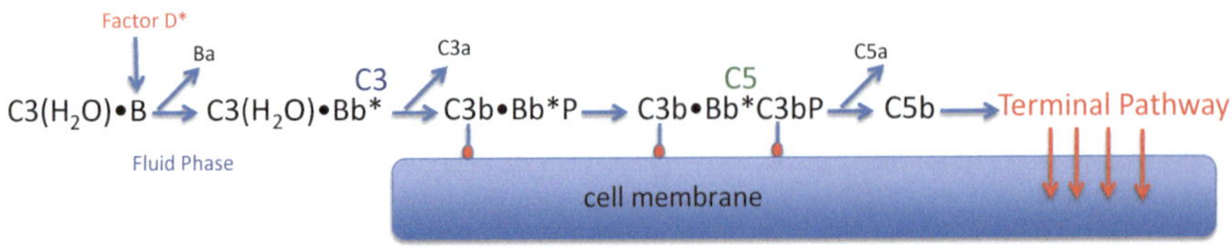

Fig. 4.2 *The alternative pathway of complement* (*APC*). The APC is constitutively active due to the "tick-over" phenomenon. Hydrolysis of the internal thioester bond of C3 forms C3(H_2O), a process that induces a conformational change that exposes a magnesium-dependent binding site for factor B. C3(H_2O)-bound factor B is activated enzymatically by factor D, forming the C3 convertase in the fluid phase (i.e., in the plasma). Subsequent activation of C3 to C3b by Bb induces a conformational change that exposes the internal thioester bond resulting in covalent binding of C3b to a protein or glycoprotein on the membrane surface of the cell. Binding of C3b serves as the nidus for formation of the C3 convertase (C3bBbP). Binding of factor B to C3b is magnesium dependent. Factor P (formerly properdin) stabilizes the C3 convertase. The APC C5 convertase is formed when a second molecule of C3b binds in close proximity to the C3 convertase. The second molecule of C3b serves as the binding site for C5. Activation of C5 by the Bb component of the C5 convertase initiates formation of the terminal pathway of complement that generates the cytolytic MAC. C3a and C5a are anaphylatoxins. * indicates enzymatic activity; • indicates magnesium-dependent binding

are structurally similar and closely associated in the MHC region of chromosome 6, suggesting that the C2 and factor B arose by gene duplication. Spontaneous fluid-phase activation of the APC is restricted by factor H that inhibits the formation and stability of the C3(H_2O)Bb complex.

Activation of the APC on erythrocytes is initiated when C3 binds to C3(H_2O)Bb (Fig. 4.2). The subsequent enzymatic cleavage of C3a from C3 bound to C3(H_2O) in the C3(H_2O)Bb complex by Bb induces a conformational change in the resulting C3b molecule such that the internal thioester becomes exposed. By acyl transfer, nascent C3b binds covalently to glycophorin A, the major erythrocyte sialoglycoprotein [90] (Fig. 4.3). Although both ester and imidoester bonds can form, the majority of C3b on erythrocytes is bound via an ester bond to the carbohydrate moiety of glycophorin A [91]. The cell surface C3 convertase is formed when factor B binds to C3b in a magnesium-dependent reaction (Fig. 4.2). Factor B is activated by factor D, and the amplification C3 convertase (C3bBb) is stabilized by factor P (properdin) [31] (Fig. 4.2).

Both plasma factors and membrane proteins control the formation and stability of the APC C3 convertase (Fig. 4.3). Factor H regulates the formation and stability of the convertase in the following three ways: first, by binding to C3b, it inhibits factor B binding; second, by binding to C3b in the C3bBb complex, it displaces Bb from the complex; third, by binding to C3b, it acts as a cofactor for the enzymatic degradation of C3b to iC3b by factor I [73, 83, 132] (Fig. 4.3). DAF is the erythrocyte membrane constituent that is primarily responsible for regulating the activity of the APC C3 convertase (Fig. 4.3). It binds to C3b in the C3bBb complex causing the enzymatic subunit to dissociate [76]. CR1 also controls C3 convertase activity (Fig. 4.3). Using isolated complement components, purified CR1 has been shown to

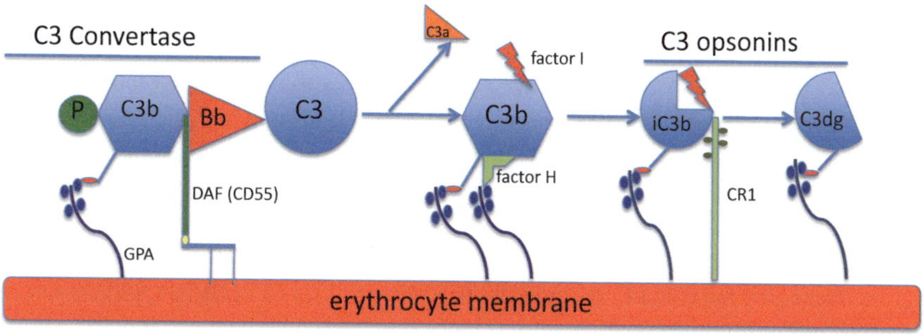

Fig. 4.3 *Regulation of the APC on human erythrocytes*. Activated C3 (C3b) binds covalently via an ester bond to sialic acid residues on glycophorin A. Membrane bound C3b serves as the nidus for formation of the C3 convertase (C3bBbP) of the APC. The formation and stability of the C3 convertase is regulated by DAF (CD55), a glycosylphosphatidylinositol-anchored protein that is deficient in PNH. Enzymatic cleavage of C3 by Bb generates C3a and C3b. Activated C3b binds covalently to glycophorin A. Glycophorin A is the primary sialoglycoprotein of human erythrocytes and serves as the binding site for factor H, the primary plasma inhibitor of the APC. Like DAF, factor H has decay-accelerating activity for the APC C3 convertase, and it also serves as a cofactor for the enzymatic cleavage of C3b by factor I, generating an inactive form of C3b called iC3b. Further degradation of iC3b by factor I requires binding of complement receptor 1 (CR1) to C3b or iC3b, resulting in generation of C3dg through enzymatic cleavage by factor I. C3b, iC3b, and C3dg are opsonins. Opsonized erythrocytes are phagocytosed by reticuloendothelial cells bearing specific receptors for C3b, iC3b, and C3dg

accelerate the decay of the APC C3 convertase in vitro [29]. In vivo, however, it appears likely that erythrocyte CR1 functions primarily as a factor I cofactor rather than as a regulator of the C3 convertase because blocking CR1 function does not enhance APC C3 convertase activity when serum is used as the complement source [133] (Fig. 4.3). Further, available evidence suggests that CR1 exerts its activity intercellularly (binding to C3b on neighboring cells), while DAF functions as an intracellular regulator of the convertase (binding to C3bBb on the same cell) [68].

Once covalently bound to the erythrocyte surface, C3b is rapidly degraded to iC3b and then to C3dg by the concert actions of factor H, CR1, and factor I (Fig. 4.3). These activation and degradation products of C3 are recognized by specific complement receptors (CR1, CR2, and CR3) expressed by cells of the reticuloendothelial system. Binding to reticuloendothelial cells induces phagocytosis of complement-opsonized erythrocytes resulting in extravascular hemolysis. Extravascular hemolysis is not observed in patients with PNH (unless they are treated with eculizumab) because the cells are destroyed intravascularly by complement-mediated cytolysis (see below, eculizumab and treatment of the hemolysis of PNH).

The C5 convertase of the APC consists of C3bBbC3bP, with one of the C3b molecules acting as the binding site for Bb and the other molecule serving to position C5 for cleavage by Bb [20] (Fig. 4.2). As is the case for the C3 convertase, the C5 convertase is stabilized by factor P, and the same plasma and membrane constituents that regulate the C3 convertase control the activity of the C5 convertase

(Fig. 4.3). Generation of C5b as a result of enzymatic cleavage of C5 by Bb releases C5a and activates the terminal pathway of complement (Fig. 4.2).

As an aside, the properties of the APC explain some interesting observations about the relationship between complement and the hemolysis of PNH. Lysis of PNH erythrocytes in acidified serum is explained by the fact that both the formation and activity of the APC C3 and C5 convertases are enhanced at pH 6.4 [35]. Thus, the greater activity of the APC under mildly acidic conditions explains the seminal observations of Ham and others. As noted in the Introduction section, early investigators dismissed the role of complement in the hemolysis of PNH in acidified serum because, although the hemolytic activity was inactivated by heating, it could not be restored by adding a small amount of unheated serum to the heat-inactivated sample. As is the case with C2, factor B is a thermolabile protein, thus explaining the loss of APC hemolytic activity when heat-treated serum is used as the complement source. However, unlike classical pathway-mediated lysis that is sustained despite using serum (as the complement source) at high dilutions (dilutions of >1:100), a characteristic feature of APC-mediated lysis is that activity is no longer observed following modest dilutions (1:4 or 1:8) of serum. This difference explains why heat-inactivated serum repleted with amounts of serum known to support classical pathway-mediated lysis did not restore the hemolytic activity of acidified serum.

The Complement Anaphylatoxins Enzymatic cleavage of C4, C3, and C5 by their respective convertases (Figs. 4.1 and 4.2) generates small peptides of approximately 10 kDa (C4a, C3a, and C5a, respectively) that are biologically active [34, 38, 43, 54]. When produced in large amounts (in animal model systems), they induce a generalized circulatory collapse, producing a shock-like syndrome similar to that seen in a systemic allergic reaction involving IgE antibodies. Such a reaction is termed anaphylactic shock, and these small complement fragments are therefore referred to as anaphylatoxins. The complement anaphylatoxins C3a and C5a mediate their activity by binding to specific G-protein-coupled receptors [2, 42]. All three anaphylatoxins induce smooth muscle contraction and vascular permeability. In addition to being potent anaphylatoxins, C5a and to a lesser extent C3a mediate a variety of pro-inflammatory events [53]. Both C3a and C5a act on the endothelial cells lining blood vessels to induce expression of adhesion molecules for inflammatory cells. In addition, C3a and C5a activate mast cells populating submucosal tissues to release inflammatory mediators including histamine and TNF-α. C5a also acts directly on neutrophils and monocytes to increase the expression of complement receptors 1 and 3 (CR1 and CR3) on the cell surface and to enhance their adherence to vessel walls, their migration toward sites of antigen deposition, and their capacity to ingest particulate matter [44].

The Terminal Pathway of Complement After the generation of C5b, no further enzymatic activity is involved in either the formation or the cytolytic activity of the MAC of complement that consists of C5b, C6, C7, C8, and C9 (C5b-9) (Fig. 4.4). Components C6, C7, and C9 are single-chain polypeptides [12, 13, 17, 24–26, 98]. C5b is a disulfide-linked heterodimer that is the product of a single gene. C8 con-

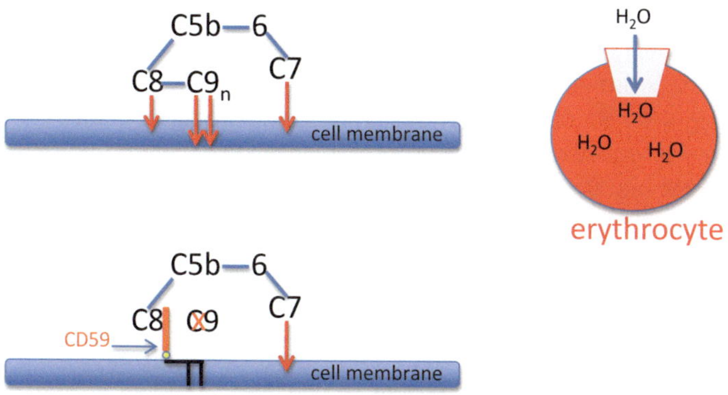

Fig. 4.4 *The terminal pathway of complement.* Formation of the cytolytic MAC is initiated when C5 is cleaved by the C5 convertase of the classical lectin or APC. Nascent C5b binds specifically to C6, forming a stable, hydrophilic complex. Binding to the C5b6 complex induces a conformational change in C7 that exposes a labile membrane-binding site and causes the molecule to undergo a hydrophilic-amphiphilic transition. This process allows the trimolecular C5b67 complex to integrate into the lipid bilayer of the erythrocyte (*top*, *left*). Once inserted into the cell, the complex is stable. Binding of C8 to the C5b67 complex induces a conformational rearrangement that allows the α-chain of C8 to insert into the hydrophobic core of the lipid bilayer and exposes a single binding site for C9 (*top*, *left*). Binding to C8α within the C5b-8 complex causes C9 to unfold. This conformational change exposes hydrophobic regions that allow the molecule to insert into membrane and exposes a binding site for an additional C9 molecule. Binding to C5b-9_1 causes the second C9 molecule to undergo the same conformational change as the first C9 molecule, and in this way, multiple molecules of C9 become incorporated into the MAC (C5b-9_n) (*top*, *left*). The C9 molecules undergo polymerization, and this process forms the ring-like structure that appears as the classical torous (doughnut) lesion visualized by electron microscopy (*top*, *right*). Disruption of the integrity of the lipid bilayer of the erythrocyte by the MAC creates an osmotic gradient because small ions can traverse the damaged membrane, but large cytoplasmic components such as hemoglobin cannot (*top*, *right*). The consequent inflow of water causes the cell to expand rapidly. If damage is great enough, the cell ruptures, releasing hemoglobin into the plasma (a process called colloid osmotic lysis). The glycosylphosphytidylinositol-anchored protein, CD59, inhibits formation of the MAC by binding to C8, blocking C9 binding, and limiting C9 multiplicity (*bottom*)

sists of three nonidentical peptide chains [122]. The α and γ chains comprise a disulfide-linked unit that is noncovalently associated with the β chain. The three polypeptide chains that comprise C8 are the products of separate genes [75]. There are structural and antigenic similarities among four of the components (C6, C7, C8, and C9), and at the nucleotide level, modest homology is observed for C7, C8α, C8β, and C9 [73].

Formation of the MAC is initiated when nascent C5b (i.e., still complexed with C3b) binds specifically to C6, forming a stable, hydrophilic complex [99, 135]. Binding to the C5b6 complex induces a conformational change in C7 that exposes a labile membrane-binding site and causes the molecule to undergo a hydrophilic-amphiphilic transition [23, 101]. This process allows the trimolecular C5b67 complex to integrate into the lipid bilayer of the erythrocyte (Fig. 4.4). Once inserted into the cell, the complex is stable. Binding of C8 to the C5b67 complex is mediated through the β chain that has a specific recognition site for C5b [125, 126]. Binding to C5b67 induces a conformational rearrangement that allows the α-chain of C8 to insert into the hydrophobic core of the lipid bilayer and exposes a single binding site for C9 (Fig. 4.4). Binding to C8α within the C5b-8 complex causes C9 to unfold [126]. This conformational change exposes hydrophobic regions that allow the molecule to insert into the membrane and exposes a binding site for an additional C9 molecule. Binding to $C5b\text{-}9_1$ causes the second C9 molecule to undergo the same conformational change as the first C9 molecule, and in this way, multiple molecules of C9 become incorporated into the MAC ($C5b\text{-}9_n$) [73] (Fig. 4.4). The C9 molecules undergo polymerization, and this process forms the ring-like structure that appears as the classic torus (doughnut) lesion visualized by electron microscopy [8, 15]. Individual MACs are heterogeneous in size due to differences in C9 composition [7, 9, 97]. Thus, the stoichiometry of the MAC is $C5b_1$, $C6_1$, $C7_1$, $C8_1$, and $C9_n$ where n ranges from 2–18 depending upon the experimental conditions. On normal human erythrocytes that have undergone hemolysis, the average C8:C9 ratio is 1:3, whereas on PNH erythrocytes that have undergone lysis, the average C8:C9 ratio is 1:6 [92]. These results predicted that PNH erythrocytes are deficient in a membrane constituent that regulates the formation of the MAC (see below).

Disruption of the integrity of the lipid bilayer of the erythrocyte by the MAC creates an osmotic gradient because small ions can traverse the damaged membrane, but large cytoplasmic components such as hemoglobin cannot (Fig. 4.4). The consequent inflow of water causes the cell to expand rapidly. If damage is great enough, the cell ruptures, releasing hemoglobin into the plasma (a process called colloid osmotic lysis). The mechanism by which the MAC produces cell lysis is debated. According to the "leaky patch" hypothesis, insertion of the hydrophobic elements of the MAC causes local disruption of the integrity of the phospholipid bilayer [28]. The proponents of the competing "pore" hypothesis argue that the polar surfaces of the MAC components aggregate, forming a hydrophilic channel through the membrane [10]. Data in support of both hypotheses has been presented, suggesting that both processes may be operative depending upon the experimental conditions.

Plasma proteins including vitronectin [99] and apolipoproteins (particularly clusterin) have been shown to inhibit the activity of the MAC in vitro [57, 99, 100, 106, 130, 131]. The importance of these plasma constituents in regulating the lytic actions of complement in vivo, however, has not been established unequivocally. Erythrocytes are protected from lytic action of the MAC by CD59 [49]. This glycosylphosphatidylinositol-anchored protein inhibits MAC formation primarily by binding to C8, thereby restricting the subsequent binding and polymerization of C9 [64, 70, 105].

4.3 Differences in Complement Sensitivity Identified the Phenotypic Mosaicism of PNH

In discussing the acidified serum lysis test, Professor John Dacie commented in his 1963 review of PNH that "Even if the serum is changed several times there appear to be always some cells which resist hemolysis"[19]. As had Ham and Dingle, Dacie observed that PNH erythrocytes were abnormally sensitive to lysis when complement was activated by antibody in vitro, but again, complete hemolysis was never observed. These observations suggested the existence either of one population of cells that varied in sensitivity to lysis or of two populations, one more sensitive to complement than the other.

Based in a large part on a biphasic red cell survival pattern for transfused PNH erythrocytes (the curve showed a steep slope early suggesting a population with a very short life span and a less steep slope subsequently that approximated that observed for normal erythrocytes), Dacie favored the hypothesis that the erythrocytes of PNH consisted of two discrete populations [19]. Compared to normal erythrocytes, Dacie also hypothesized that the greater sensitivity of PNH erythrocytes to antibody-initiated lysis was due to aberrant interactions with complement. In the early 1960s, the pioneering work of Manfred Mayer made possible quantitative analysis of complement activity. Working with Dacie, Rosse modified the technique that Mayer had developed in order to quantify the complement sensitivity of PNH erythrocytes [113]. The results of those studies demonstrated for the first time the magnitude of the difference in sensitivity between PNH and normal erythrocytes and clearly separated the erythrocytes of patients with PNH into two quantitatively definable populations.

In the complement lysis sensitivity (CLS) assay of Rosse and Dacie, erythrocytes were incubated with an excess of sensitizing antibody and with incremental concentrations of serum as the complement source [113]. Subsequently, lysis was quantitated based on hemoglobin released (determined spectrophotometrically). When the results were plotted as the logarithm of the fraction of cells lysed/fraction of cells unlysed vs. the logarithm of the complement concentration, a straight line was observed for normal erythrocytes [113]. In contrast, when erythrocytes from patients with PNH were analyzed, the plot showed two connected, nearly parallel straight lines. These findings were interpreted to mean that the peripheral blood of patients with PNH consisted of two populations of cells that differed in susceptibility to complement-mediated lysis with the complement-sensitive population requiring ~4 % as much serum for an equal degree of lysis as normal cells.

The seminal studies of Rosse and Dacie demonstrated conclusively for the first time that the erythrocytes of PNH are a mosaic [113]. Rosse and Dacie also interpreted their results as establishing unequivocally that abnormal sensitivity to complement underlies the greater hemolysis of PNH erythrocytes "regardless of the factors responsible for the initiation of the immune reaction." This conclusion was strongly supported by the observation that the cells that underwent hemolysis in the acidified serum lysis test (Ham's test) were the same as the sensitive population defined by the complement lysis sensitivity assay [113].

By examining the erythrocytes from 11 patients, the variation in the proportion of complement-sensitive cells was also demonstrated (the range was from 4 to 80 %) [113]. This observation provided a plausible explanation for the variability among patients in the severity of the hemolytic component of the disease, illuminating another important characteristic feature of the disease.

The studies of Rosse and Dacie represented a major conceptual advance and defined many of the fundamental characteristics of PNH. These studies also greatly influenced future investigation. In particular, the recognition that the basic defect underlying the disease was represented in the complement-sensitive population provided a means for assessing whether a particular observation was fundamentally related to PNH. According to this paradigm, if a process is specific for PNH erythrocytes, it should be observed in the complement-sensitive population but not in the complement-insensitive population. By separating cell populations into complement-sensitive and complement-insensitive groups, the importance of the deficiency of erythrocyte acetylcholinesterase in PNH was firmly established [4, 60]. Although 25 years past between the time the acetylcholinesterase deficiency in PNH was identified and the time the basis of the deficiency became apparent, the association between erythrocyte acetylcholinesterase deficiency and PNH led ultimately to an understanding of the fundamental abnormality of the disease (i.e., that all of the proteins deficient in PNH are glycosylphosphatidylinositol anchored) [22]. Studies indicating that the complement-sensitive erythrocytes were monoclonal while the complement-insensitive cells were polyclonal provided critically important experimental support for the hypothesis that somatic mutations account for the phenotypic mosaicism characteristic of PNH [19, 81]. In 1969, Aster and Enright demonstrated that platelets and neutrophils from PNH patients are abnormally sensitive to complement-mediated lysis [3]. These studies were consistent with the hypotheses that the somatic mutation occurs in a primitive hematopoietic stem cell. (Inasmuch as the existence of a pluripotent stem cell was still an issue of active debate at that time, these studies also supported those who hypothesized the existence of a bone marrow cell that could differentiate along erythrocytic, myelocytic, and megakaryocytic lines.) By using a modification of the complement lysis sensitivity assay, Stern and Rosse confirmed that like the erythrocytes, the granulocytes of PNH are also a mosaic [124].

As noted above, the red cells of patients with PNH were initially divided into two groups (sensitive and insensitive) based on susceptibility to hemolysis by complement. According to this classification, the insensitive population was on average approximately twice as sensitive to complement-induced hemolysis as normal erythrocytes. However, with more experience using the assay, it became apparent that the complement-insensitive population was heterogeneous [110]. Careful analysis of the data generated by the complement lysis sensitivity assay showed that three populations of erythrocytes could be identified in some patients with PNH. Based on these observations, Rosse, in 1974, proposed the following phenotypic classification: type I, normal complement sensitivity; type II, moderate complement sensitivity (3–4 times more sensitive than normal); and type III, marked complement sensitivity (15–20 time more sensitive than normal) [112]. In the majority of patients, a population of cells with complement sensitivity equivalent to that of normal cells was observed along with a variable proportion of abnormally sensitive cells. Erythrocytes of intermediate sensitivity (the PNH II phenotype) could be identified coexisting with cells of normal sensitive (the PNH I phenotype), marked sensitivity (the PNH III phenotype), or both [109–112]. The finding that three different red cell phenotypes could be identified in the peripheral blood of patients challenged the hypothesis that PNH arose by monoclonal expansion [110]. The functional basis of the variability in complement sensitivity of PNH erythrocytes was delineated in 1989, and in 1996, the molecular basis of the phenotypic mosaicism was defined [27, 52]. The pathophysiological pressure that selects for the abnormal stem cells, however, remains enigmatic. Any hypothesis that attempts to explain PNH must account for this remarkable feature of the disease that was defined originally by careful analysis of complement sensitivity of the erythrocytes.

4.4 Functional Basis of the Abnormal Sensitivity of the Erythrocytes of PNH to Complement-Mediated Lysis

Overview In a pivotal paper published in 1973, Logue et al. reported that PNH erythrocytes bound more C3 than normal erythrocytes when complement was activated by either the classical or the APC [66]. Those investigators also observed that, for a given amount of C3 bound, PNH erythrocytes lysed to a much greater degree than normal cells. These results suggested that both quantitative and qualitative differences in complement interactions with PNH erythrocytes mediated the greater lytic sensitivity. The interpretation of these elegant experiments provided the conceptual framework for subsequent studies aimed at delineating the aberrant interactions of complement with PNH red cells. By analyzing the relationship between the extent of lysis and the amount of C3 bound, Rosse and colleagues demonstrated differences between PNH II and PNH III erythrocytes [112]. They found that while both phenotypes bound equivalent, supernormal amounts of C3, the type III cells underwent more lysis per C3 molecule bound when compared with type II cells. These results suggested that either PNH III cells had an additional defect that was not shared by PNH II cells or that the abnormality was the same for both types but that the type III cells were more severely affected than the type II cells.

Rouault and colleagues presented compelling evidence in 1978 that, compared to normal erythrocytes, the MAC is more efficient at inducing lysis of PNH III [116]. Those investigators subjected normal and PNH III erythrocytes (PNH II cells were not analyzed in this study) to hemolysis induced by the classical pathway. By varying the concentration of antibody, conditions were designed so that the normal and

PNH III cells lysed to the same extent. Next, the number of MAC lesions formed on the lysed cells was counted using electron microscopy to identify the characteristic lesion. For the same extent of lysis, approximately ten times more MAC lesions were observed on normal erythrocytes compared to PNH III erythrocytes. These studies demonstrated that greater lytic efficiency of the terminal complement pathway when activated on PNH III cells contributes to their abnormal susceptibility to complement-mediated lysis. The efficacy of the MAC on PNH erythrocytes was also investigated by Packman et al., who reported that type III cells were abnormally susceptible to reactive lysis, whereas type II cells were not [82]. In reactive lysis systems (also known as passive or bystander lysis), the entire complement cascade is not activated directly on the surface of the erythrocyte as it is when hemolysis is induced either by the classical pathway (e.g., in the complement lysis sensitivity assay) or by the APC (e.g., in the acidified serum lysis test). Rather, the C3 convertase step is bypassed in reactive lysis systems, and the terminal complement pathway is activated in the fluid phase, thereby generating the MAC directly on the cell surface (Fig. 4.4). Thus, in reactive lysis systems, the effects of the MAC are examined directly. The studies of Packman and colleagues provided additional evidence of aberrant regulation of terminal complement pathway on PNH erythrocytes and suggested that the greater lytic susceptibility of PNH III erythrocytes compared to PNH II cells was due primarily to the greater efficiency with which the MAC induced lysis of the type III cells. The basis of this difference between the type II and type III cells and the nature of the abnormal regulation of the terminal pathway on type III cells, however, remained enigmatic.

Identification of Erythrocyte Membrane Proteins that Regulate the C3 Convertase The studies of Logue et al., Rosse et al., and Packman and colleagues demonstrated that both PNH II and PNH III erythrocytes bound more C3b than normal erythrocytes when complement was activated by either the classical or the APC [66, 82, 112]. These results suggested that regulation of the C3 convertases of both pathways might be abnormal on PNH erythrocytes. During the 1970s methods for purifying components of the complement cascade became available, and by 1980, it was possible to assemble the entire C3 convertase of the APC using isolated components. The switch from using whole serum as the complement source to using the purified components allowed a more precise view of the influence of the cell surface on the assembly and stability of the convertase complex. Using isolated components of the APC C3 convertase, Parker et al. and Pangburn et al. demonstrated that the activity, formation, and stability of the convertase are enhanced on PNH cells [86, 89]. Those findings provided a clear explanation for the greater binding of activated C3 to PNH erythrocytes but did not define the molecular basis of the abnormal convertase activity.

In 1979, Fearon reported the isolation of a protein from normal human erythrocytes that inhibited the activity of the C3 convertase of the APC [29]. By binding to cell-associated C3b, the protein prevented the formation of the amplification convertase. This regulatory factor also accelerated the decay of formed convertases (C3bBb) by binding to C3b and thereby dissociating the enzymatic subunit (Bb). In addition, the isolated erythrocyte membrane protein was shown to act as a cofactor for factor I in the enzymatic degradation of C3b (Fig. 4.3). Subsequent studies by Fearon demonstrated that the inhibitory factor was the membrane receptor for C3b known as complement receptor type I (CR1) [30].

The functional properties of CR1 (CD35) suggested that its absence from erythrocytes could result in greater binding of C3b to cells because the formation and stability of the C3 convertase would be enhanced. Accordingly, studies designed to characterize CR1 on PNH erythrocytes were undertaken. The functional activity of CR1 on PNH erythrocytes was found to be normal, and blocking CR1 activity on normal erythrocytes by using specific antibodies did not enhance the susceptibility of the cells to complement-mediated lysis [104]. Studies that quantitated CR1 showed that PNH erythrocytes expressed subnormal amounts of the protein [91, 108]. The deficiency, however, appeared to be an epiphenomenon resulting from exposure of the erythrocytes to complement activation in vivo and was not specific for PNH cells [91, 108].

A decade earlier (1969), Hoffmann published the results of a series of rigorous experiments showing that an *n*-butanol extract prepared from human erythrocyte stroma contained a factor or factors that inhibited complement-mediated hemolysis [46, 47]. He also showed that a portion (~20 %) of the active material possessed the capacity to bind to the indicator cell and remained functionally active. Subsequently, Hoffmann used the name "decay-accelerating factor" (DAF) to describe the functional property of the extract because the material enhanced the rate at which the activity of the classical pathway C3 convertase diminished over time [48].

In 1982, one of the complement regulatory proteins contained in the *n*-butanol extract described by Hoffmann was purified to homogeneity by Nicholson-Weller and colleagues [76]. This protein was named decay-accelerating factor of stroma (DAF-S). The term DAF-S was introduced to distinguish the membrane-derived factor from plasma-derived factors with decay-accelerating activity (e.g., factor H) that were being characterized at the same time by others. The DAF-S designation did not endure, however, and the protein isolated by Nicholson-Weller and colleagues quickly became known simply as DAF. In addition to its capacity to restrict the activity of the classical pathway C3 convertase, DAF was found to inhibit the activity of the APC C3 convertase. Thus, the functional properties of DAF suggested that its absence from erythrocytes would lead to greater C3 convertase activity and hence to greater C3b deposition on the cell surface whether complement was activated by the classical or the APC. The absence of DAF could therefore account for the observed differences between PNH and normal erythrocytes. That PNH erythrocytes were deficient in DAF was reported by Nicholson-Weller and colleagues in 1983 [77]. Those investigators also presented data suggesting that PNH II cells were partially deficient, while PNH III cells were completely DAF deficient. Almost simultaneously, Pangburn et al. presented both functional and immunochemical evidence of DAF deficiency in PNH [85]. The discovery of this deficiency was a milestone in the journey toward understanding the basis of the hemolysis of PNH that began with the observations of Strübing, Hijmans van den Berg, and Ham in the late nineteenth and early twentieth century.

DAF is a 70 kDa single-chain glycoprotein. DAF contains four short consensus repeat units that are homologous to domains found in other complement regulatory proteins (e.g., CR1-, CR2-, C4b-binding proteins, factor H, and membrane cofactor protein). The DAF gene maps to chromosome 1 (band q32) and forms part of the regulators of complement activation locus that includes the genes that encode CR1, CR2, C4b-binding proteins, factor H, and membrane cofactor protein. DAF destabilizes the C3 convertases of both the classical and APCs. It does not inhibit either binding of C2 to C4b or binding of factor B to C3b. Rather, once the convertase is formed (Fig. 4.3), DAF causes the catalytic subunit (C2b in the case of the classical pathway and Bb in the case of the APC) to dissociate [40] (Fig. 4.3).

The deficiency of DAF provided a logical explanation for the greater binding of C3b to PNH erythrocytes when complement was activated either by antibody (classical pathway) or by acidification of serum (APC), and a causal role for DAF in the pathophysiology of PNH was readily accepted. But could DAF deficiency explain all of the aberrant interactions of complement with PNH erythrocytes? As noted above, compelling evidence indicated that regulation of the terminal complement pathway was abnormal on PNH erythrocytes. Thus, if DAF deficiency alone were sufficient to account for the lytic sensitivity of PNH erythrocytes, DAF would have to play a role (direct or indirect) in the regulation of the MAC. Detailed studies, however, demonstrated that DAF had no inhibitory activity in the process of reactive lysis [67, 119]. These results implied that another protein that functioned as a regulator of the terminal complement pathway must also be deficient in PNH.

The idea that more than one protein was deficient in PNH was supported by previous work that had shown that erythrocyte acetylcholinesterase was also expressed abnormally in PNH and that the acetylcholinesterase deficiency correlated with the proportion of complement-sensitive cells [4, 60]. Earlier studies had also shown that neutrophils from patients with PNH were deficient in alkaline phosphatase, and again, the severity of the deficiency appeared to be concordant with the severity of the disease (based on the proportion of complement-sensitive erythrocytes) [6, 65].

That multiple proteins were deficient in PNH made remote the probability that discrete mutations affecting each gene individually accounted for the abnormality. Conceivably, a large deletion could affect the loss of multiple proteins if the genes were in relatively close proximity on the same chromosome. Arguing against this mechanism, however, was the absence of consistent karyotypic abnormalities in PNH. A more feasible explanation for the deficiency of multiple proteins in PNH was that the affected membrane constituents shared a common posttranslational modification and that some step in the processing of this modification was abnormal. A tenet of this hypothesis was that the genes that encode the deficient proteins in PNH are structurally and functionally normal. As anticipated, that neither mutations nor abnormalities in DAF gene expression are found in PNH was reported in 1988 [121]. Meanwhile, the posttranslational modification (the glycosylphosphatidylinositol anchor) that is shared by all of the proteins that are deficient in PNH was identified in 1986 [22].

Identification of Erythrocyte Membrane Proteins that Inhibit the MAC Inasmuch as DAF deficiency could not account for the abnormal regulation of the MAC on PNH erythrocytes, attention was focused on identifying an erythrocyte membrane protein that inhibited the lytic activity of the terminal complement pathway (C5b-9). Using a reactive lysis system in which whole serum complement was activated by cobra venom factor (CVF), Parker et al. demonstrated in 1985 that PNH III erythrocytes bound much greater amounts of C9 than either PNH II or normal cells [92]. These findings confirmed that PNH erythrocytes lacked a membrane factor or factors that regulated assembly of the MAC.

In 1989, Holguin et al. reported the isolation of a protein from normal human erythrocytes that inhibited CVF-initiated lysis of PNH erythrocytes [49]. This protein, that they named membrane inhibitor of reactive lysis (MIRL), was shown by immunohistochemical studies to be deficient on PNH III erythrocytes. MIRL was observed to incorporate into the membrane of PNH III erythrocytes and protect them from reactive lysis. The capacity of the isolated protein to reincorporate into the cell suggested that, like other proteins that are deficient in PNH, MIRL was glycosylphosphatidylinositol anchored. Finally, by blocking MIRL function with antibody, normal erythrocytes could be made susceptible to reactive lysis. Together, the studies of Holguin et al. provided compelling evidence that MIRL deficiency is an important component of the pathophysiology of PNH.

Nearly simultaneously, the protein was identified independently by several groups, although none of those investigators were attempting to identify the factor that accounted for the abnormal sensitivity of PNH erythrocytes to reactive lysis [21, 78, 80, 123]. A number of different names have been proposed for the protein (e.g., CD59, protectin, MACIF, HRF 20, MEM-43, H19). The International Complement Society recognizes CD59 as the official term for this protein that regulates the terminal pathway of complement. CD59 is an 18 kDa glycosylphosphatidylinositol-anchored protein with wide tissue distribution [51]. It inhibits the lytic activity of the MAC primarily by binding to the C8 component of the C5b-8 complex and to the C9 component of the C5b-9 complex (Fig. 4.4). Binding to C5b-8 inhibits C9 binding, and binding to C9 within the C5b-9 complex restricts C9 multiplicity [64, 70, 105]. Normal human erythrocytes express 25,000–30,000 copies of CD59/RBC (there are approximately ten times more copies of CD59 than DAF per RBC).

In the case of DAF, determination of the primary sequence provided insight into the functional properties of the protein because DAF was found to share a common structural motif (the short consensus repeat unit) with other proteins that bind to activated C3 and C4. In the case of CD59, however, delineation of the primary structure revealed no significant homology with any other complement regulatory factors. CD59 shares modest homology with a number of other proteins, including members of the murine Ly-6 multigene family, a squid protein, the receptor for urokinase plasminogen activator, and snake α-neurotoxins [21, 79, 93, 95, 96, 123, 127, 134]. Obviously these proteins are functionally diverse. The common feature that ties these proteins together is the conservation of the Cys residues. CD59 is a prototypic example, containing ten Cys that are paired to form five intrachain disulfide bonds. As a result of these disulfides, the locked loop structures that are characteristic of this group of proteins are generated. By using NMR, the three-dimensional structure of CD59 has been determined [36, 37, 59, 127]. The molecule appears disc-shaped and flat. It consists of two antiparallel β-sheet regions, a short helical region, and a carboxy-terminal region devoid of secondary structure. CD59 contains a single, large N-linked carbohydrate moiety that accounts for approximately one-third of the mass of the molecule. The structure of the N-linked sugar is heterogeneous and complex, but it is not required for the terminal pathway regulatory activity of CD59 [185–188] [1, 14, 115, 117]. The gene that encodes CD59 [177, 189] is located on the short arm of chromosome 11 (p14-p13) [11, 93].

4.5 Molecular Basis of the Erythrocyte Phenotypes of PNH

As discussed above, PNH III erythrocytes had been shown to be susceptible to reactive lysis, whereas PNH II erythrocytes were resistance to this process. Either of two hypotheses seemed plausible as explanations for the molecular basis of the differences between the PNH II and the PNH III phenotypes. According to the first hypothesis, the two phenotypes have the same basic defect with the PNH III cells being more severely affected. According to the second hypothesis, PNH III erythrocytes have two independent defects. One deficiency (that of DAF) accounts for the intermediate complement sensitivity resulting from the greater activity of the C3/C5 convertase, and this defect is shared by both PNH II and PNH III cells. The absence of a second complement regulatory factor (i.e., CD59) is responsible for the greater susceptibility of PNH III cells to reactive lysis, and that factor is normal on PNH II cells, accounting for their resistance to that process. Compelling data showed that the first hypothesis is correct [52]. Using immunochemical techniques, DAF and CD59 were quantitated on PNH II and PNH III erythrocytes. As anticipated, the PNH III cells were almost completely deficient in both regulatory proteins. PNH II erythrocytes were also shown to be markedly deficient in both regulatory proteins, but the deficiency was less severe in comparison with PNH III cells. Thus, these results demonstrate that the erythrocytes that are classified as PNH II have an amount of CD59 that is abnormally low but still above the threshold that provides protection against reactive lysis (Fig. 4.5). On PNH erythrocytes, the deficiency of DAF and CD59 are concordant (Fig. 4.5). In general, PNH II cells have approximately 10 % of the amount of DAF and CD59 expressed by normal erythrocytes (Fig. 4.5). Thus, PNH II cells express about 250–300 copies of DAF and about 2500–3000 copies of CD59. This amount of CD59 is sufficient to inhibit the lytic activity of the MAC in reactive lysis systems, but this amount of DAF is insufficient to control the activity of the C3 convertase when complement is activated by either the classical or the APC. Currently, the erythrocyte phenotypes of PNH are defined by flow cytometric analysis using anti-CD59 as the primary antibody [114] (Fig. 4.5). This technique is particularly informative because it clearly separates the different phenotypes and depicts the mosaicism that is characteristic of PNH (Fig. 4.5).

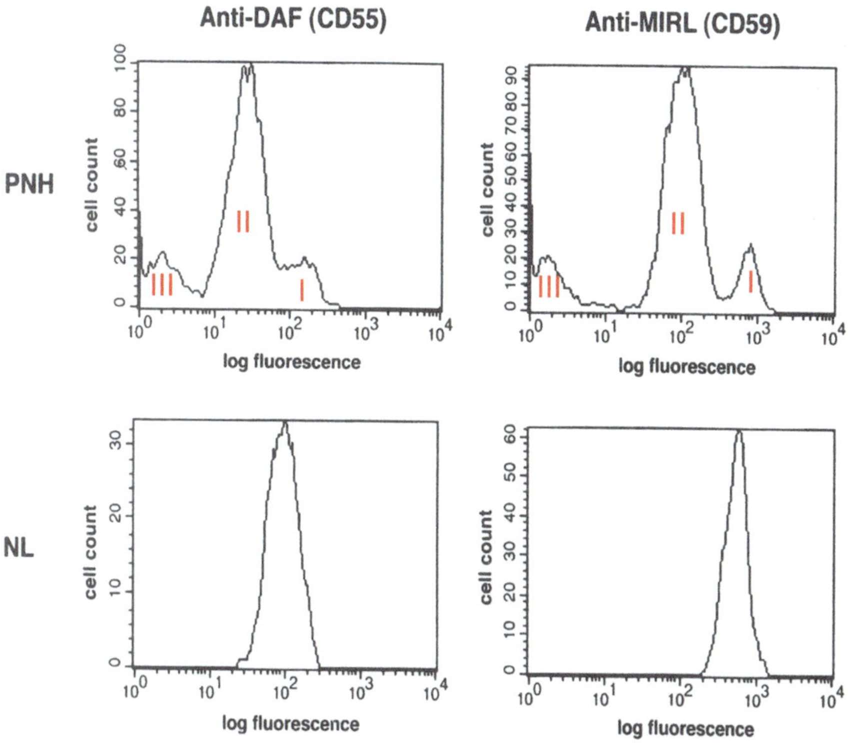

Fig. 4.5 *Phenotypic mosaicism of PNH based on flow cytometric analysis.* The phenotypic mosaicism of PNH was first recognized by Rosse and Dacie who demonstrated that the peripheral blood of patients with PNH was composed of a population of complement-sensitive (type III) and complement-insensitive (type I) cells. Rosse subsequently found that some PNH patients had a population of erythrocytes that were intermediately sensitive to complement-mediated lysis (type II cells). Discovery of the basis of the complement sensitivity of PNH erythrocytes showed that the type III cells were completely deficient in the complement regulatory proteins DAF and CD59, while the erythrocytes of intermediate sensitivity (type II) were partially deficient in DAF and CD59 (*top*). The type III and the type II cells are derived from different stem cells with discrete *PIGA* gene mutations. The type I cells express normal amounts of DAF and CD59 (top panels compared to bottom panels) and are the product of hematopoietic stem cells without mutant *PIGA* (i.e., the residual normal stem cells). In this example, the peripheral blood erythrocytes of a patient with PNH (*top*) were incubated with fluorescently labeled anti-DAF (*top, left*) or anti-MIRL (CD59) (*top, right*) and analyzed by flow cytometry. Normal (NL) erythrocytes (bottom) were analyzed simultaneous to demonstrate, for comparison, normal expression of DAF (*bottom, left*) and MIRL (CD59) (*bottom, right*)

Isolated Deficiencies of CD55 and CD59 Of the two complement regulatory proteins, CD59 is more important than DAF in protecting cells from complement-mediated lysis in vivo. Antigens of the Cromer-related blood group complex are located on DAF, and rare cases of a null phenotype called Inab have been reported [50, 71, 120, 128, 129]. Like PNH cells, Inab erythrocytes are deficient in DAF, but unlike PNH erythrocytes, CD59 expression is normal on Inab red cells [50]. Although Inab erythrocytes bind more activated C3 when exposed to acidified serum, they undergo little or no hemolysis [50]. Further, subjects with the Inab phenotype have no clinical hematological abnormalities, and in particular, they have no laboratory evidence of hemolysis [71, 128]. These observations show that isolated deficiency of DAF does not produce the PNH syndrome.

In contrast, a patient with an inherited, isolated deficiency of CD59 had a syndrome that was indistinguishable from PNH [72, 136]. Clinically, the patient experienced recurrent episodes of hemoglobinuria, suggesting that CD59 is essential for protecting erythrocytes against complement-mediated lysis in vivo. Recurrent thromboembolic events were also observed in this patient. That patient had normal DAF expression, but in vitro, his cells were susceptible to hemolysis in acidified serum, implying that CD59 deficiency accounts primarily for the positive Ham's test in PNH [133].

More recently, Nevo and colleagues reported on five patients, from four unrelated families, who presented in infancy with symmetric muscle weakness accompanied by hypotonia and absent deep tendon reflexes involving the legs more than the arms [74]. The neurological disease was classified as chronic inflammatory demyelinating polyneuropathy. Symptomatic episodes were accompanied by hemolytic anemia characterized by reticulocytosis, negative direct antiglobulin test, elevated serum lactate dehydrogenase concentration, and low serum haptoglobin concentration. There was no report of thrombotic complications, although the oldest of the patients in the study was 5 years old. Whole exome sequencing of DNA from one of the patients identified a homozygous missense mutation in the gene that encodes CD59. Subsequent studies identified the same mutation in the other four patients. The mutation segregated with the disease in the families and had a carrier rate of 1:66 among Jewish subjects of North African origin. Cell surface expression of CD59 was absent from the erythrocytes of patients, while expression of CD55 was normal. Together, these studies confirm the importance of CD59 in the pathophysiology of the complement-mediated hemolysis of PNH and suggest an important pathological role for aberrant regulation of the cytolytic MAC in chronic inflammatory demyelinating polyneuropathy and perhaps other diseases characterized by loss of myelin and axonal integrity.

While the above studies provide interesting insights into the individual function of DAF and CD59 in vivo, it is important to remember that, in PNH, both proteins are deficient. Therefore, it is the combined deficiency of DAF and CD59 that results in the markedly abnormal susceptibility of the red cells of PNH to complement-mediated lysis.

4.6 Eculizumab and Treatment of the Hemolysis of PNH

Eculizumab is a humanized monoclonal antibody that binds to C5 and thereby prevents proteolytic conversion of C5 into C5a and C5b fragments by the C5 convertase of the APC [87] (Fig. 4.6). Consequently activation of the terminal pathway of

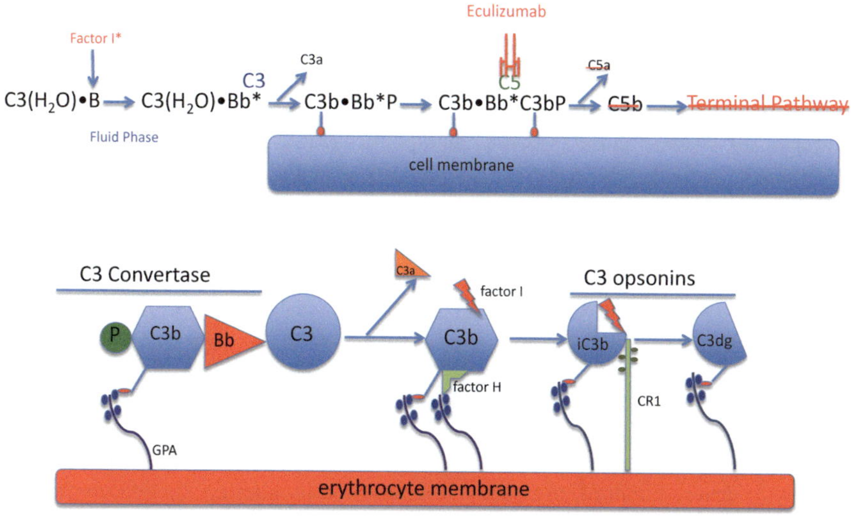

Fig. 4.6 *Effects of treatment with eculizumab.* Binding of eculizumab to C5 blocks activation of the terminal pathway by the APC C5 convertase thereby protecting PNH erythrocytes against complement-mediated intravascular hemolysis (*top*). Eculizumab has no inhibitory effect against the activity of the APC C3 convertase; however, due to deficiency of DAF and CD59, convertase activity is relatively unrestricted. Consequently, PNH erythrocytes become opsonized with activation and degradation products of C3 (*bottom*), resulting in extravascular hemolysis mediated by reticuloendothelial cells that express receptors for C3b, iC3b, and C3dg

complement is inhibited, and there is no generation of the C5a anaphylatoxin. Eculizumab is a highly effective inhibitor of the intravascular hemolysis of PNH, but it does not prevent the formation of the APC C3 convertase that readily forms on PNH erythrocytes because of DAF deficiency (Fig. 4.6). PNH erythrocytes that are protected by terminal pathway-mediated lysis by eculizumab become opsonized by activation and degradation fragments of C3 (Fig. 4.6) and consequently undergo extravascular hemolysis mediated by reticuloendothelial cells that express receptors for C3b, iC3b, and C3dg [102]. In some patients, the rate of extravascular hemolysis is clinically significant [103]. Interestingly, unlike the erythrocytes of patients with PNH treated with eculizumab, the erythrocytes of patients with an isolated deficiency of DAF [the Inab (null) phenotype of the Cromer blood group] do not become opsonized with C3 activation and degradation products [50]. This observation suggests that CD59 deficiency in addition to DAF deficiency is necessary for in vivo complement opsonization to occur. Support for this hypothesis was reported by Holguin and colleagues who showed that blocking CD59 expression on Inab erythrocytes resulted in an approximately 200-fold increase in the amount of membrane-bound C3 products when the APC was activated by acidification of serum [50].

Based on the success of eculizumab in treating complement-mediated diseases (particularly PNH and atypical hemolytic uremic syndrome), new drug development targeting C5 (C5 antibodies recognizing various epitopes, small molecule inhibitors of C5, naturally occurring inhibitors of C5, and siRNA technology targeting hepatic C5 RNA) and components of the APC (including an orally available small molecule inhibitor of factor D and small peptide inhibitors of C3) are underway with some of these reagents now being tested in phase I–II clinical trial in humans. If proven safe and effective, therapeutic options may soon be available for treatment of patients who respond suboptimally to eculizumab.

4.7 Conclusions

Investigation of the hemolysis of PNH has provided numerous insights into the basic physiology of the complement system, especially in relationship to regulation of both the APC and the terminal pathway on human erythrocytes. A detailed understanding of the pathophysiologic basis of intravascular hemolysis of PNH leads directly to development of an effective therapy, and by altering the hemolytic phenotype, the treatment itself provided a greater understanding of APC C3 convertase regulation in vivo. Much of the current complement research as it relates to PNH is focused on developing new approaches to inhibiting both intravascular and extravascular hemolysis. In addition to benefiting patients with PNH, this research has the potential to ameliorate the clinical manifestation of other complement-mediated diseases [63, 88].

References

1. Akami T, Arakawa K, Okamoto M, Akioka K, Fujiwara I, Nakai I, Mitsuo M, Sawada R, Naruto M, Oka T (1994) Enhancement of the complement regulatory function of CD59 by site-directed mutagenesis at the N-glycosylation site. Transplant Proc 26(3):1256–1258
2. Ames RS, Li Y, Sarau HM, Nuthulaganti P, Foley JJ, Ellis C, Zeng Z, Su K, Jurewicz AJ, Hertzberg RP, Bergsma DJ, Kumar C (1996) Molecular cloning and characterization of the human anaphylatoxin C3a receptor. J Biol Chem 271(34):20231–20234
3. Aster RH, Enright SE (1969) A platelet and granulocyte membrane defect in paroxysmal nocturnal hemoglobinuria: usefulness for the detection of platelet antibodies. J Clin Invest 48(7):1199–1210. doi:10.1172/JCI106084
4. Auditore JV, Hartmann RC (1959) Paroxysmal nocturnal hemoglobinuria II. erythrocyte acetylcholinesterase defect. Am J Med 27:401–410
5. Barilla-LaBarca ML, Liszewski MK, Lambris JD, Hourcade D, Atkinson JP (2002) Role of membrane cofactor protein (CD46) in regulation of C4b and C3b deposited on cells. J Immunol 168(12):6298–6304
6. Beck WS, Valentine WN (1951) Biochemical studies on leucocytes. II. Phosphatase activity in chronic lymphatic leukemia, acute leukemia, and miscellaneous hematologic conditions. J Lab Clin Med 38:245–253
7. Bhakdi S, Bjerrum OJ, Bhakdi-Lehnen B, Tranum-Jensen J (1978) Complement lysis: evidence for an amphiphilic nature of the terminal membrane C5b-9 complex of human complement. J Immunol 121(6):2526–2532

8. Bhakdi S, Tranum-Jensen J (1978) Molecular nature of the complement lesion. Proc Natl Acad Sci U S A 75(11):5655–5659
9. Bhakdi S, Tranum-Jensen J (1984) On the cause and nature of C9-related heterogeneity of terminal complement complexes generated on target erythrocytes through the action of whole serum. J Immunol 133(3):1453–1463
10. Bhakdi S, Tranum-Jensen J (1991) Complement lysis: a hole is a hole. Immunol Today 12(9):318–320. doi:10.1016/0167-5699(91)90007-G; discussion 321
11. Bickmore WA, Longbottom D, Oghene K, Fletcher JM, van Heyningen V (1993) Colocalization of the human CD59 gene to 11p13 with the MIC11 cell surface antigen. Genomics 17(1):129–135
12. Biesecker G, Gerard C, Hugli TE (1982) An amphiphilic structure of the ninth component of human complement. Evidence from analysis of fragments produced by alpha-thrombin. J Biol Chem 257(5):2584–2590
13. Biesecker G, Muller-Eberhard HJ (1980) The ninth component of human complement: purification and physicochemical characterization. J Immunol 124(3):1291–1296
14. Bodian DL, Davis SJ, Morgan BP, Rushmere NK (1997) Mutational analysis of the active site and antibody epitopes of the complement-inhibitory glycoprotein, CD59. J Exp Med 185(3):507–516
15. Borsos T, Dourmashkin RR, Humphrey JH (1964) Lesions in erythrocyte membranes caused by immune haemolysis. Nature 202:251–252
16. Capel PJ, Groeneboer O, Grosveld G, Pondman KW (1978) The binding of activated C3 to polysaccharides and immunoglobulins. J Immunol 121(6):2566–2572
17. Chakravarti DN, Chakravarti B, Parra CA, Muller-Eberhard HJ (1989) Structural homology of complement protein C6 with other channel-forming proteins of complement. Proc Natl Acad Sci U S A 86(8):2799–2803
18. Cooper NR (1985) The classical complement pathway: activation and regulation of the first complement component. Adv Immunol 37:151–216
19. Dacie JV (1963) Paroxsymal nocturnal haemoglobinuria. Proc R Soc Med 56:587–596
20. Daha MR, Fearon DT, Austen KF (1976) C3 requirements for formation of alternative pathway C5 convertase. J Immunol 117(2):630–634
21. Davies A, Simmons DL, Hale G, Harrison RA, Tighe H, Lachmann PJ, Waldmann H (1989) CD59, an LY-6-like protein expressed in human lymphoid cells, regulates the action of the complement membrane attack complex on homologous cells. J Exp Med 170(3):637–654
22. Davitz MA, Low MG, Nussenzweig V (1986) Release of decay-accelerating factor (DAF) from the cell membrane by phosphatidylinositol-specific phospholipase C (PIPLC). Selective modification of a complement regulatory protein. J Exp Med 163(5):1150–1161
23. DiScipio RG (1992) Formation and structure of the C5b-7 complex of the lytic pathway of complement. J Biol Chem 267(24):17087–17094
24. DiScipio RG, Chakravarti DN, Muller-Eberhard HJ, Fey GH (1988) The structure of human complement component C7 and the C5b-7 complex. J Biol Chem 263(1):549–560
25. Discipio RG, Gagnon J (1982) Characterization of human complement components C6 and C7. Mol Immunol 19(11):1425–1431
26. DiScipio RG, Gehring MR, Podack ER, Kan CC, Hugli TE, Fey GH (1984) Nucleotide sequence of cDNA and derived amino acid sequence of human complement component C9. Proc Natl Acad Sci U S A 81(23):7298–7302
27. Endo M, Ware RE, Vreeke TM, Singh SP, Howard TA, Tomita A, Holguin MH, Parker CJ (1996) Molecular basis of the heterogeneity of expression of glycosyl phosphatidylinositol anchored proteins in paroxysmal nocturnal hemoglobinuria. Blood 87(6):2546–2557
28. Esser AF (1991) Big MAC attack: complement proteins cause leaky patches. Immunol Today 12(9):316–318. doi:10.1016/0167-5699(91)90006-F; discussion 321
29. Fearon DT (1979) Regulation of the amplification C3 convertase of human complement by an inhibitory protein isolated from human erythrocyte membrane. Proc Natl Acad Sci U S A 76(11):5867–5871

30. Fearon DT (1980) Identification of the membrane glycoprotein that is the C3b receptor of the human erythrocyte, polymorphonuclear leukocyte, B lymphocyte, and monocyte. J Exp Med 152(1):20–30
31. Fearon DT, Austen KF (1975) Properdin: binding to C3b and stabilization of the C3b-dependent C3 convertase. J Exp Med 142(4):856–863
32. Fearon DT, Austen KF (1980) Current concepts in immunology: the alternative pathway of complement–a system for host resistance to microbial infection. N Engl J Med 303(5):259–263. doi:10.1056/NEJM198007313030505
33. Fearon DT, Ruddy S, Schur PH, McCabe WR (1975) Activation of the properdin pathway of complement in patients with gram-negative of bacteremia. N Engl J Med 292(18):937–940. doi:10.1056/NEJM197505012921802
34. Fernandez HN, Hugli TE (1978) Primary structural analysis of the polypeptide portion of human C5a anaphylatoxin. Polypeptide sequence determination and assignment of the oligosaccharide attachment site in C5a. J Biol Chem 253(19):6955–6964
35. Fishelson Z, Horstmann RD, Muller-Eberhard HJ (1987) Regulation of the alternative pathway of complement by pH. J Immunol 138(10):3392–3395
36. Fletcher CM, Harrison RA, Lachmann PJ, Neuhaus D (1993) Sequence-specific 1H-NMR assignments and folding topology of human CD59. Protein sci A Publ Protein Soc 2(12):2015–2027. doi:10.1002/pro.5560021203
37. Fletcher CM, Harrison RA, Lachmann PJ, Neuhaus D (1994) Structure of a soluble, glycosylated form of the human complement regulatory protein CD59. Structure 2(3):185–199
38. Frank MM, Fries LF (1991) The role of complement in inflammation and phagocytosis. Immunol Today 12(9):322–326. doi:10.1016/0167-5699(91)90009-I
39. Fries LF, Gaither TA, Hammer CH, Frank MM (1984) C3b covalently bound to IgG demonstrates a reduced rate of inactivation by factors H and I. J Exp Med 160(6):1640–1655
40. Fujita T, Inoue T, Ogawa K, Iida K, Tamura N (1987) The mechanism of action of decay-accelerating factor (DAF). DAF inhibits the assembly of C3 convertases by dissociating C2a and Bb. J Exp Med 166(5):1221–1228
41. Fujita T, Tamura N (1983) Interaction of C4-binding protein with cell-bound C4b. A quantitative analysis of binding and the role of C4-binding protein in proteolysis of cell-bound C4b. J Exp Med 157(4):1239–1251
42. Gerard C, Gerard NP (1994) C5A anaphylatoxin and its seven transmembrane-segment receptor. Annu Rev Immunol 12:775–808. doi:10.1146/annurev.iy.12.040194.004015
43. Gerard C, Hugli TE (1981) Identification of classical anaphylatoxin as the des-Arg form of the C5a molecule: evidence of a modulator role for the oligosaccharide unit in human des-Arg74-C5a. Proc Natl Acad Sci U S A 78(3):1833–1837
44. Guo RF, Ward PA (2005) Role of C5a in inflammatory responses. Annu Rev Immunol 23:821–852. doi:10.1146/annurev.immunol.23.021704.115835
45. Ham TH, Dingle JH (1939) Studies on destruction of Red blood cells. Ii. Chronic hemolytic anemia with paroxysmal nocturnal hemoglobinuria: certain immunological aspects of the hemolytic mechanism with special reference to serum complement. J Clin Invest 18(6):657–672. doi:10.1172/JCI101081
46. Hoffmann EM (1969) Inhibition of complement by a substance isolated from human erythrocytes. II. Studies on the site and mechanism of action. Immunochemistry 6(3):405–419
47. Hoffmann EM (1969) Inhibition of complement by a substrate isolated from human erythrocytes: I. Extraction from human erythrocyte stromata. Immunochemistry 6:391–403
48. Hoffmann EM, Cheng WC, Tomeu EJ, Renk CM (1974) Resistance of sheep erythrocytes to immune lysis by treatment of the cells with a human erythrocyte extract: studies on the site of inhibition. J Immunol 113(5):1501–1509
49. Holguin MH, Fredrick LR, Bernshaw NJ, Wilcox LA, Parker CJ (1989) Isolation and characterization of a membrane protein from normal human erythrocytes that inhibits reactive lysis of the erythrocytes of paroxysmal nocturnal hemoglobinuria. J Clin Invest 84(1):7–17

50. Holguin MH, Martin CB, Bernshaw NJ, Parker CJ (1992) Analysis of the effects of activation of the alternative pathway of complement on erythrocytes with an isolated deficiency of decay accelerating factor. J Immunol 148(2):498–502
51. Holguin MH, Parker CJ (1992) Membrane inhibitor of reactive lysis. Curr Top Microbiol Immunol 178:61–85
52. Holguin MH, Wilcox LA, Bernshaw NJ, Rosse WF, Parker CJ (1989) Relationship between the membrane inhibitor of reactive lysis and the erythrocyte phenotypes of paroxysmal nocturnal hemoglobinuria. J Clin Invest 84(5):1387–1394
53. Hugli TE (1984) Structure and function of the anaphylatoxins. Springer Semin Immunopathol 7(2–3):193–219
54. Hugli TE, Vallota EH, Muller-Eberhard HJ (1975) Purification and partial characterization of human and porcine C3a anaphylatoxin. J Biol Chem 250(4):1472–1478
55. Iida K, Nussenzweig V (1981) Complement receptor is an inhibitor of the complement cascade. J Exp Med 153(5):1138–1150
56. Isenman DE, Young JR (1986) Covalent binding properties of the C4A and C4B isotypes of the fourth component of human complement on several C1-bearing cell surfaces. J Immunol 136(7):2542–2550
57. Jenne D, Stanley KK (1985) Molecular cloning of S-protein, a link between complement, coagulation and cell-substrate adhesion. EMBO J 4(12):3153–3157
58. Kerr MA, Porter RR (1978) The purification and properties of the second component of human complement. Biochem J 171(1):99–107
59. Kieffer B, Driscoll PC, Campbell ID, Willis AC, van der Merwe PA, Davis SJ (1994) Three-dimensional solution structure of the extracellular region of the complement regulatory protein CD59, a new cell-surface protein domain related to snake venom neurotoxins. Biochemistry 33(15):4471–4482
60. Kunstling TR, Rosse WF (1969) Erythrocyte acetylcholinesterase deficiency in paroxysmal nocturnal hemoglobinuria (PNH). A comparison of the complement-sensitive and insensitive populations. Blood 33(4):607–616
61. Law SK, Lichtenberg NA, Holcombe FH, Levine RP (1980) Interaction between the labile binding sites of the fourth (C4) and fifth (C5) human complement proteins and erythrocyte cell membranes. J Immunol 125(2):634–639
62. Law SK, Lichtenberg NA, Levine RP (1979) Evidence for an ester linkage between the labile binding site of C3b and receptive surfaces. J Immunol 123(3):1388–1394
63. Legendre CM, Licht C, Muus P, Greenbaum LA, Babu S, Bedrosian C, Bingham C, Cohen DJ, Delmas Y, Douglas K, Eitner F, Feldkamp T, Fouque D, Furman RR, Gaber O, Herthelius M, Hourmant M, Karpman D, Lebranchu Y, Mariat C, Menne J, Moulin B, Nurnberger J, Ogawa M, Remuzzi G, Richard T, Sberro-Soussan R, Severino B, Sheerin NS, Trivelli A, Zimmerhackl LB, Goodship T, Loirat C (2013) Terminal complement inhibitor eculizumab in atypical hemolytic-uremic syndrome. N Engl J Med 368(23):2169–2181. doi:10.1056/NEJMoa1208981
64. Lehto T, Meri S (1993) Interactions of soluble CD59 with the terminal complement complexes. CD59 and C9 compete for a nascent epitope on C8. J Immunol 151(9):4941–4949
65. Lewis SM, Dacie JV (1965) Neutrophil (leucocyte) alkaline phosphatase in paroxysmal nocturnal haemoglobinuria. Br J Haematol 11(5):549–556
66. Logue GL, Rosse WF, Adams JP (1973) Mechanisms of immune lysis of red blood cells in vitro. I. Paroxysmal nocturnal hemoglobinuria cells. J Clin Invest 52(5):1129–1137
67. Medof ME, Gottlieb A, Kinoshita T, Hall S, Silber R, Nussenzweig V, Rosse WF (1987) Relationship between decay accelerating factor deficiency, diminished acetylcholinesterase activity, and defective terminal complement pathway restriction in paroxysmal nocturnal hemoglobinuria erythrocytes. J Clin Invest 80(1):165–174. doi:10.1172/JCI113043
68. Medof ME, Kinoshita T, Nussenzweig V (1984) Inhibition of complement activation on the surface of cells after incorporation of decay-accelerating factor (DAF) into their membranes. J Exp Med 160(5):1558–1578

69. Medof ME, Nussenzweig V (1984) Control of the function of substrate-bound C4b-C3b by the complement receptor Cr1. J Exp Med 159(6):1669–1685
70. Meri S, Morgan BP, Davies A, Daniels RH, Olavesen MG, Waldmann H, Lachmann PJ (1990) Human protectin (CD59), an 18,000–20,000 MW complement lysis restricting factor, inhibits C5b-8 catalysed insertion of C9 into lipid bilayers. Immunology 71(1):1–9
71. Merry AH, Rawlinson VI, Uchikawa M, Daha MR, Sim RB (1989) Studies on the sensitivity to complement-mediated lysis of erythrocytes (Inab phenotype) with a deficiency of DAF (decay accelerating factor). Br J Haematol 73(2):248–253
72. Motoyama N, Okada N, Yamashina M, Okada H (1992) Paroxysmal nocturnal hemoglobinuria due to hereditary nucleotide deletion in the HRF20 (CD59) gene. Eur J Immunol 22(10):2669–2673
73. Muller-Eberhard HJ (1988) Molecular organization and function of the complement system. Annu Rev Biochem 57:321–347. doi:10.1146/annurev.bi.57.070188.001541
74. Nevo Y, Ben-Zeev B, Tabib A, Straussberg R, Anikster Y, Shorer Z, Fattal-Valevski A, Ta-Shma A, Aharoni S, Rabie M, Zenvirt S, Goldshmidt H, Fellig Y, Shaag A, Mevorach D, Elpeleg O (2013) CD59 deficiency is associated with chronic hemolysis and childhood relapsing immune-mediated polyneuropathy. Blood 121(1):129–135. doi:blood-2012-07-441857 [pii] 10.1182/blood-2012-07-441857
75. Ng SC, Rao AG, Howard OM, Sodetz JM (1987) The eighth component of human complement: evidence that it is an oligomeric serum protein assembled from products of three different genes. Biochemistry 26(17):5229–5233
76. Nicholson-Weller A, Burge J, Fearon DT, Weller PF, Austen KF (1982) Isolation of a human erythrocyte membrane glycoprotein with decay-accelerating activity for C3 convertases of the complement system. J Immunol 129(1):184–189
77. Nicholson-Weller A, March JP, Rosenfeld SI, Austen KF (1983) Affected erythrocytes of patients with paroxysmal nocturnal hemoglobinuria are deficient in the complement regulatory protein, decay accelerating factor. Proc Natl Acad Sci U S A 80(16):5066–5070
78. Nose M, Katoh M, Okada N, Kyogoku M, Okada H (1990) Tissue distribution of HRF20, a novel factor preventing the membrane attack of homologous complement, and its predominant expression on endothelial cells in vivo. Immunology 70(2):145–149
79. Okada H, Nagami Y, Takahashi K, Okada N, Hideshima T, Takizawa H, Kondo J (1989) 20 KDa homologous restriction factor of complement resembles T cell activating protein. Biochem Biophys Res Commun 162(3):1553–1559
80. Okada N, Harada R, Fujita T, Okada H (1989) Monoclonal antibodies capable of causing hemolysis of neuraminidase-treated human erythrocytes by homologous complement. J Immunol 143(7):2262–2266
81. Oni SB, Osunkoya BO, Luzzatto L (1970) Paroxysmal nocturnal hemoglobinuria: evidence for monoclonal origin of abnormal red cells. Blood 36(2):145–152
82. Packman CH, Rosenfeld SI, Jenkins DE Jr, Thiem PA, Leddy JP (1979) Complement lysis of human erythrocytes. Differing susceptibility of two types of paroxysmal nocturnal hemoglobinuria cells to C5b-9. J Clin Invest 64(2):428–433
83. Pangburn MK, Schreiber RD, Muller-Eberhard HJ (1977) Human complement C3b inactivator: isolation, characterization, and demonstration of an absolute requirement for the serum protein beta1H for cleavage of C3b and C4b in solution. J Exp Med 146(1):257–270
84. Pangburn MK, Schreiber RD, Muller-Eberhard HJ (1981) Formation of the initial C3 convertase of the alternative complement pathway. Acquisition of C3b-like activities by spontaneous hydrolysis of the putative thioester in native C3. J Exp Med 154(3):856–867
85. Pangburn MK, Schreiber RD, Muller-Eberhard HJ (1983) Deficiency of an erythrocyte membrane protein with complement regulatory activity in paroxysmal nocturnal hemoglobinuria. Proc Natl Acad Sci U S A 80(17):5430–5434
86. Pangburn MK, Schreiber RD, Trombold JS, Muller-Eberhard HJ (1983) Paroxysmal nocturnal hemoglobinuria: deficiency in factor H-like functions of the abnormal erythrocytes. J Exp Med 157(6):1971–1980

87. Parker C (2009) Eculizumab for paroxysmal nocturnal haemoglobinuria. Lancet 373(9665):759–767. doi:10.1016/S0140-6736(09)60001-5
88. Parker CJ (2011) Thanks for the complement (inhibitor). Blood 118:4503–4504
89. Parker CJ, Baker PJ, Rosse WF (1982) Increased enzymatic activity of the alternative pathway convertase when bound to the erythrocytes of paroxysmal nocturnal hemoglobinuria. J Clin Invest 69(2):337–346
90. Parker CJ, Soldato CM, Rosse WF (1984) Abnormality of glycophorin-alpha on paroxysmal nocturnal hemoglobinuria erythrocytes. J Clin Invest 73(4):1130–1143. doi:10.1172/JCI111299
91. Parker CJ, Soldato CM, Telen MJ (1984) Increased efficiency of binding of nascent C3b to the erythrocytes of chronic cold agglutinin disease. J Clin Invest 74(3):1050–1062. doi:10.1172/JCI111472
92. Parker CJ, Wiedmer T, Sims PJ, Rosse WF (1985) Characterization of the complement sensitivity of paroxysmal nocturnal hemoglobinuria erythrocytes. J Clin Invest 75(6):2074–2084. doi:10.1172/JCI111927
93. Philbrick WM, Palfree RG, Maher SE, Bridgett MM, Sirlin S, Bothwell AL (1990) The CD59 antigen is a structural homologue of murine Ly-6 antigens but lacks interferon inducibility. Eur J Immunol 20(1):87–92. doi:10.1002/eji.1830200113
94. Pillemer L, Blum L, Lepow IH, Ross OA, Todd EW, Wardlaw AC (1954) The properdin system and immunity. I. Demonstration and isolation of a new serum protein, properdin, and its role in immune phenomena. Science 120(3112):279–285
95. Ploug M, Ellis V (1994) Structure-function relationships in the receptor for urokinase-type plasminogen activator. Comparison to other members of the Ly-6 family and snake venom alpha-neurotoxins. FEBS Lett 349(2):163–168
96. Ploug M, Kjalke M, Ronne E, Weidle U, Hoyer-Hansen G, Dano K (1993) Localization of the disulfide bonds in the NH2-terminal domain of the cellular receptor for human urokinase-type plasminogen activator. A domain structure belonging to a novel superfamily of glycolipid-anchored membrane proteins. J Biol Chem 268(23):17539–17546
97. Podack ER (1984) Molecular composition of the tubular structure of the membrane attack complex of complement. J Biol Chem 259(13):8641–8647
98. Podack ER, Kolb WP, Esser AF, Muller-Eberhard HJ (1979) Structural similarities between C6 and C7 of human complement. J Immunol 123(3):1071–1077
99. Podack ER, Kolb WP, Muller-Eberhard HJ (1978) The C5b-6 complex: formation, isolation, and inhibition of its activity by lipoprotein and the S-protein of human serum. J Immunol 120(6):1841–1848
100. Podack ER, Muller-Eberhard HJ (1978) Binding of desoxycholate, phosphatidylcholine vesicles, lipoprotein and of the S-protein to complexes of terminal complement components. J Immunol 121(3):1025–1030
101. Preissner KT, Podack ER, Muller-Eberhard HJ (1985) The membrane attack complex of complement: relation of C7 to the metastable membrane binding site of the intermediate complex C5b-7. J Immunol 135(1):445–451
102. Risitano AM, Notaro R, Luzzatto L, Hill A, Kelly R, Hillmen P (2010) Paroxysmal nocturnal hemoglobinuria–hemolysis before and after eculizumab. N Engl J Med 363(23):2270–2272. doi:10.1056/NEJMc1010351 [doi]
103. Risitano AM, Notaro R, Marando L, Serio B, Ranaldi D, Seneca E, Ricci P, Alfinito F, Camera A, Gianfaldoni G, Amendola A, Boschetti C, Di Bona E, Fratellanza G, Barbano F, Rodeghiero F, Zanella A, Iori AP, Selleri C, Luzzatto L, Rotoli B (2009) Complement fraction 3 binding on erythrocytes as additional mechanism of disease in paroxysmal nocturnal hemoglobinuria patients treated by eculizumab. Blood 113(17):4094–4100. doi:blood-2008-11-189944 [pii] 10.1182/blood-2008-11-189944 [doi]
104. Roberts WN, Wilson JG, Wong W, Jenkins DE Jr, Fearon DT, Austen KF, Nicholson-Weller A (1985) Normal function of CR1 on affected erythrocytes of patients with paroxysmal nocturnal hemoglobinuria. J Immunol 134(1):512–517

105. Rollins SA, Zhao J, Ninomiya H, Sims PJ (1991) Inhibition of homologous complement by CD59 is mediated by a species-selective recognition conferred through binding to C8 within C5b-8 or C9 within C5b-9. J Immunol 146(7):2345–2351
106. Rosenfeld SI, Packman CH, Leddy JP (1983) Inhibition of the lytic action of cell-bound terminal complement components by human high density lipoproteins and apoproteins. J Clin Invest 71(4):795–808
107. Ross GD (1992) Complement receptor type 1. Curr Top Microbiol Immunol 178:31–44
108. Ross GD, Yount WJ, Walport MJ, Winfield JB, Parker CJ, Fuller CR, Taylor RP, Myones BL, Lachmann PJ (1985) Disease-associated loss of erythrocyte complement receptors (CR1, C3b receptors) in patients with systemic lupus erythematosus and other diseases involving autoantibodies and/or complement activation. J Immunol 135(3):2005–2014
109. Rosse WF (1972) The complement sensitivity on PNH cells. Ser Haematol 5(3):101–114
110. Rosse WF (1973) Variations in the red cells in paroxysmal nocturnal haemoglobinuria. Br J Haematol 24(3):327–342
111. Rosse WF (1980) Paroxysmal nocturnal hemoglobinuria–present status and future prospects. West J Med 132(3):219–228
112. Rosse WF, Adams JP, Thorpe AM (1974) The population of cells in paroxysmal nocturnal haemoglobinuria of intermediate sensitivity to complement lysis: significance and mechanism of increased immune lysis. Br J Haematol 28(2):181–190
113. Rosse WF, Dacie JV (1966) Immune lysis of normal human and paroxysmal nocturnal hemoglobinuria (PNH) red blood cells. I. The sensitivity of PNH red cells to lysis by complement and specific antibody. J Clin Invest 45(5):736–748. doi:10.1172/JCI105388
114. Rosse WF, Hoffman S, Campbell M, Borowitz M, Moore JO, Parker CJ (1991) The erythrocytes in paroxysmal nocturnal haemoglobinuria of intermediate sensitivity to complement lysis. Br J Haematol 79(1):99–107
115. Rother RP, Zhao J, Zhou Q, Sims PJ (1996) Elimination of potential sites of glycosylation fails to abrogate complement regulatory function of cell surface CD59. J Biol Chem 271(39):23842–23845
116. Rouault TA, Rosse WF, Bell S, Shelburne J (1978) Differences in the terminal steps of complement lysis of normal and paroxysmal nocturnal hemoglobinuria red cells. Blood 51(2):325–330
117. Rudd PM, Morgan BP, Wormald MR, Harvey DJ, van den Berg CW, Davis SJ, Ferguson MA, Dwek RA (1997) The glycosylation of the complement regulatory protein, human erythrocyte CD59. J Biol Chem 272(11):7229–7244
118. Scharfstein J, Ferreira A, Gigli I, Nussenzweig V (1978) Human C4-binding protein. I. Isolation and characterization. J Exp Med 148(1):207–222
119. Shin ML, Hansch G, Hu VW, Nicholson-Weller A (1986) Membrane factors responsible for homologous species restriction of complement-mediated lysis: evidence for a factor other than DAF operating at the stage of C8 and C9. J Immunol 136(5):1777–1782
120. Spring FA, Judson PA, Daniels GL, Parsons SF, Mallinson G, Anstee DJ (1987) A human cell-surface glycoprotein that carries Cromer-related blood group antigens on erythrocytes and is also expressed on leucocytes and platelets. Immunology 62(2):307–313
121. Stafford HA, Tykocinski ML, Lublin DM, Holers VM, Rosse WF, Atkinson JP, Medof ME (1988) Normal polymorphic variations and transcription of the decay accelerating factor gene in paroxysmal nocturnal hemoglobinuria cells. Proc Natl Acad Sci U S A 85(3):880–884
122. Steckel EW, York RG, Monahan JB, Sodetz JM (1980) The eighth component of human complement. Purification and physicochemical characterization of its unusual subunit structure. J Biol Chem 255(24):11997–12005
123. Stefanova I, Hilgert I, Kristofova H, Brown R, Low MG, Horejsi V (1989) Characterization of a broadly expressed human leucocyte surface antigen MEM-43 anchored in membrane through phosphatidylinositol. Mol Immunol 26(2):153–161
124. Stern M, Rosse WF (1979) Two populations of granulocytes in paroxysmal nocturnal hemoglobinuria. Blood 53(5):928–934

125. Stewart JL, Kolb WP, Sodetz JM (1987) Evidence that C5b recognizes and mediates C8 incorporation into the cytolytic complex of complement. J Immunol 139(6):1960–1964
126. Stewart JL, Sodetz JM (1985) Analysis of the specific association of the eighth and ninth components of human complement: identification of a direct role for the alpha subunit of C8. Biochemistry 24(17):4598–4602
127. Sugita Y, Tobe T, Oda E, Tomita M, Yasukawa K, Yamaji N, Takemoto T, Furuichi K, Takayama M, Yano S (1989) Molecular cloning and characterization of MACIF, an inhibitor of membrane channel formation of complement. J Biochem 106(4):555–557
128. Telen MJ, Green AM (1989) The Inab phenotype: characterization of the membrane protein and complement regulatory defect. Blood 74(1):437–441
129. Telen MJ, Hall SE, Green AM, Moulds JJ, Rosse WF (1988) Identification of human erythrocyte blood group antigens on decay-accelerating factor (DAF) and an erythrocyte phenotype negative for DAF. J Exp Med 167(6):1993–1998
130. Tschopp J, Chonn A, Hertig S, French LE (1993) Clusterin, the human apolipoprotein and complement inhibitor, binds to complement C7, C8 beta, and the b domain of C9. J Immunol 151(4):2159–2165
131. Tschopp J, Masson D, Schafer S, Peitsch M, Preissner KT (1988) The heparin binding domain of S-protein/vitronectin binds to complement components C7, C8, and C9 and perforin from cytolytic T-cells and inhibits their lytic activities. Biochemistry 27(11):4103–4109
132. Whaley K, Ruddy S (1976) Modulation of the alternative complement pathways by beta 1 H globulin. J Exp Med 144(5):1147–1163
133. Wilcox LA, Ezzell JL, Bernshaw NJ, Parker CJ (1991) Molecular basis of the enhanced susceptibility of the erythrocytes of paroxysmal nocturnal hemoglobinuria to hemolysis in acidified serum. Blood 78(3):820–829
134. Williams AF, Tse AG, Gagnon J (1988) Squid glycoproteins with structural similarities to Thy-1 and Ly-6 antigens. Immunogenetics 27(4):265–272
135. Yamamoto KI, Gewurz G (1978) The complex of C5b and C6: isolation, characterization, and identification of a modified form of C5b consisting of three polypeptide chains. J Immunol 120(6):2008–2015
136. Yamashina M, Ueda E, Kinoshita T, Takami T, Ojima A, Ono H, Tanaka H, Kondo N, Orii T, Okada N et al (1990) Inherited complete deficiency of 20-kilodalton homologous restriction factor (CD59) as a cause of paroxysmal nocturnal hemoglobinuria. N Engl J Med 323(17):1184–1189
137. Yongqing T, Drentin N, Duncan RC, Wijeyewickrema LC, Pike RN (2012) Mannose-binding lectin serine proteases and associated proteins of the lectin pathway of complement: two genes, five proteins and many functions? Biochim Biophys Acta 1824(1):253–262. doi:10.1016/j.bbapap.2011.05.021
138. Ziccardi RJ, Dahlback B, Muller-Eberhard HJ (1984) Characterization of the interaction of human C4b-binding protein with physiological ligands. J Biol Chem 259(22):13674–13679

Part II
Clinical Sciences in PNH

Chapter 5
Epidemiology in PNH: The PNH Global Registry

Robert A. Brodsky

Abstract Advances in the clinical and scientific underpinnings of paroxysmal nocturnal hemoglobinuria (PNH) have had a profound impact on the natural history of PNH. Over the past 25 years, novel diagnostics and therapeutic agents have refined the definition of the disease and improved clinical outcomes. These achievements have set the stage for developing an International PNH Registry that is an ongoing worldwide, noninterventional study collecting safety, effectiveness, and quality-of-life data from patients with a confirmed PNH diagnosis or a detectable PNH clone ($\geq$0.01 %). This registry is the first PNH Registry to collect data on the disease burden from the patient's perspective and is the first to collect data on the natural history of PNH patients treated with eculizumab.

Keywords Paroxysmal nocturnal hemoglobinuria • Natural history • Epidemiology • Registry • Eculizumab

5.1 Introduction

Paroxysmal nocturnal hemoglobinuria (PNH) is a rare clonal hematopoietic stem cell disorder that manifests with hemolytic anemia, bone marrow failure, and thrombosis [3, 4, 23]. The epidemiology and natural history of PNH has evolved, especially over the last three decades, because of improved diagnostic reagents, better understanding of the cellular and molecular underpinnings of PNH, and, most recently, development of effective drug therapy in the form of terminal complement inhibition.

One of the earliest descriptions of PNH was by Dr. Paul Strübing in the late 1800s, but it was Enneking, in 1925, who introduced the term *paroxysmal nocturnal*

R.A. Brodsky, M.D. (✉)
Division of Hematology, Department of Medicine, Johns Hopkins University School of Medicine, Ross Research Building, Room 1025, 720 Rutland Avenue, Baltimore, MD 21205-2196, USA
e-mail: brodsro@jhmi.edu

Y. Kanakura et al. (eds.), *Paroxysmal Nocturnal Hemoglobinuria*,
DOI 10.1007/978-4-431-56003-6_5

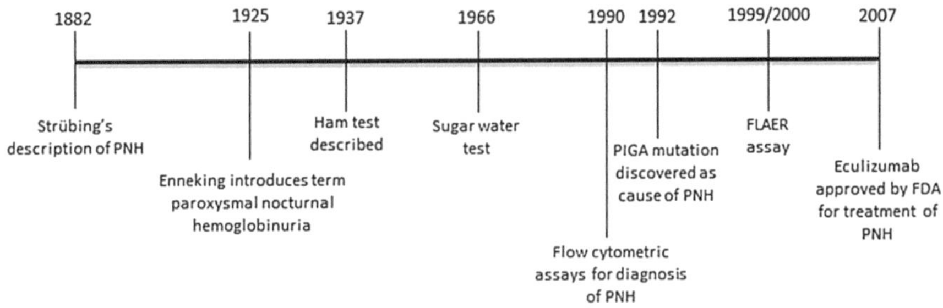

Fig. 5.1 Abbreviated timeline of key discoveries that influence epidemiologic and natural history studies of PNH

hemoglobinuria [10]. In 1937, Thomas Ham reported that PNH erythrocytes were hemolyzed when incubated with normal, acidified serum [11]. This seminal discovery resulted in the first diagnostic test for PNH, the acidified serum (Ham) test. In the 1980s it was discovered that PNH cells display a global deficiency of glycosylphosphatidylinositol (GPI)-anchored proteins (GPI-AP). In the 1990s, red cell assays for PNH like the sugar water test [13] and the Ham test were replaced by flow cytometric assays using reagents like monoclonal antibodies that bind the protein portion of individual GPI-APs (e.g., CD55 and CD59) [28, 31] and eventually fluorescent proaerolysin variants (FLAER) that binds to the glycan portion of the GPI anchor of all GPI-APs [5, 6]. These newer assays were more sensitive and specific than the red cell-based assays and also made it possible to measure the percentage of cells from different hematopoietic cells (red cells, granulocytes, monocytes, etc.) that were GPI-AP deficient. Before flow cytometric-based assays, fewer than 15 % of patients with aplastic anemia had a positive assay (Ham or sugar water test) at diagnosis. After the development of more sensitive flow cytometry-based assays, it became clear that more than 50 % of patients with newly diagnosed acquired, but not inherited, aplastic anemia have an expanded PNH clone at diagnosis [21, 33]. Also in the 1990s, a genetic mutation (*PIGA*) responsible for the GPI-anchored protein deficiency was discovered [1, 18, 19, 30], and about a decade ago, a humanized monoclonal antibody, eculizumab, that inhibits terminal complement activation was shown to ameliorate hemolysis and thrombosis (heretofore the leading cause of death) and improve quality of life in PNH patients [25]. This abbreviated timeline of the history of PNH (Fig. 5.1) is important to keep in mind when studying the epidemiology/natural history of PNH several reasons. First, accuracy of diagnosis in patients diagnosed before the 1990s cannot be assured. Second, the impact of PNH clone size on natural history could not be assessed with red cell-based assays. Third, before the 1990s, patients tended to present later in the course of disease due to delay in diagnosis and failure to detect small PNH clones in most patients with acquired SAA. Finally, the development of eculizumab has increased awareness of PNH and appears to have changed the natural history of the disease by practically eliminating the thrombosis risk. Before eculizumab, thrombosis was the leading cause of death from PNH. These tremendous advances in the diagnosis and treatment of PNH highlight the importance of the PNH global registry. While it is important to understand the historical impact of the disease, it is even more important to understand the epidemiology and natural history in the era of modern diagnostics and therapeutics.

5.2 Epidemiology Before Modern Diagnostic Assays

In 1995, Hillmen et al. published a large retrospective study of 80 PNH patients who were referred to the Hammersmith Hospital in London between the years 1940 and 1970 [14]. The diagnosis of PNH was established using Ham's test, and the patients were managed with supportive care that included blood transfusions and anticoagulation as indicated. The median age was 42 (range, 16–75) years and the median survival was 10 years with a wide range; however, the onset of symptoms often preceded the diagnosis by several years in most cases. A diagnosis of aplastic anemia preceded the diagnosis of PNH in 29 % of the cases. At the time of publication, 60 patients had died. In 12 cases, the cause of death was unknown; in 28 of the remaining 48 patients, death was attributable to either venous thrombosis (leading cause of death) or hemorrhage. Interestingly, 12 patients (15 % overall) reportedly achieved spontaneous recovery, but given that the PNH diagnosis was based on Ham's tests, this high percentage may be an overestimate.

In 1996, Socie et al. performed a retrospective study of 220 French PNH patients who were diagnosed with Ham's test between 1950 and 1995 [29]. Like the English study above, therapy was largely supportive with blood transfusions, anticoagulation, steroids, and androgens; four patients were managed with bone marrow transplantation. The median survival was 14.6 years and the 8-year cumulative incidence of thrombosis, pancytopenia, MDS, and AML was 28 %, 15 %, 5 %, and 1 %, respectively. Poor survival was associated with thrombosis, pancytopenia, evolution to MDS/AML, age greater than 55 at diagnosis, thrombocytopenia at diagnosis, and need for additional treatment. Patients who presented with thrombosis had a 40 % survival rate at 4 years.

PNH is rare in children and when it occurs, it is often in the setting of acquired aplastic anemia. While rare cases of PNH in the setting of inherited bone marrow failure have been reported [32], the finding of a PNH in clone in the setting of aplastic anemia virtually assures that the bone marrow failure is acquired rather than inherited [9, 16]. Ware et al. published a retrospective study of pediatric PNH patients seen at Duke University between 1966 and 1990 [34]. The median survival was 13.5 years and 15 (58 %) of the patients had bone marrow failure at diagnosis.

5.3 Epidemiology After Modern Diagnostic Assays

Before 1990, the diagnosis of PNH was established using complement-based red cell assays such as the Ham's test and the sugar water test. Complement-based assays cannot detect small PNH populations and may be falsely negative in patients requiring frequent red cell transfusions. Thus, PNH natural history studies where patients were diagnosed before 1990 were likely to have excluded patients with small to moderate PNH clones. Another advantage of flow cytometric assays is that they can measure the percentage of cells from different lineages that are GPI-anchored protein deficient. In the late 1990s, Brodsky et al. demonstrated that the GPI anchor is the receptor for the bacterial pore-forming toxin proaerolysin [6]. In collaboration with J. Thomas Buckley, he developed a novel diagnostic flow cytometric assay using a fluorescein-labeled inactive proaerolysin variant known as FLAER [5]. FLAER binds with high affinity and specificity to the glycan portion of all GPI anchors and in conjunction with fluorescein-labeled monoclonal antibodies is used routinely for the diagnosis of PNH [2].

In 2004, Moyo performed the first natural history study of PNH using modern diagnostic assays [20]. In this study of 49 PNH patients, the diagnosis was based on FLAER in 44 cases and monoclonal antibodies in 5. The median age was 34.2 (range, 6.3–80.7) years and the median duration of disease was 2 years. There were nine deaths – six from thrombosis, one from ovarian cancer, one from leukemia, and one from sepsis. The authors found that patients with large PNH granulocyte clones (>60 % PNH cells) were more likely to develop complications such as thrombosis, abdominal pain, hemoglobinuria, esophageal spasm, and male erectile dysfunction. At the time of publication, 12/22 (54.5 %) of patients with >60 % PNH granulocytes developed a thrombus; no patient with fewer than 60 % PNH granulocytes developed a thrombus. There was no increased incidence of other PNH symptoms (headache and fatigue) in patients with large PNH granulocyte clones compared to patients with small PNH clones.

The French updated their previous retrospective series in 2008 [7]. This time they included 460 PNH patients from 58 French hematology centers from 1950 to 2008 and stratified them into two groups on the basis of peripheral blood counts or whether they experienced a thrombosis at presentation. The diagnosis was established by Ham's test or flow cytometry. Obviously, most of the more recent patients (after ~1990) were diagnosed using flow cytometry. Patients with thrombosis at presentation and not cytopenias other than anemia were classified as classical PNH ($n = 113$), patients without thrombosis and with evidence of multilineage cytopenias ($n = 224$) were classified as AA-PNH, and those that did not fit in either of the category ($n = 93$) were classified as intermediate. The median follow-up was 6.8 years. Median survival for the entire group was 22 years but just 16 years for the 113 patients with classical PNH. MDS developed in 5.2 % of patients and acute leukemia developed in 2.4 %. The improved overall survival in this study was likely a function of more sensitive diagnostic assays as the earlier French study and the

English study relied on Ham's test for diagnosis. Ham's tests are not as sensitive in detecting smaller PNH clones, especially in heavily transfused patients. This may have resulted in lead time bias.

Nishimura et al. reported on the clinical course and flow cytometric data of PNH patients in the United States and Japan [22]. There were 164 PNH patients seen at Duke University with complete flow cytometry data and 233 Japanese patients included in this retrospective analysis. The diagnosis of PNH was established or confirmed using at least one of the following: Ham's test, sugar water test, complement lysis sensitivity test, or flow cytometry. In both cohorts, a larger PNH clone was associated with classical PNH symptoms, while a smaller clone was associated with marrow aplasia. Thrombosis was significantly prevalent in white patients than Asian patients. Japanese patients had a longer mean survival time (32 years vs 19 years). A PNH granulocyte clone greater than 50 % was associated with a greater risk for thrombosis. Significantly more Duke patients had classical PNH symptoms, while Japanese patients had more evidence of bone marrow aplasia. The most striking difference between the two cohorts related to thrombosis rates. The Duke patients accounted for 46 % of the patients but 76 % of those with thrombosis. It's hard to know whether this is due to genetic or environmental factors or whether the differences in referral patterns and diagnostic methods contributed may have contributed to these differences.

5.4 Epidemiology and Natural History of Small PNH Clones

PNH and aplastic anemia are closely related disorders. Indeed, the autoimmune attack that accompanies most forms of acquired aplastic anemia seems to provide a conditional survival advantage to *PIGA* mutant stem cells [12]. This explains why small PNH clones are found in most cases of acquired but not inherited forms of aplastic anemia [9, 16]. This may also explain why AA-PNH had a better prognosis in the recent French series than classical PNH. Most forms of acquired aplastic anemia can be successfully treated with BMT or immunosuppressive therapy. BMT will cure the disease and eradicate the PNH clone. Immunosuppressive therapy does not usually eliminate the PNH clone; however, it may take over a decade for the PNH clone to expand enough to cause severe hemolysis and life-threatening problems such as thrombosis. Several groups have now reported that the presence of a PNH clone in the setting of aplastic anemia is associated with low morbidity and mortality [24, 26]. Pu et al. found that an erythrocyte clone of 3–5 % and a granulocyte clone of 23 % were the thresholds to predict intravascular hemolysis as measured by an elevated LDH. In addition, AA patients with <15 % PNH granulocytes at diagnosis were less likely to develop signs and symptoms of intravascular hemolysis. At a median follow-up of almost 6 years after treatment, the PNH clone expanded in roughly 50 % of patients and remained stable or decreased in the other 50 %.

5.5 Epidemiology of PNH in the Era of Terminal Complement Inhibition

There is a paucity of long-term follow-up data of PNH patients treated with eculizumab at this time. Hillmen et al. evaluated the "long-term" safety and efficacy of eculizumab in 195 clinical trial patients over 66 months [15]. All patients experienced a reduction in LDH levels that was sustained over the course of treatment (median reduction 87 % at 36 months), and 96.4 % of the patients have remained free of thromboembolic events. Stabilization or improvement in renal function at 36 months was observed in 93 % of patients, and transfusion independence was increased by 90 % from baseline with the number or red cell transfusions decreasing by 54.7 %. There was no evidence of cumulative drug toxicity. Investigators from Leeds, England, reported long-term outcomes of 79 consecutive patients treated with eculizumab between May 2002 and July 2010 and reported that survival was similar to age-matched controls [17]. Transfusion independence was achieved by 40 of 61 (66 %) patients who were on eculizumab for greater than 12 months. A more recent study from the United States performed a single center, retrospective study of 30 PNH patients treated with eculizumab and categorized them with respect to hemoglobin response [8]. A complete response (CR) was defined as transfusion independence with normal hemoglobin for age and sex, no PNH symptoms, and an LDH < 1.5× the upper limit of normal. A good partial response (GPR) was defined as decreased transfusions from pretreatment and lactate dehydrogenase <1.5 upper limit of normal, and a suboptimal response was defined as unchanged transfusion needs and persistent PNH symptoms. Four patients achieved a CR, 16 achieved a GPR, and ten had a suboptimal response over 863 patient-months of treatment. Complete responders had a decrease in red cell clone size, while good partial responders had an increase. The authors demonstrated that eculizumab responses can vary in PNH and may depend on underlying marrow failure, underlying inflammatory conditions and red cell clone size following treatment. Normalization of hemoglobin with decrease in red cell clone size seems to predict for CR.

5.6 The PNH Global Registry

The International PNH Registry is an ongoing worldwide, noninterventional study collecting safety, effectiveness, and quality-of-life data from patients with a confirmed PNH diagnosis or a detectable PNH clone (≥0.01 %). This is the first PNH Registry that is collecting data on the disease burden of PNH from the patient's perspective. In addition, it will be the first and largest registry to collect data on the natural history of PNH patients treated with eculizumab. The first publication on this data set reported on patients from 273 centers in 25 countries although more than 90 % were from North America or Europe and more than 87 % of patients were Caucasian [27]. Data in this inaugural manuscript is through June 30, 2012. Median age is 42 (range, 3–99) years and median disease duration is 4.6 years; 53.2 % of the patients are female. Median granulocyte clone was 68.1 (range, 0.01–100) percent. At enrollment, 43.5 % had a history of aplastic anemia or hypoplastic anemia, 15.5 % had experienced a thrombotic event, and 13 % had a history of impaired renal function. The most commonly administered therapies have been anticoagulation (31 %), eculizumab (25 %), and immunosuppressive therapy (19 %). The most common reported symptoms include fatigue (80 %), dyspnea (64 %), hemoglobinuria (62 %), abdominal pain (44 %), and chest pain (33 %). Hospitalization due to PNH-related complications was reported by 23 % of the patients and 17 % of patients attributed PNH as the reason they were unable to work. This large, global registry will continue to prospectively collect data to evaluate disease burden and long-term natural history of PNH and treatment outcomes. Some of the more important clinical questions to be addressed by the global registry will relate to pregnancy outcomes, thrombosis risk, long-term survival, risk for Neisserial infections, and impact of underlying bone marrow failure in PNH patients in the era of terminal complement inhibition.

References

1. Bessler M, Mason PJ, Hillmen P, Miyata T, Yamada N, Takeda J, Luzzatto L, Kinoshita T (1994) Paroxysmal nocturnal haemoglobinuria (PNH) is caused by somatic mutations in the PIG-A gene. EMBO J 13:110–117
2. Borowitz MJ, Craig FE, DiGiuseppe JA, Illingworth AJ, Rosse W, Sutherland DR, Wittwer CT, Richards SJ (2010) Guidelines for the diagnosis and monitoring of paroxysmal nocturnal hemoglobinuria and related disorders by flow cytometry. Cytometry B Clin Cytom 78(4):211–230
3. Brodsky RA (2008) Narrative review: paroxysmal nocturnal hemoglobinuria: the physiology of complement-related hemolytic anemia. Ann Intern Med 148(8):587–595
4. Brodsky RA (2014) Paroxysmal nocturnal hemoglobinuria. Blood 124(18):2804–2811
5. Brodsky RA, Mukhina GL, Li S, Nelson KL, Chiurazzi PL, Buckley JT, Borowitz MJ (2000) Improved detection and characterization of paroxysmal nocturnal hemoglobinuria using fluorescent aerolysin. Am J Clin Pathol 114(3):459–466
6. Brodsky RA, Mukhina GL, Nelson KL, Lawrence TS, Jones RJ, Buckley JT (1999) Resistance of paroxysmal nocturnal hemoglobinuria cells to the glycosylphosphatidylinositol-binding toxin aerolysin. Blood 93(5):1749–1756
7. de Latour RP, Mary JY, Salanoubat C, Terriou L, Etienne G, Mohty M, Roth S, de Guibert S, Maury S, Cahn JY, Socie G (2008) Paroxysmal nocturnal hemoglobinuria: natural history of disease subcategories. Blood 112(8):3099–3106
8. DeZern AE, Dorr D, Brodsky RA (2013) Predictors of hemoglobin response to eculizumab therapy in paroxysmal nocturnal hemoglobinuria. Eur J Haematol 90(1):16–24. doi:10.1111/ejh.12021
9. Dezern AE, Symons HJ, Resar LS, Borowitz MJ, Armanios MY, Brodsky RA (2014) Detection of paroxysmal nocturnal hemoglobinuria clones to exclude inherited bone marrow failure syndromes. Eur J Haematol. doi:10.1111/ejh.12299
10. Enneking J (1928) Eine neue form intermittierender haemoglobinurie (Haemoglobinuria paroxysmalis nocturia). Klin Wochenschr 7:2045

11. Ham T (1937) Chronic hemolytic anemia with paroxysmal nocturnal hemoglobinuria. A study of the mechanism of hemolysisin relation to acid–base equilibrium. N Engl J Med 217:915–917
12. Hanaoka N, Nakakuma H, Horikawa K, Nagakura S, Tsuzuki Y, Shimanuki M, Kojima K, Yonemura Y, Kawaguchi T (2009) NKG2D-mediated immunity underlying paroxysmal nocturnal haemoglobinuria and related bone marrow failure syndromes. Br J Haematol 146(5):538–545. doi:10.1111/j.1365-2141.2009.07795.x
13. Hartmann RC, Jenkins DE (1966) The "sugar-water" test for paroxysmal nocturnal hemoglobinuria. N Engl J Med 275(3):155–157
14. Hillmen P, Lewis SM, Bessler M, Luzzatto L, Dacie JV (1995) Natural history of paroxysmal nocturnal hemoglobinuria. N Engl J Med 333:1253–1258
15. Hillmen P, Muus P, Roth A, Elebute MO, Risitano AM, Schrezenmeier H, Szer J, Browne P, Maciejewski JP, Schubert J, Urbano-Ispizua A, de Castro C, Socie G, Brodsky RA (2013) Long-term safety and efficacy of sustained eculizumab treatment in patients with paroxysmal nocturnal haemoglobinuria. Br J Haematol 162(1):62–73. doi:10.1111/bjh.12347
16. Keller P, Debaun MR, Rothbaum RJ, Bessler M (2002) Bone marrow failure in Shwachman-Diamond syndrome does not select for clonal haematopoiesis of the paroxysmal nocturnal haemoglobinuria phenotype. Br J Haematol 119(3):830–832
17. Kelly RJ, Hill A, Arnold LM, Brooksbank GL, Richards SJ, Cullen M, Mitchell LD, Cohen DR, Gregory WM, Hillmen P (2011) Long-term treatment with eculizumab in paroxysmal nocturnal hemoglobinuria: sustained efficacy and improved survival. Blood 117(25):6786–6792. doi:10.1182/blood-2011-02-333997
18. Miyata T, Takeda J, Iida Y, Yamada N, Inoue N, Takahashi M, Maeda K, Kitani T, Kinoshita T (1993) The cloning of PIG-A, a component in the early step of GPI-anchor biosynthesis. Science 259:1318–1320
19. Miyata T, Yamada N, Iida Y, Nishimura J, Takeda J, Kitani T, Kinoshita T (1994) Abnormalities of PIG-A transcripts in granulocytes from patients with paroxysmal nocturnal hemoglobinuria. N Engl J Med 330:249–255
20. Moyo VM, Mukhina GL, Garrett ES, Brodsky RA (2004) Natural history of paroxysmal nocturnal hemoglobinuria using modern diagnostic assays. Br J Haematol 126:133–138
21. Mukhina GL, Buckley JT, Barber JP, Jones RJ, Brodsky RA (2001) Multilineage glycosylphosphatidylinositol anchor deficient hematopoiesis in untreated aplastic anemia. Br J Haematol 115:476–482
22. Nishimura J, Kanakura Y, Ware RE, Shichishima T, Nakakuma H, Ninomiya H, DeCastro CM, Hall S, Kanamaru A, Sullivan KM, Mizoguchi H, Omine M, Kinoshita T, Rosse WF (2004) Clinical course and flow cytometric analysis of paroxysmal nocturnal hemoglobinuria in the United States and Japan. Medicine (Baltimore) 83(3):193–207
23. Parker CJ (2002) Historical aspects of paroxysmal nocturnal haemoglobinuria: 'defining the disease'. Br J Haematol 117(1):3–22
24. Pu JJ, Mukhina G, Wang H, Savage WJ, Brodsky RA (2011) Natural history of paroxysmal nocturnal hemoglobinuria clones in patients presenting as aplastic anemia. Eur J Haematol 87(1):37–45. doi:10.1111/j.1600-0609.2011.01615.x
25. Rother RP, Rollins SA, Mojcik CF, Brodsky RA, Bell L (2007) Discovery and development of the complement inhibitor eculizumab for the treatment of paroxysmal nocturnal hemoglobinuria. Nat Biotechnol 25(11):1256–1264
26. Scheinberg P, Marte M, Nunez O, Young NS (2010) Paroxysmal nocturnal hemoglobinuria clones in severe aplastic anemia patients treated with horse anti-thymocyte globulin plus cyclosporine. Haematologica 95(7):1075–1080. doi:10.3324/haematol.2009.017889
27. Schrezenmeier H, Muus P, Socie G, Szer J, Urbano-Ispizua A, Maciejewski JP, Brodsky RA, Bessler M, Kanakura Y, Rosse W, Khursigara G, Bedrosian C, Hillmen P (2014) Baseline characteristics and disease burden in patients in the international paroxysmal nocturnal hemoglobinuria registry. Haematologica. doi:10.3324/haematol.2013.093161

28. Schubert J, Alvarado M, Uciechowski P, Zielinska-Skowronek M, Freund M, Vogt H, Schmidt RE (1991) Diagnosis of paroxysmal nocturnal haemoglobinuria using immunophenotyping of peripheral blood cells. Br J Haematol 79:487–492
29. Socie G, Mary JY, de Gramont A, Rio B, Leporrier M, Rose C, Heudier P, Rochant H, Cahn JY, Gluckman E (1996) Paroxysmal nocturnal haemoglobinuria: long-term follow-up and prognostic factors. French Society of Haematology. Lancet 348(9027):573–577
30. Takeda J, Miyata T, Kawagoe K, Iida Y, Endo Y, Fujita T, Takahashi M, Kitani T, Kinoshita T (1993) Deficiency of the GPI anchor caused by a somatic mutation of the PIG-A gene in paroxysmal nocturnal hemoglobinuria. Cell 73:703–711
31. Vanderschoot CE, Huizinga TWJ, Van't Veer-Korthof E, Wijmans R, Pinkster J, von dem Borne AEGK (1990) Deficiency of glycosyl-phosphatidylinositol-linked membrane glycoproteins of leukocytes in paroxysmal nocturnal hemoglobinuria, description of a new diagnostic cytoflourometric assay. Blood 76(9):1853–1859
32. Wainwright L, Brodsky RA, Erasmus LK, Poyiadjis S, Naidu G, MacKinnon D (2003) Paroxysmal nocturnal hemoglobinuria arising from fanconi anemia. J Pediatr Hematol Oncol 25(2):167–168
33. Wang H, Chuhjo T, Yamazaki H, Shiobara S, Teramura M, Mizoguchi H, Nakao S (2001) Relative increase of granulocytes with a paroxysmal nocturnal haemoglobinuria phenotype in aplastic anaemia patients: the high prevalence at diagnosis. Eur J Haematol 66(3):200–205
34. Ware RE, Hall SE, Rosse WF (1991) Paroxysmal nocturnal hemoglobinuria with onset in childhood and adolescence. N Engl J Med 325:991–996

Chapter 6
Epidemiology in PNH: Clinical Epidemiological Studies in Korea

Jong Wook Lee

Abstract A retrospective analysis was performed on 301 PNH patients from the South Korean National PNH Registry to describe disease burden and identify the associated risk factors for thromboembolism (TE) and mortality. A multivariate analysis showed that PNH patients with elevated hemolysis (LDH levels ≥1.5 times the upper limit of normal [ULN]) at diagnosis were at significantly higher risk for TE than patients with LDH <1.5 × ULN (odds ratio [OR] 7.0; $P = 0.013$). The combination of LDH ≥1.5 × ULN at diagnosis with the clinical symptoms of abdominal pain, chest pain, dyspnea, or hemoglobinuria was associated with a greater increased risk for TE than elevated hemolysis or clinical symptoms alone. TE (OR 7.11; 95 % confidence interval [CI] (3.052–16.562), impaired renal function (OR 2.953; 95 % CI 1.116–7.818), and PNH-cytopenia (OR 2.547;95 % CI 1.159–5.597) are independent risk factors for mortality, with mortality rates 14-fold ($P < 0.001$), 8-fold ($P < 0.001$), and 6.2-fold ($P < 0.001$) greater than that of the age- and sex-matched general population, respectively.

Early identification of risk factors related to TE and mortality is crucial for the management of high-risk PNH patients.

Keywords Disease burden • Thrombosis • Mortality • Risk factor • PNH

6.1 Disease Burden

The Aplastic Anemia (AA) Working Party of the Korean Society of Hematology has established a web-based nationwide registry of PNH patients. Patient data included in the Korean PNH Registry were captured using an electronic case reporting form (eCRF) registered by the responsible physician of each institution. This registry is a resource for long-term PNH disease observation, and it includes recently collected

J.W. Lee, M.D., Ph.D. (✉)
Division of Hematology, Seoul St. Mary's Hospital, College of Medicine, The Catholic University of Korea, 222 Banpo-daero, Seocho-gu, Seoul 06591, South Korea
e-mail: jwlee@catholic.ac.kr

Y. Kanakura et al. (eds.), *Paroxysmal Nocturnal Hemoglobinuria*,
DOI 10.1007/978-4-431-56003-6_6

Table 6.1 Patient demographics and disease burden from Korean National PNH Registry

Patient demographics and disease characteristics	*N* = 301
Age, years	
Median (range)	37 (8–88)
Mean (SD)	39.3 (15.4)
Patients <40 years, *n* (%)	172 (57.1)
Gender, female, *n* (%)	149 (49.5)
Additional bone marrow disorder, *n* (%)	
Aplastic anemia	121 (40.2)
Myelodysplastic syndrome	19 (6.3)
PNH granulocyte clone size, % (*n* = 195)	
Median (range)	48.8 (0–100)
Mean (SD)	49.5 (30.8)
PNH RBC clone size, % (*n* = 199)	
Median	28.1 (0–99.8)
Mean (SD)	33.2 (27.8)
LDH, fold above ULN (*n* = 224)	
Median (range)	4.10 (0.2–36.3)
Mean (SD)	5.6 (5.5)
≥1.5 × ULN, *n* (%)	171 (76.3)
Follow-up since diagnosis, years	
Median (range)	6.6 (0–28.8)
Mean (SD)	7.8 (6.0)
Symptoms and signs, *n* (%)	
TE	54 (17.9)
Venous	37 (68.5[a])
Arterial	17 (31.5[a])
Impaired renal function	51 (17)
Hemoglobinuria	169 (56.1)
Abdominal pain	141 (46.8)
Dyspnea	111 (36.9)
Chest pain	39 (13.0)
Pain	169 (56.1)
Treatment, *n* (%)	
Corticosteroids	233 (77.4)
RBC transfusions	178 (59.1)
NSAIDs	66 (21.9)
Immunosuppressive treatment	62 (20.6)
Anticoagulation	44 (14.6)
Opioids	39 (13.0)
Bone marrow transplant	37 (12.3)

[a]% of patients with TE.

LDH lactate dehydrogenase, *NSAID* nonsteroidal anti-inflammatory drugs, *PNH* paroxysmal nocturnal hemoglobinuria, *RBC* red blood cell, *SD* standard deviation, *TE* thromboembolism, *ULN* upper limit of normal laboratory and clinical parameters. Data from this registry provided a representative profile of PNH disease course and outcomes.

Three hundred-one patients were enrolled in the Korean PNH Registry. The median age at diagnosis was 37 years (range: 8–88 years), median follow-up time from diagnosis was 6.6 years (range: 0–28.8 years), and there was an approximately equal number of male and female patients. Forty percent of patients had a history of AA and 6.3 % a history of myelodysplastic syndrome (MDS). Overall, 47.2 % of patients ($n = 142$) were categorized as having PNH-cytopenia.

The median granulocyte and erythrocyte clone sizes were 48.8 % and 28.1 %, respectively (Table 6.1). At diagnosis, 171 of 224 patients (76.3 %) with recorded LDH levels had values ≥1.5 times the upper limit of normal (ULN). The most frequently reported clinical symptoms were hemoglobinuria (56 %), pain (56 %), and abdominal pain (47 %) (Table 6.1) [1, 2]. The reports of hemoglobinuria were most likely self-reported macroscopic hemoglobinuria, as this symptom was not objectively assessed.

Thromboembolism (TE) was reported in 54 patients (18 %), of whom 19 (35.2 %) had multiple TE events. Similar percentages of patients reported TE irrespective of if they had underlying AA (16.8 %) or not (18.8 %). Fifty-one patients (17 %) reported impaired renal function (IRF), defined as a history of acute renal failure (ARF) requiring dialysis or estimated glomerular filtration rate (eGFR) of <60 mL/min/1.73 m^2 captured before or after diagnosis of PNH. Forty-four patients (14.6 %) had a recorded history of ARF, and 8.6 % ($n = 26$) had chronic eGFR <60 mL/min/1.73 m^2. One-third of patients who reported IRF had both history of ARF at diagnosis and eGFR <60 mL/min/1.73 m^2.

Corticosteroids (77.4 %), transfusions (59.1 %), and nonsteroidal anti-inflammatory drugs (NSAIDs) (21.9 %) represented the most common supportive care provided. Anticoagulation therapy was administered to 14.6 % of patients and immunosuppressive therapy (IST) to 20.6 % (Table 6.1) [1, 2]. Medical intervention was required in 66 of 169 of patients (39.1 %) reporting pain; the most common interventions were NSAIDs, administered to 37 of these 66 patients (56.1 %), and opioids to 22 of them (33.3 %). Twelve percent ($n = 37$) received bone marrow transplant (BMT) from related or unrelated donors. No patient received treatment with the terminal complement inhibitor eculizumab.

6.2 PNH with Bone Marrow Failure

Although PNH clone may be detected in patients with MDS, AA is the most frequently associated BM failure disorder in the patients with PNH. Although eculizumab, a monoclonal antibody to complement 5a, can be effective in controlling intravascular hemolysis in both classic PNH and PNH-cytopenia, it does not improve underlying cytopenia related with BM failure. Especially, the risk of serious infection and/or bleeding is very high in patients with compatible hematologic values to severe aplastic anemia (SAA). Therefore, the patients with PNH-cytopenia

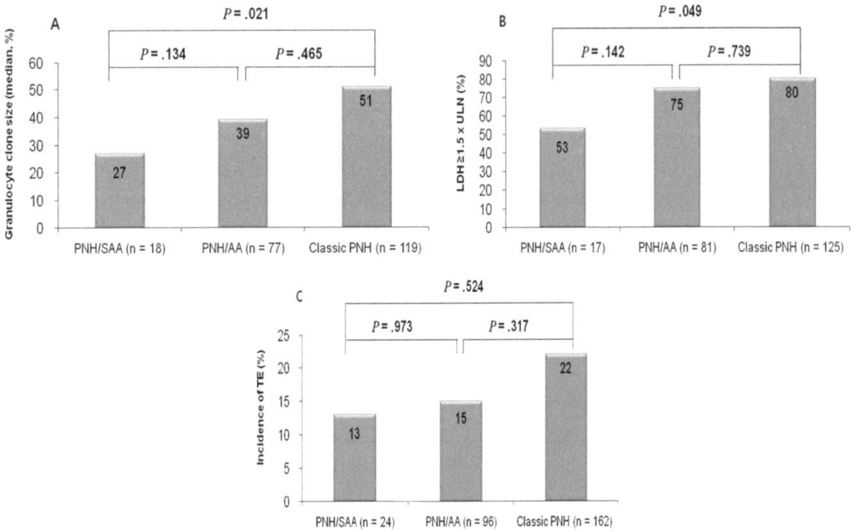

Fig. 6.1 Clinical characteristics in three subgroups. (**a**) The median PNH clone sizes of granulocyte, (**b**) incidence of elevated hemolysis (LDH levels ≥ 1.5 times ULN), and (c) incidence of the first TE per patient

should be further subdivided into PNH patients with concomitant severe aplastic anemia (PNH/SAA) and PNH with non-SAA (PNH/AA) according to the severity of cytopenia because patients with PNH/SAA require treatment such as IST or allogeneic BMT.

Therefore, we analyzed to identify the clinical characteristics of patients with PNH-cytopenia according to the severity of cytopenia. Among the 282 patients with hematological values at diagnosis, there were 24 patients with PNH/SAA (at least two of the following three criteria: hemoglobin ≤8 g/dL, absolute neutrophil count (ANC) $<0.5 \times 10^9$/L, platelet count $<20 \times 10^9$/L), 96 patients with PNH/AA (at least two of the following three criteria: hemoglobin 8–10 g/dL, ANC 0.5–1.5 × 10^9/L, platelet count 20–100 × 10^9/L) and 162 classic PNH patients with hemolytic sign and not categorized into PNH/SAA or PNH/AA [3].

Median granulocyte PNH clone sizes were 26.7 % in PNH/SAA, 39.0 % in PNH/AA, and 50.8 % in classic PNH patients. Post hoc analyses showed that the median clone size was significantly lower in the PNH/SAA subgroup compared with the classic PNH subgroup (P = 0.021, Fig. 6.1a). The percentage of the patients with a high granulocyte PNH clone size (>50 %) was reported in 4 patients with PNH/SAA (22.2 %), 33 patients with PNH/AA (42.9 %), and 60 patients with classic PNH (50.4 %) with the differences between subgroups being statistically significant for the PNH/SAA versus the classic PNH subgroups (P = 0.039) but not between the PNH/SAA versus the PNH/AA subgroups (P = 0.165) and the PNH/AA versus the classic PNH subgroups (P = 0.578). At diagnosis, LDH levels were significantly lower in the PNH/SAA subgroup compared with the classic PNH subgroup (1.8-fold

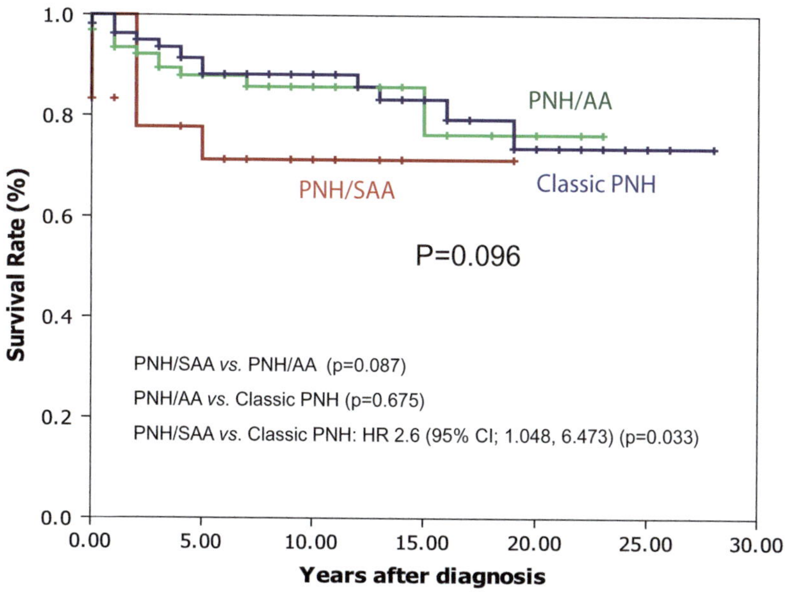

Fig. 6.2 Kaplan-Meier survival curves in three PNH subgroups

versus 4.5-fold greater than ULN; $P = 0.008$) but was not statistically significant in any of the other subgroup comparisons [3, 4]. The percentages of patients with elevated levels of hemolysis (LDH levels ≥ 1.5 times ULN) at diagnosis were also significantly lower in the PNH/SAA subgroup than in the classic PNH subgroup ($P = 0.049$, Fig. 6.1b). TE events were reported in 12.5 % of patients with PNH/SAA ($n = 3$), 14.6 % of patients with PNH/AA ($n = 14$), and 22.2 % of patients with classic PNH ($n = 36$) with no significant differences between the subgroups (Fig. 6.1c) [3].

Among 282 patients, 39 patients (13.8 %) died during the median follow-up time from diagnosis of 6.6 years (range 0–28.8 years). Six patients (25.0 %) with PNH/SAA, 12 (12.5 %) with PNH/AA, and 21 (13.0 %) with classic PNH died. The overall survival rate was not different between the three subgroups of PNH ($P = 0.096$). However, the overall survival was significantly lower in the PNH/SAA subgroup than in the classic PNH subgroup ($P = 0.033$). The hazard ratio comparing the PNH/SAA subgroup to the classic PNH subgroup was 2.6 (95 % confidence interval [CI] 1.048–6.473, Fig. 6.2). The most common cause of death was infection or critical bleeding related with underlying cytopenia in the PNH/SAA subgroup (5/6, 83.3 %) and the PNH/AA subgroup (6/12, 50.0 %). Two patients with PNH/SAA died from bleeding complications (one intracerebral hemorrhage and one pulmonary hemorrhage). However, TE was the most common cause of death in the classic PNH subgroup (5/21, 23.8 %) [3].

Therefore, the identification of the PNH/SAA subgroup among the patients with PNH-cytopenia should be required because the PNH/SAA subgroup showed different clinical manifestations and poor outcome [3]. Treatment strategy should be individualized in patients with PNH-cytopenia based on severity of cytopenia, age, availability of transplant donor, comorbidities, etc. Our suggested criteria for PNH/SAA or PNH/AA can be used as a tool to select appropriate PNH patients who may benefit from BMT or IST. However, an individualization of treatment strategies using these criteria still requires more robust investigations.

6.3 Clinical Symptoms and Sign Associated with Risk of Thrombosis

6.3.1 Characteristics of TE

TE occurred at both venous (69.1 %) and arterial (30.9 %) sites. TE was found in typical sites, including deep vein, pulmonary vein, and renal vein, as well as in atypical sites, including cerebral vein and renal artery. Fifty-three percent of the TE events were reported in patients with classic PNH and 47 % in patients with PNH-cytopenia ($P = 0.981$). In patients with a reported TE and granulocyte clone ($n = 37$), TE was recorded in all three clone size categories assessed (<20, 20–50, and >50 %), with the prevalence of TE being 16, 19, and 20 %, respectively; there was no evidence of any association between clone size category and the risk of experiencing a TE ($P = 0.843$) (Fig. 6.3) [1].

Five of 16 patients receiving prophylactic anticoagulant therapy (31.3 %) experienced a first thrombosis, and 12 of 21 patients receiving therapeutic anticoagulant treatment (57.1 %) experienced subsequent TE events during anticoagulant treatment.

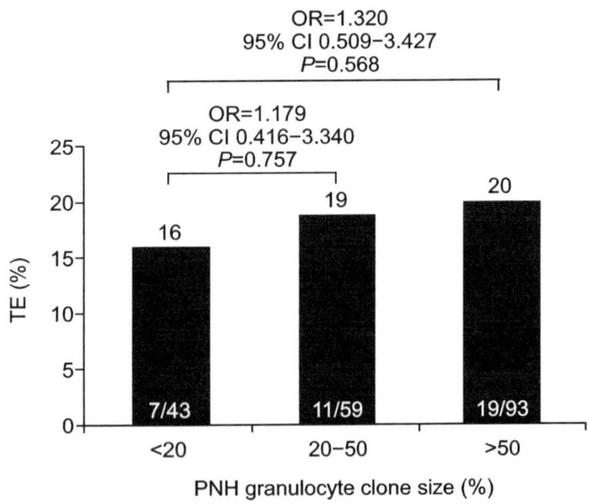

Fig. 6.3 Incidence of TE in PNH granulocyte clone size categories. Overall test of association between clone size and TE ($P = 0.843$)

6.3.2 Risk Factors Associated with TE

6.3.2.1 Elevated LDH

Median LDH at diagnosis was higher in patients with TE than in those without TE, the difference between the two groups bordering on statistical significance (P = 0.05). Age, history of bone marrow disorders, PNH granulocyte clone size, platelet count, and hemoglobin did not differ significantly in patients with or without TE.

Univariate analysis showed patients with LDH ≥1.5 × ULN at diagnosis had a significantly increased incidence of TE (43 of 171 [25.1 %]) compared with patients with LDH <1.5 × ULN (2 of 53 [3.8 %]; OR 8.57; 95 % CI 2.00–36.68; $P < 0.001$) [1, 6]. Adjusting for age, gender, and bone marrow failure (BMF), multivariate analyses confirmed that elevated LDH ≥1.5 × ULN at diagnosis was independently associated with increased odds of experiencing TE (OR 7.0; 95 % CI 1.5–32; P = 0.013; Fig. 6.4) [1, 2, 4].

A receiver operating characteristic (ROC) analysis was performed to determine which LDH value would represent the most sensitive threshold to detect TE (Fig. 6.5). This analysis demonstrated that LDH ≥1.5 × ULN as a threshold detected 96 % of the patients with TE and also showed that an LDH threshold of ≥3.0 × ULN or ≥5.0 × ULN at diagnosis detected only 67 or 47 % of the population with TE, respectively. Furthermore, logistic regression analysis demonstrated that neither LDH ≥3.0 × ULN nor LDH ≥5.0 × ULN were independently associated with risk of TE (≥3.0 × ULN: OR 1.5, 95 % CI 0.78–3.07, P = 0.208; ≥5.0 × ULN: OR 1.3, 95 % CI 0.66–2.45, P = 0.476) [1, 7].

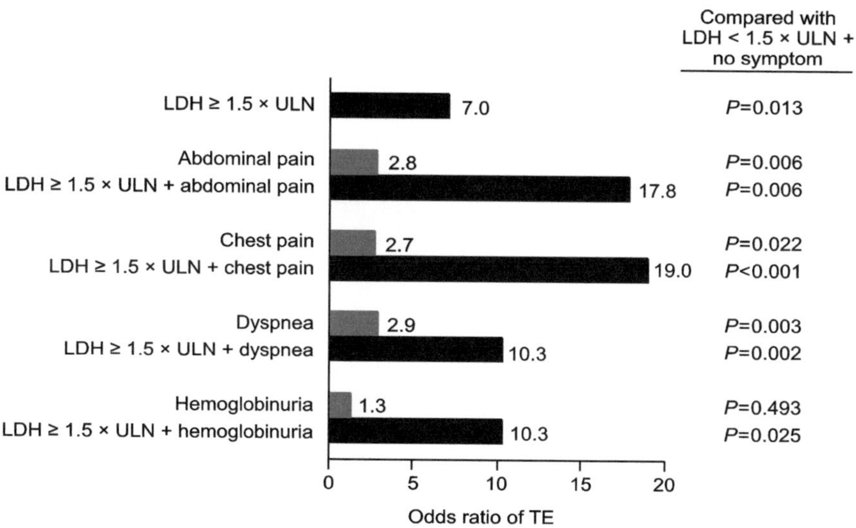

Fig. 6.4 Multivariate analysis of the effect of LDH ≥1.5 × ULN and clinical symptoms on associated risk of TE

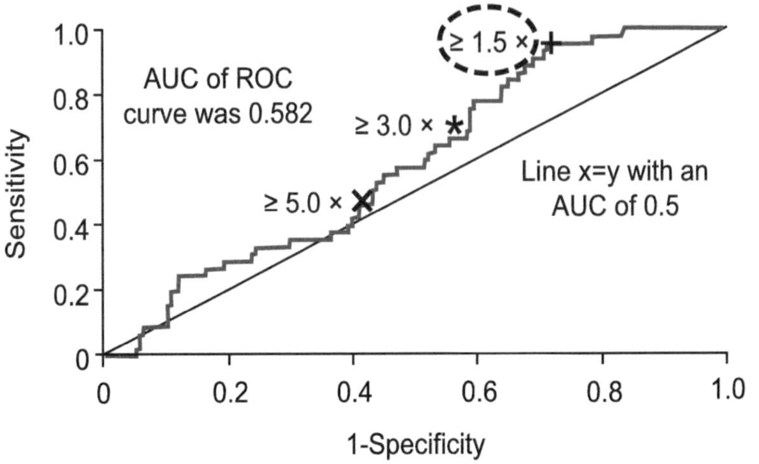

Fig. 6.5 Receiver operating characteristic (ROC) curve of LDH cutoff for detecting TE

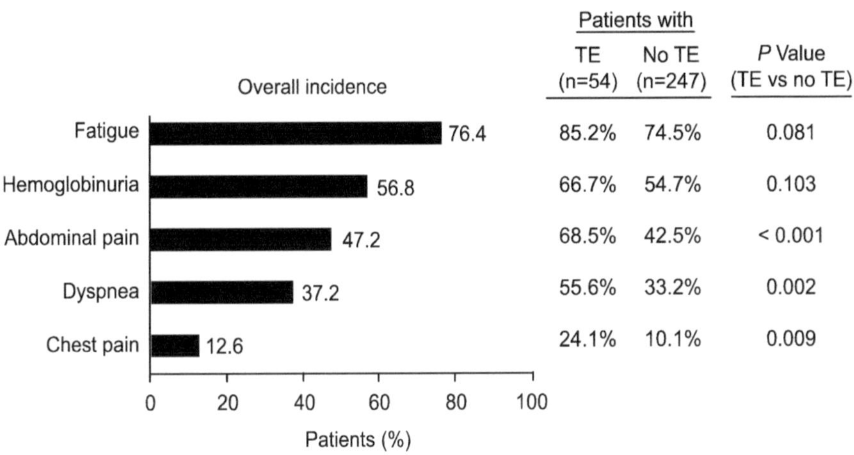

Fig. 6.6 Incidence of clinical symptoms in the overall patient population and in patients with or without TE

6.3.2.2 Clinical Symptoms

The incidences of abdominal pain, chest pain, and dyspnea were significantly increased in patients with TE compared with those without TE (Fig. 6.6) [1, 2, 6]. Multivariate analysis demonstrated that patients with abdominal pain, chest pain, and dyspnea had significantly increased odds of experiencing a TE compared with patients with no symptom (Fig. 6.4) [1, 2, 4]. Patients with LDH ≥1.5 × ULN at diagnosis were at increased risk of experiencing TE; the odds of a TE were further increased when patients presented with LDH ≥1.5 × ULN at diagnosis and any of the clinical symptoms of abdominal pain, chest pain, dyspnea, or hemoglobinuria

(Fig. 6.4). This was particularly pronounced for abdominal pain (OR 17.79; 95 % CI 2.33–36.01) and chest pain (OR 19.04; 95 % CI 3.74–96.99) ($P \leq 0.006$), but it was also seen in patients with dyspnea (OR 10.35; 95 % CI 2.31–46.45) and hemoglobinuria (OR 10.28; 95 % CI 1.34–79.02) ($P \leq 0.025$) [1].

6.4 Predictive Factors for Mortality

During the median follow-up of 6.6 years (range 0–28.8), 43 of the 301 patients (14.3 %) had died. There were significantly more patient deaths reported in PNH patients with LDH ≥1.5 × ULN at diagnosis ($n = 28$; 16.4 %) compared with patients with LDH <1.5 × ULN ($n = 2$; 3.7 %; $p = 0.009$) [2, 6].

Twenty-three out of 54 patients with a history of TE died after the median time of 8 months (range 1 day −17 years) from the occurrence of TE. Multiple TE events were reported in ten deceased patients (43.4 %), and 13 patients experienced one TE event during the disease course before dying. Patients with multiple TE events were significantly associated with poor survival (HR 6.3; 95 % CI 2.96–13.55; $p < 0.001$), and one TE event also had a significantly increased risk of mortality (HR 4.5; 95 % CI 2.3–9.1; $p < 0.001$) compared with patients without TE [5].

Univariate analyses showed that significant predictors of mortality were TE ($p < 0.001$), IRF ($p = 0.001$), LDH ≥1.5 × ULN ($p = 0.009$), PNH-cytopenia ($p = 0.023$), abdominal pain ($p = 0.026$), and dyspnea/chest pain ($p = 0.026$) (Table 6.2). Multivariate analyses indicated that TE, IRF, and PNH-cytopenia were significantly associated with an increased risk of mortality ($p < 0.001$, $p = 0.029$ and $p = 0.020$, respectively) (Table 6.2) [8, 9]. Elevated levels of LDH were not an independent risk factor for mortality in the multivariate regression analysis ($p = 0.159$; Table 6.2).

Table 6.2 Univariate and multivariate analysis of risk factors of mortality

	Univariate analysis		Multivariate analysis	
Risk factor for mortality	*p* value	Odds ratio (95 % CI)	*p* value	Odds ratio (95 % CI)
TE	<0.001	8.42 (4.15–17.08)	<0.001	7.110 (3.052–16.562)
IRF	0.001	3.41 (1.66–7.02)	0.029	2.953 (1.116–7.818)
PNH-cytopenia	0.023	2.17 (1.11–4.21)	0.020	2.547 (1.159–5.597)
LDH ≥1.5 × ULN	0.009	4.99 (1.15–21.70)	0.159	3.204 (0.633–16.230)
Abdominal pain	0.026	2.10 (1.08–4.08)	0.162	1.828 (0.785–4.256)
Dyspnea/chest pain	0.026	2.09 (1.086–4.024)	0.855	1.077 (0.487–2.381)
Hemoglobinuria	0.636	0.86 (0.45–1.63)	0.073	0.449 (0.187–1.077)
Clone size	0.391	1.01 (0.99–1.02)	0.744	0.995 (0.967–1.024)

CI confidence interval, *IRF* impaired renal function, *LDH* lactate dehydrogenase, *TE* thromboembolism, *ULN* upper limit of normal

6.5 Prognostic Factors for Survival

Table 6.3 presents the calculated standard mortality ratio (SMR) for this population of PNH patients. SMR is the ratio of the observed mortality rate in the PNH population to the expected mortality rate of the age-sex-matched cohort from the Korean population.

Overall, a diagnosis of PNH increased the risk of mortality by 3.9-fold ($p < 0.001$). The greatest risk factor for mortality was a TE, which increased mortality by 13.9-fold compared with the general population ($p < 0.001$, Fig. 6.7a). Other significant risk factors, compared with an age- and gender-matched population ($p < 0.001$ in each case), included IRF (7.8-fold increase), PNH-cytopenia (6.2-fold increase), classic PNH (4.4-fold increase), and LDH ≥1.5 × ULN (4.8-fold increase) (Fig. 6.7b–d). Patients without evidence of elevated hemolysis (LDH <1.5 × ULN) were the only subset of patients with a mortality rate similar to that of the age- and gender-matched population (SMR = 1.17; $p = 0.824$). Symptomatic risk factors for higher mortality rates compared with the general population included abdominal pain (SMR = 4.92; $p < 0.001$), dyspnea (SMR = 4.48; $p < 0.001$), and chest pain (SMR = 4.29; $p < 0.001$). Patients with both of these symptoms and LDH ≥1.5 × ULN at diagnosis had SMR values that were approximately 25 % (dyspnea) or 33 %

Table 6.3 Standard mortality ratio according to risk factors

	SMR vs age- and sex-matched general population	
Patient population	SMR (95 % CI)	p value
Total PNH patients (*n* = 301)	3.89 (2.73–5.05)	<0.001
No TE (*n* = 247)	2.13 (1.19–3.06)	<0.001
TE (*n* = 54)	13.92 (8.23–19.61)	<0.001
LDH <1.5× ULN (*n* = 53)	1.17 (0.00–2.79)	0.824
LDH ≥1.5 × ULN (*n* = 171)	4.81 (3.03–6.59)	<0.001
No IRF(*n* = 251)	3.06 (1.93–4.20)	<0.001
IRF (*n* = 50)	7.81 (3.86–11.77)	<0.001
Classic PNH (*n* = 157)	4.4 (2.72–6.23)	<0.001
PNH-cytopenia (*n* = 107)	6.2 (4.71–9.34).	<0.001
No abdominal pain (*n* = 159)	2.87 (1.46–4.28)	<0.001
Abdominal pain (*n* = 142)	4.92 (3.06–6.77)	<0.001
LDH ≥1.5 × ULN + abdominal pain (*n* = 92)	6.55 (3.60–9.49)	<0.001
No dyspnea (*n* = 189)	3.42 (1.95–4.88)	<0.001
Dyspnea (*n* = 112)	4.48 (2.61–6.35)	<0.001
LDH ≥1.5× ULN + dyspnea (*n* = 58)	5.58 (2.85–8.32)	<0.001
No chest pain (*n* = 263)	3.82 (2.57–5.06)	<0.001
Chest pain (*n* = 38)	4.29 (1.11–7.47)	<0.001
LDH ≥1.5 × ULN + chest pain (*n* = 24)	5.72 (0.71–10.73)	<0.001

SMR standard mortality ratio, *CI* confidence interval, *PNH* paroxysmal nocturnal hemoglobinuria, *LDH* lactate dehydrogenase, *ULN* upper limit of normal, *TE* thromboembolism, *IRF* impaired renal function

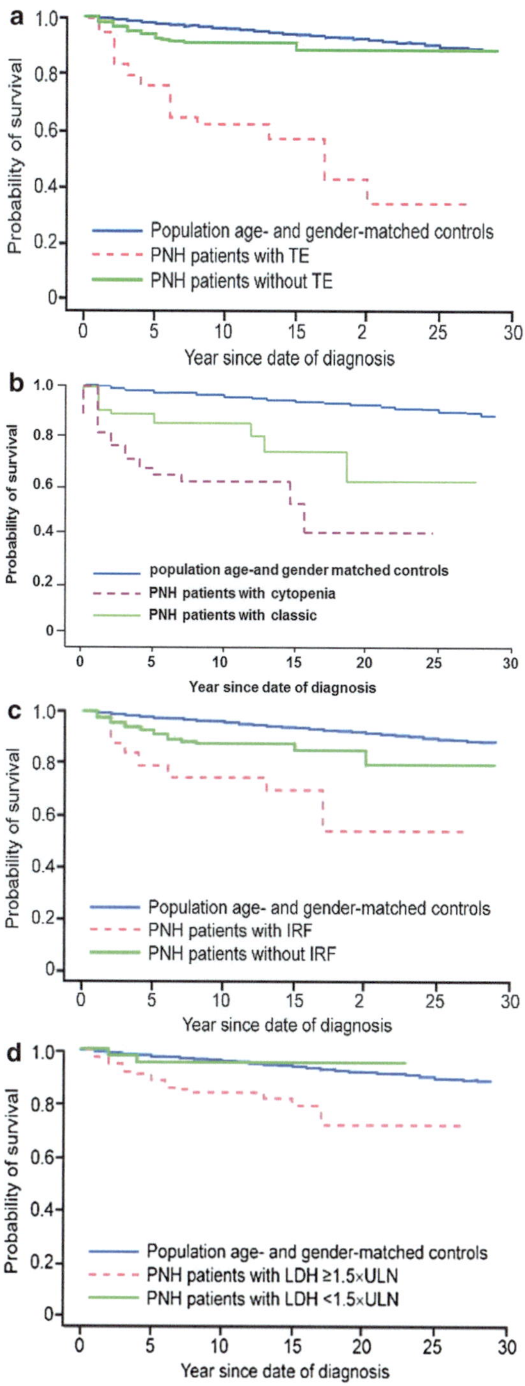

Fig. 6.7 Kaplan-Meier survival of PNH patients compared with age- and gender-matched general population. (**a**) Patients with TE had a 14-fold higher mortality rate compared with the general population (standard mortality ratio [SMR] = 13.9; 95 % confidence interval [CI], 8.2-19.6; P < 0.001). (**b**) Patients with cytopenia had a mortality rate 6.2-fold greater than the age- and gender-matched general population (SMR = 6.2; 95 % CI, 4.7–9.3; *P* < 0.001). (**c**) Patients with impaired renal function (IRF) had a mortality rate 7.8-fold greater than the age- and gender-matched general population (SMR = 7.8; 95 % CI, 3.9–11.8; *P* < 0.001). (**d**) PNH patients with lactate dehydrogenase (LDH) ≥1.5 times the upper limit of normal (ULN) had a 5.0-fold greater risk for mortality compared with patients with LDH <1.5 × ULN (95 % CI, 1.15–21.70; *P* = 0.009). PNH patients with LDH ≥1.5 × ULN had a 4.8-fold higher mortality rate compared with the general population (SMR = 4.8; 95 % CI, 3.0–6.6; *P* < 0.001)

(abdominal pain and chest pain) higher than for the overall subset of patients with these individual symptoms alone (Table 6.3) [9].

References

1. Lee JW, Jang JH, Kim JS et al (2013) Clinical signs and symptoms associated with increased risk for thrombosis in patients with paroxysmal nocturnal hemoglobinuria from a Korean Registry. Int J Hematol 97(6):749–757
2. Lee JW, Jang JH, Lee JH, Yoon SS, Kim JS, Kim YK, Cho DY, Sohn SK, Chung JS (2010) Clinical symptoms of hemolysis are predictive of disease burden and mortality in Asian patients with paroxysmal nocturnal hemoglobinuria(PNH). Haematologica 95(Suppl. 2):206, abs. 0506
3. Kim JS, Jang JH, Yoon SS, Lee JH, Kim YK, Jo DY, Chung JS, Sohn SK, Lee JW (2016) Distinct subgroups of paroxysmal nocturnal hemoglobinuria (PNH) with cytopenia: results from South Korean National PNH Registry. Ann Hematol 95:125–133
4. Kim JS, Lee JW, Yoon SS, Lee JH, Jo DY, Jang JH, Kim YK, Chung JS, Sohn SK (2010) Association between elevated hemolysis at diagnosis and early mortality and risk of thrombosis in paroxysmal nocturnal hemoglobinuria (PNH) patients with cytopenia. Blood 116(21), abs. 4241
5. Lee JW, Jang JH, Lee JH, Yoon SS, Kim JS, Kim YK, Cho DY, Sohn SK, Chung JS (2010) High prevalence and mortality associated with thromboembolism in Asian patients with paroxysmal nocturnal hemoglobinuria(PNH). Haematologica 95(Suppl. 2):205, abs. 0505
6. Lee JW, Jang JH, Kim JS, Yoon SS, Lee JH, Kim YK, Jo DY, Chung JS, Sohn SK (2011) Uncontrolled complement activation and the resulting chronic hemolysis as measured by LDH serum level at diagnosis as predictor of thrombotic complications and mortality in a large cohort of patients with paroxysmal nocturnal hemoglobinuria(PNH). Blood 118(21), abs. 3166
7. Lee JW, Jang JH, Kim JS, Yoon SS, Lee JH, Kim YK, Jo DY, Chung JS, Sohn SK (2012) LDH = 1.5x above normal is a sensitive and specific marker to identify patients at risk of clinical complications and mortality associated with paroxysmal nocturnal hemoglobinuria. Haematologica 97(s1):579–580, abs. 1454
8. Kim JS, Jang JH, Lee JW, Yoon SS, Lee JH, Kim YK (2011) Renal impairment is a risk factor for early mortality in patients with paroxysmal nocturnal hemoglobinuria (PNH). Haematologica 96:112, abs. 0271
9. Jang JH, Kim JS, Yoon SS, Lee JH, Kim YK, Jo DY, Chung JS, Sohn SK, Lee JW (2016) Predictive factors of mortality in population of patients with paroxysmal nocturnal hemoglobinuria: results from a Korean PNH Registry. J Korean Med Sci 31:214–221

Chapter 7
Haemolysis in PNH: Depletion of Nitric Oxide

Anita Hill

Abstract The lack of complement regulation on paroxysmal nocturnal hemoglobinuria (PNH) red cells renders these cells extremely sensitive to complement-mediated lysis resulting in free haemoglobin release. Nitric oxide induces a coordinated programme of cellular events that promote blood flow and maintain smooth muscle tone. Nitric oxide reacts with haem groups quickly and irreversibly. In situations of intravascular haemolysis, as seen in PNH, nitric oxide will be rapidly depleted leading to systemic symptoms and complications. These include symptoms of smooth muscle dystonia such as abdominal pain, dysphagia and erectile dysfunction. It is also likely to contribute to significant fatigue. Complications such as thrombosis and pulmonary hypertension can also occur due to the contribution of depletion of nitric oxide.

Keywords PNH • Haemolysis • Nitric oxide • LDH • Pulmonary hypertension

7.1 The Relationship of Free Haemoglobin with Nitric Oxide Depletion (Fig. 7.1)

The lack of complement regulation on the paroxysmal nocturnal hemoglobinuria (PNH) red cell surface renders these cells extremely sensitive to complement-mediated lysis resulting in systemic haemoglobin release [39].

Nitric oxide (NO) is a soluble diatomic gas molecule, much like carbon monoxide. Because of its unpaired electron, NO is a free radical, providing it with unique reactivities and biological properties [113]. It has a half-life of seconds and is continuously synthesised in endothelial cells from the amino acid L-arginine by isoforms of the NO synthase enzyme. There is oxygen-dependent conversion of L-arginine to citrulline [79]. Once produced, NO can diffuse in a paracrine fashion to adjacent smooth muscle, where it binds avidly to the haem moiety of soluble

A. Hill, MBChB (Hons), Ph.D. (✉)
Department of Haematology, St. James' University Hospital,
Beckett Street, Leeds, West Yorkshire LS9 7TF, UK
e-mail: anitahill@nhs.net

Y. Kanakura et al. (eds.), *Paroxysmal Nocturnal Hemoglobinuria*,
DOI 10.1007/978-4-431-56003-6_7

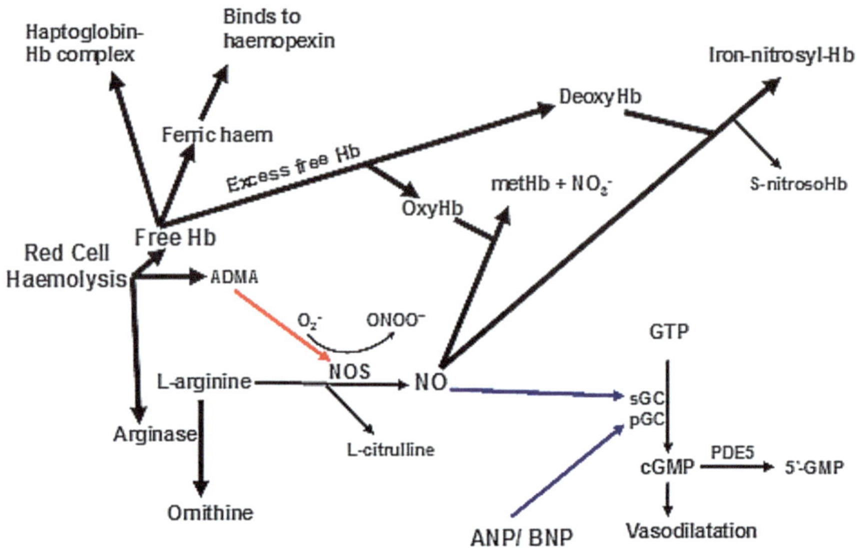

Fig. 7.1 The relationship of free haemoglobin and nitric oxide (the explanation below the title of the figure is to give help understand the diagram)

guanylate cyclase resulting in increased intracellular cyclic guanosine monophosphate (cGMP) [42, 43]. Cyclic GMP activates cGMP-dependent kinases (through allosteric modification) that decrease intracellular calcium concentration in smooth muscle, producing relaxation, vasodilatation and increased regional blood flow [1, 25, 41, 60, 79]. Indeed, NO is one of the most potent vasodilators known [60] and is essential to vascular homeostasis and maintenance of vasomotor tone.

In addition to this vasodilatation, which is tonic in nature and controls approximately 25 % of our resting blood flow, NO induces a coordinated programme of cellular events that promote blood flow, primarily by suppressing platelet aggregation [41, 60, 79], expression of cell adhesion molecules on endothelial cells and secretion of procoagulant proteins [29, 87, 90, 109]. It also limits platelet aggregation and ischaemia-reperfusion injury [46], modulates endothelial proliferation [30] and has anti-inflammatory properties [80].

Importantly, NO also reacts with the oxygenated and deoxygenated haem groups of haemoglobin (oxyhaemoglobin and deoxyhaemoglobin) at nearly diffusion-limited rates (10^7 M^{-1} s^{-1}) to produce methaemoglobin and bio-inactive nitrate and iron-nitrosyl-haemoglobin, respectively [13, 22, 31, 57, 77].

The reaction of nitric oxide with oxyhaemoglobin is so fast (10^7 M^{-1} s^{-1}) and irreversible; it would be expected that nitric oxide produced by endothelium would not survive long enough as it would be immediately scavenged by haemoglobin and would therefore be incapable of paracrine diffusion from endothelium to vascular smooth muscle [77, 95]. However, under normal physiological conditions, this effect is severely limited by compartmentalisation of the haemoglobin inside the erythrocyte [11, 55], laminar flowing blood, and the plasma haemoglobin scavenging systems that limit extravasation of free plasma haemoglobin into the interstitial space [95]. This compartmentalisation of haemoglobin from endothelium creates two diffusional barriers, in addition to the sub-membrane network of proteins [40, 106]: an erythrocyte-free diffusion barrier along the endothelium in laminar flowing blood [54, 107] and an unstirred bulk diffusional barrier surrounding the erythrocyte membrane [55]. In this context, the evolution of the erythrocyte can be considered as a mechanism to ensure separation of the critical respiratory transport machinery from the endothelium in order to reduce direct toxicity while maintaining efficient oxygen delivery [15, 54, 55]. Understanding the role of such barriers and the requirement for a physical separation of haemoglobin from the source of NO production in endothelium helps explain the remarkable morbidity and mortality associated with the use of stroma-free haemoglobin-based blood substitutes and many of the clinical manifestations of haemolytic disease [77, 87, 90].

Lactate dehydrogenase (LDH) catalyses the reversible reduction of pyruvate to lactate by nicotinamide adenine dinucleotide (NADH). Red blood cells contain large amounts of LDH, which is released into the plasma during haemolysis, and levels of serum LDH are generally elevated in patients with intravascular haemolysis [102]. Importantly, in vitro studies have shown that total LDH levels are significantly and linearly correlated with the red cell haemoglobin content over a very broad range of haemoglobin concentrations. Quantitation of total LDH and haemoglobin in osmotically lysed red cells shows a near uniform correlation between these parameters [105].

In a setting of intravascular haemolysis, where lactate dehydrogenase levels can easily exceed 2–3 times their normal levels, free haemoglobin would be expected to obtain concentrations of 0.8–1.6 g/L [105]. Further, total LDH is an accurate measure of free haemoglobin in vivo as LDH levels correlate well with free plasma haemoglobin levels [35].

Plasma haemoglobin levels in patients with PNH are commonly in the range of 0.05–0.2 g/dL and can exceed 1.0 g/dL during severe haemolytic episodes [28, 35]. In comparison, plasma haemoglobin levels range from 0.001 to 0.033 g/dL in sickle cell disease and can exceed 0.041 g/dL during vaso-occlusive crisis [74, 87]. The occurrence of steady-state intravascular haemolysis in diseases such as PNH and sickle cell disease typically generates sufficient plasma haemoglobin to completely deplete haptoglobin.

A further consequence of extracellular haemoglobin is the promotion of highly oxidative reactions involving iron, the haem porphyrin ring and oxygen radicals that produce endothelial dysfunction. The resulting reactive oxygen species can then react with NO, further reducing its bioavailability and producing the highly oxidative peroxynitrite. Free haemoglobin also directly impairs endothelial function [3, 19, 90]. Although not linked directly to haemolysis, NO also appears to be consumed by reactive oxygen species generated by the high levels of xanthine oxidase activity and NADPH oxidase activity that accompany sickle cell disease [2–4, 27, 86, 114].

7.2 The Relationship of L-Arginine and Arginase with Nitric Oxide Depletion

In addition to haemoglobin decompartmentalisation and NO scavenging [87], haemolysis also releases erythrocyte arginase, an enzyme that converts L-arginine, the substrate for NO synthesis, to ornithine, thereby further reducing the systemic availability of NO [5, 66, 67, 96] (see Fig. 7.1). Arginase is an intracellular enzyme that appears in plasma only after cell damage or death. Arginase activity is particularly abundant in immature or young red blood cells and reticulocytes [5], both of which are plentiful in conditions of rapid erythrocyte turnover. Elevated erythrocyte arginase activity has also been reported in patients with megaloblastic anaemia [5] and thalassaemia patients [88]. The enzyme is released into blood plasma as those cells lyse, depleting the plasma pool of arginine. Plasma arginase levels are highest in those patients with markers of accelerated haemolytic rate [57].

L-arginine is an important amino acid in the endogenous production of NO. Arginine is taken up into cells via a cationic amino acid transporter and is converted to NO via a family of enzymes termed the NO synthases (NOS) [60]. Arginine can be broken down into ornithine via the enzyme arginase and ultimately converted into proline and polyamines. Pathological release of erythrocyte arginase into blood plasma from the red blood cell during haemolysis [63] and thereby decreased bioavailability of the arginine substrate through its rapid consumption [63–65] will compound the decreased NO bioavailability through NO scavenging and reactive oxygen species [57].

Since arginine and ornithine compete for the same transport system for cellular uptake [14], a decrease in the ratio of arginine to ornithine resulting from increased arginase activity could further limit arginine bioavailability for NO synthesis, even when plasma arginine concentration appears sufficient [63, 64].

Multiple systems have evolved to control the level of cell-free haemoglobin in the plasma during normal physiological haemolysis, presumably to curtail the deleterious effects of plasma haemoglobin on nitric oxide bioavailability and endothelial function. During severe bouts of haemolysis (paroxysms), haemoglobin escapes into the plasma, dimerises and can saturate these biochemical systems in place to remove it, resulting in haemoglobinuria [102]. One such biochemical system is the formation of the haptoglobin-haemoglobin complex. The occurrence of intravascular haemolysis often generates sufficient free haemoglobin to completely deplete the haptoglobin. The haptoglobin-haemoglobin complex exposes a neoepitope that is recognised by the haemoglobin scavenger receptor, CD163 on the surface of monocytes and macrophages, which binds the complex with high affinity and mediates haptoglobin-haemoglobin endocytosis (phagocytosis) and degradation in the liver [49, 59, 72]. Since haptoglobin is not recycled, the formation of large amounts of haptoglobin-haemoglobin complexes leads to rapid haptoglobin depletion [75]. Thus, in severe haemolytic diseases such as PNH and sickle cell disease, serum haptoglobin is typically undetectable [102].

Since haptoglobin can only bind approximately 0.7–1.5 g/L (10.9–23.4 μM) of haemoglobin depending on the haptoglobin allotype [52], once the capacity of this haemoglobin scavenging protein is exceeded, levels of haemoglobin and haem increase in the plasma and urine.

Ferrous haem (Fe^{II}), the oxygen-binding component of haemoglobin, can be oxidised to ferric haem (Fe^{III}), which is then released from haemoglobin and binds with high affinity to a plasma glycoprotein, haemopexin. Haem bound to haemopexin is degraded in a series of enzymatic steps in the liver. Haem oxygenase 1 (HO-1) subsequently breaks down the pro-oxidant and pro-inflammatory haem into carbon monoxide, biliverdin and iron. Carbon monoxide has vasodilatory, antiproliferative, anti-inflammatory and antioxidant properties [44, 78, 83, 91], while biliverdin is an antioxidant that is converted by biliverdin reductase to bilirubin [7, 98]. Biliverdin reductase itself has catalytic antioxidant properties [7]. The haem-derived oxidant iron is directly sequestered and inactivated by ferritin [97]. Additionally, haptoglobin-haemoglobin binding to CD163 signals anti-inflammatory IL-10 and HO-1 induction in circulating monocytes [81]. Thus, the antioxidant, anticoagulant, antiproliferative and vasodilating effects of the CD163/HO-1/biliverdin reductase systems likely represent an evolved compensation for the nitric oxide scavenging, vasoconstrictive, proliferative, inflammatory and pro-oxidant effects of extracellular haemoglobin, haem and haem-iron [90].

The best protection against NO depletion would be to stop haemolysis. In sickle cell disease, this is attempted by agents such as hydroxycarbamide. In PNH, haemolysis may be prevented with the sustained use of the complement inhibitor, eculizumab.

The rate of NO depletion correlates with the severity of haemolysis. Since LDH is a sensitive marker of changes in haemolysis in vivo and changes in LDH reflect changes in free haemoglobin, it is reasonable that LDH should also correlate with NO consumption.

7.3 Consequences of Nitric Oxide Depletion

Nitric oxide scavenging by excess plasma haemoglobin has been implicated in various clinical manifestations of intravascular haemolysis. Nitric oxide is a regulator of smooth muscle tone and platelet activation, and reductions in nitric oxide plasma levels lead to smooth muscle dystonias, including hypertension, gastrointestinal contractions and erectile dysfunction, as well as clot formation [18, 23, 71, 84]. This state of reduced NO bioavailability is associated with impaired blood flow physiology in patients and mice with sickle cell disease and also in healthy dogs with induced intravascular haemolytic anaemia [8, 20, 27, 47, 48, 58, 73]. The normal balance of vasoconstriction to vasodilation is therefore skewed toward vasoconstriction, endothelial activation and proliferation [45].

7.4 The Role of Nitric Oxide and Free Haemoglobin in the Symptoms Associated with Intravascular Haemolysis

In patients with brisk intravascular haemolysis, symptoms can include haemoglobinuria, dysphagia, recurrent abdominal pain, severe lethargy and erectile failure.

The symptoms associated with ongoing haemolysis and/or insufficient haematopoiesis have a major impact on the patient's well-being. In PNH, patients usually have acute exacerbations of haemolysis on the background of persistent lower levels of haemolysis. The acute exacerbations can occur either regularly or unpredictably and have a further adverse impact on quality of life. Anaemia and the need for transfusions to sustain haemoglobin levels occur frequently. Haemolysis has been linked to smooth muscle dystonia including abdominal pain, dysphagia and erectile dysfunction [90].

This systemic removal of NO has been shown to contribute to clinical morbidities including severe oesophageal spasm and dysphagia, abdominal pain, erectile dysfunction and thrombosis [70, 71, 76, 84, 85, 94]. In addition, the systemic release of haemoglobin is associated with pulmonary and systemic hypertension [17, 18, 32, 53, 84], decreased organ perfusion and increased mortality [17, 32, 53, 84, 101, 103, 110]. Free haemoglobin and its breakdown product haem can also directly activate endothelial cells and further promote inflammation and coagulation [33, 111].

There are dose-dependent occurrences of gastrointestinal symptoms including abdominal pain, oesophageal spasms and dysphagia [12, 50, 51, 71, 84, 92, 93, 108]. The occurrence of these symptoms is likely mediated by the systemic depletion of NO by plasma free haemoglobin. Indeed, NO inhibition in healthy human volunteers causes an increase in oesophageal peristaltic amplitude and velocity (spasms), and a decrease in gastric distension triggers transient lower oesophageal sphincter relaxation [38]. Therefore, mechanistically, haemoglobin-induced oesophageal spasms are most likely attributable to NO consumption. Further, the pathological effects of free haemoglobin-induced NO consumption on oesophageal dysmotility are supported by the clinical benefit obtained from the enhancement of NO via inhibition of phosphodiesterase type 5 (PDE5) with sildenafil in patients with oesophageal motor disorders [9, 21].

These findings are consistent with those seen in PNH, supporting the likelihood that these symptoms are associated with the excessive release of haemoglobin from the red blood cells [90].

Although thrombosis of the mesenteric venous tree has been implicated in recurrent episodes of abdominal pain [104], many such cases do not show evidence of thrombosis. Abdominal pain usually rapidly resolves when the paroxysm abates, supporting the hypothesis that nitric oxide scavenging causes intestinal dystonia and spasm.

Oesophageal spasm and dysphagia due to strong peristaltic waves are a common occurrence in PNH patients, with a reported incidence of approximately 23 % [70]. Similarly, episodes of dysphagia are most commonly associated with paroxysms and tend to resolve as the haemolysis subsides [89] although it can be chronic and disabling for some.

Free haemoglobin release during intravascular haemolysis leading to haemoglobin-mediated NO depletion and subsequent smooth muscle contractility has also been implicated in erectile dysfunction in PNH males at a frequency of at least 35 % and is closely linked to paroxysms [70], although erectile dysfunction can persist past the paroxysm and may become permanent [70, 89].

It has been well established that local NO deficiency, due to decreased synthesis, impaired release or premature destruction, is one of the major factors responsible for erectile dysfunction. The physiological mechanism responsible for erection of the penis involves the release of NO from nerve endings and endothelial cells in the corpus cavernosum during sexual stimulation. NO then activates the enzyme guanylate cyclase, which results in increased levels of cGMP. Cyclic GMP causes vascular smooth muscle relaxation in the corpus cavernosum resulting in increased penile blood flow and erection. The pathological role of free haemoglobin-associated consumption of NO in mediating this erectile dysfunction is supported by the well-described activity of drugs such as PDE5 inhibitors that promote the accumulation of NO-induced cGMP which provide dramatic benefit to patients [6, 16]. Benefit from PDE5 inhibitors in PNH patients is reported by patients to be substantially reduced when macroscopic haemoglobinuria is present. This may be explained by the excessive haemolysis seen in PNH compared with other haemolytic conditions, resulting in a greater degree of nitric oxide consumption.

It would therefore be anticipated that following eculizumab therapy, which blocks intravascular haemolysis, there would be a great improvement in all these symptoms attributed to NO depletion. Although there may be no significant change in haemoglobin level before and after eculizumab therapy (transfused to non-transfused state), there is a reassuringly definite improvement in symptoms and quality of life using the EORTC-QLQ C30 instrument, suggesting that factors other than haemoglobin level may modulate these quality life indices [34, 37]. Improvements were demonstrated in several quality of life parameters including global health, physical functioning, emotional functioning, cognitive functioning, fatigue, dyspnoea and insomnia. Interestingly, these improvements occurred despite the observation that total haemoglobin levels were unchanged during treatment, most likely due to a reduction in haemolytic rate and transfusion requirements. These observations to include clinical improvements in symptoms not captured by the QLQ-C30 instrument and that are attributed specifically to haemolysis including haemoglobinuria, abdominal pain, dysphagia and erectile dysfunction were extended [34].

7.5 The Relationship of Nitric Oxide Depletion and Free Haemoglobin with Pulmonary Hypertension

Pulmonary hypertension (PHT) is a vascular disorder of the lung in which the pulmonary artery pressure rises above normal levels, compromises oxygenation and right-heart function and can ultimately become life-threatening [24, 56, 61]. It is characterised by the obstruction of small pulmonary arteries leading to progressive right ventricular failure.

Pulmonary arterial hypertension is an increasingly recognised complication of chronic hereditary and acquired haemolytic anaemias.

Speculatively, chronic anaemia and tissue ischaemia might contribute to a proliferative vasculopathy via activation of HIF-1 (hypoxia-inducible factor)-dependent factors such as iNOS (inducible nitric oxide synthase), erythropoietin and VEGF (vascular endothelial growth factor), which has been seen in an animal model of pulmonary hypertension [99, 112]. However, consistent with a requirement for intravascular haemolysis, rather than anaemia itself, there are no case reports of pulmonary hypertension complicating iron deficiency anaemia, the most common cause of anaemia in the world [26]. The absence of this association between cardiac output and tricuspid regurgitant jet velocity in studies argues against a role for chronic anaemia and a high cardiac output state, leading to vascular remodelling and arteriopathy [26, 100].

Free haemoglobin augments hypoxic pulmonary vasoconstriction by scavenging NO [18, 58]. Indeed, experiments designed to inhibit regional NO synthesis have demonstrated the importance of endothelium-derived NO in the regulation of coronary and systemic vasodilator tone [10].

The simultaneous release of erythrocyte arginase during haemolysis [63] will limit the availability of arginine to NO synthase, resulting in a deficiency of NO. Once released into circulation, arginase will convert L-arginine (the substrate for NO synthesis) to ornithine, which in turn is the precursor to proline, an amino acid involved in collagen formation [115], lung fibrosis, airway remodelling and vascular smooth muscle proliferation [62–64, 68], common features of pulmonary dysfunction in thalassaemia [82, 117]. By creating a shift toward ornithine metabolism, arginase triggers a proliferative pathway that contributes to the pathogenesis of PHT [57, 64].

In paroxysmal nocturnal haemoglobinuria, the deficiency of CD59 from the PNH cell surface results in the unopposed assembly of the terminal complement complex on the surface of PNH red blood cells and, as a consequence, in intravascular haemolysis [69, 116]. The degree of haemolysis typically occurring in PNH surpasses that of other hereditary, acquired and iatrogenic haemolytic conditions. Chronic pulmonary thromboembolic disease may also contribute to the pathogenesis of PHT [36]. Raised pulmonary pressures have been found in a significant proportion of patients with PNH [35, 36].

Eculizumab therapy blocks intravascular haemolysis and therefore significantly reduces NO depletion, vasomotor tone and dyspnoea and improves pulmonary pressures in approximately half of the patients in one study. Importantly, these improvements occurred without significant changes in anaemia [35].

7.6 Conclusion

The intravascular haemolysis seen in PNH will rapidly result in depletion of nitric oxide levels. This can lead to significant symptoms of smooth muscle dystonia and fatigue as well as complications such as thrombosis and pulmonary hypertension. Restoring nitric oxide levels occurs with prevention of intravascular haemolysis through terminal complement blockade with eculizumab therapy.

References

1. Arnold WP, Mittal CK, Katsuki S, Murad F (1977) Nitric oxide activates guanylate cyclase and increases guanosine 3′:5′-cyclic monophosphate levels in various tissue preparations. Proc Natl Acad Sci U S A 74:3203–3207
2. Aslan M, Freeman BA (2004) Oxidant-mediated impairment of nitric oxide signaling in sickle cell disease–mechanisms and consequences. Cell Mol Biol 50:95–105
3. Aslan M, Ryan TM, Adler B, Townes TM, Parks DA, Thompson JA, Tousson A, Gladwin MT, Patel RP, Tarpey MM, Batinic-Haberle I, White CR, Freeman BA (2001) Oxygen radical inhibition of nitric oxide-dependent vascular function in sickle cell disease. Proc Natl Acad Sci U S A 98:15215–15220
4. Aslan M, Ryan TM, Townes TM, Coward L, Kirk MC, Barnes S, Alexander CB, Rosenfeld SS, Freeman BA (2003) Nitric oxide-dependent generation of reactive species in sickle cell disease. Actin tyrosine induces defective cytoskeletal polymerization. J Biol Chem 278:4194–4204
5. Azizi E, Dror Y, Wallis K (1970) Arginase activity in erythrocytes of healthy and ill children. Clin Chim Acta 28:391–396
6. Ballard SA, Gingell CJ, Tang K, Turner LA, Price ME, Naylor AM (1998) Effects of sildenafil on the relaxation of human corpus cavernosum tissue in vitro and on the activities of cyclic nucleotide phosphodiesterase isozymes. J Urol 159:2164–2171
7. Baranano DE, Rao M, Ferris CD, Snyder SH (2002) Biliverdin reductase: a major physiologic cytoprotectant. Proc Natl Acad Sci U S A 99:16093–16098
8. Belhassen L, Pelle G, Sediame S, Bachir D, Carville C, Bucherer C, Lacombe C, Galacteros F, Adnot S (2001) Endothelial dysfunction in patients with sickle cell disease is related to selective impairment of shear stress-mediated vasodilation. Blood 97:1584–1589
9. Bortolotti M, Pandolfo N, Giovannini M, Mari C, Miglioli M (2002) Effect of Sildenafil on hypertensive lower oesophageal sphincter. Eur J Clin Invest 32:682–685
10. Cannon RO, Schechter AN, Panza JA, Ognibene FP, Pease-Fye ME, Waclawiw MA, Shelhamer JH, Gladwin MT (2001) Effects of inhaled nitric oxide on regional blood flow are consistent with intravascular nitric oxide delivery. J Clin Invest 108:279–287
11. Carlsen E, Comroe JH Jr (1958) The rate of uptake of carbon monoxide and of nitric oxide by normal human erythrocytes and experimentally produced spherocytes. J Gen Physiol 42:83–107

12. Carmichael FJ, Ali AC, Campbell JA, Langlois SF, Biro GP, Willan AR, Pierce CH, Greenburg AG (2000) A phase I study of oxidized raffinose cross-linked human hemoglobin. Crit Care Med 28:2283–2292
13. Cassoly R, Gibson Q (1975) Conformation, co-operativity and ligand binding in human hemoglobin. J Mol Biol 91:301–313
14. Closs EI (2002) Expression, regulation and function of carrier proteins for cationic amino acids. Curr Opin Nephrol Hypertens 11:99–107
15. Coin JT, Olson JS (1979) The rate of oxygen uptake by human red blood cells. J Biol Chem 254:1178–1190
16. Corbin JD, Francis SH, Webb DJ (2002) Phosphodiesterase type 5 as a pharmacologic target in erectile dysfunction. Urology 60:4–11
17. de Figueiredo LF, Mathru M, Solanki D, MacDonald VW, Hess J, Kramer GC (1997) Pulmonary hypertension and systemic vasoconstriction may offset the benefits of acellular hemoglobin blood substitutes. J Trauma 42:847–854
18. Deem S, Kim JU, Manjula BN, Acharya AS, Kerr ME, Patel RP, Gladwin MT, Swenson ER (2002) Effects of S-nitrosation and cross-linking of hemoglobin on hypoxic pulmonary vasoconstriction in isolated rat lungs. Circ Res 91:626–632
19. Dias-Da-Motta P, Arruda VR, Muscara MN, Saad ST, De NG, Costa FF, Condino-Neto A (1996) The release of nitric oxide and superoxide anion by neutrophils and mononuclear cells from patients with sickle cell anaemia. Br J Haematol 93:333–340
20. Eberhardt RT, McMahon L, Duffy SJ, Steinberg MH, Perrine SP, Loscalzo J, Coffman JD, Vita JA (2003) Sickle cell anemia is associated with reduced nitric oxide bioactivity in peripheral conduit and resistance vessels. Am J Hematol 74:104–111
21. Eherer AJ, Schwetz I, Hammer HF, Petnehazy T, Scheidl SJ, Weber K, Krejs GJ (2002) Effect of sildenafil on oesophageal motor function in healthy subjects and patients with oesophageal motor disorders. Gut 50:758–764
22. Eich RF, Li T, Lemon DD, Doherty DH, Curry SR, Aitken JF, Mathews AJ, Johnson KA, Smith RD, Phillips GN Jr, Olson JS (1996) Mechanism of NO-induced oxidation of myoglobin and hemoglobin. Biochemistry 35:6976–6983
23. Erhart SM, Cole DJ, Patel PM, Drummond JC, Burhop KE (2000) Effect of alpha-alpha diaspirin crosslinked hemoglobin (DCLHb) on the potency of sodium nitroprusside and nitroglycerine to decrease blood pressure in rats: a dose–response study. Artif Cells Blood Substit Immobil Biotechnol 28:385–396
24. Farber HW, Loscalzo J (2004) Pulmonary arterial hypertension. N Engl J Med 351:1655–1665
25. Furchgott RF, Zawadzki JV (1980) The obligatory role of endothelial cells in the relaxation of arterial smooth muscle by acetylcholine. Nature 288:373–376
26. Gladwin MT, SachdevV JML, ShizukudaY PJF, Minter K, Brown B, Coles WA, Nichols JS, Ernst I, Hunter LA, Blackwelder WC, Schechter AN, Rodgers GP, Castro O, Ognibene FP (2004) Pulmonary hypertension as a risk factor for death in patients with sickle cell disease. N Engl J Med 350:886–895
27. Gladwin MT, Schechter AN, Ognibene FP, Coles WA, Reiter CD, Schenke WH, Csako G, Waclawiw MA, Panza JA, Cannon RO III (2003) Divergent nitric oxide bioavailability in men and women with sickle cell disease. Circulation 107:271–278
28. Hartmann RC, Jenkins DE Jr, McKee LC, Heyssel RM (1966) Paroxysmal nocturnal hemoglobinuria: clinical and laboratory studies relating to iron metabolism and therapy with androgen and iron. Medicine (Baltimore) 45:331–363
29. Hebbel RP (1985) Auto-oxidation and a membrane-associated 'Fenton reagent': a possible explanation for development of membrane lesions in sickle erythrocytes. Clin Haematol 14:129–140
30. Hebbel RP, Osarogiagbon R, Kaul D (2004) The endothelial biology of sickle cell disease: inflammation and a chronic vasculopathy. Microcirculation 11:129–151

31. Herold S, Exner M, Nauser T (2001) Kinetic and mechanistic studies of the NO*-mediated oxidation of oxymyoglobin and oxyhemoglobin. Biochemistry 40:3385–3395
32. Hess JR, MacDonald VW, Brinkley WW (1993) Systemic and pulmonary hypertension after resuscitation with cell-free hemoglobin. J Appl Physiol 74:1769–1778
33. Hill A, Kelly RJ, Hillmen P (2013) Thrombosis in paroxysmal nocturnal hemoglobinuria. Blood 121:4985–4996
34. Hill A, Rother RP, Hillmen P (2005) Improvement in the symptoms of smooth muscle dystonia during eculizumab therapy in paroxysmal nocturnal hemoglobinuria. Haematologica 90:ECR40
35. Hill A, Rother RP, Wang X, Morris SM Jr, Quinn-Senger K, Kelly R, Richards SJ, Bessler M, Bell L, Hillmen P, Gladwin MT (2010) Effect of eculizumab on haemolysis-associated nitric oxide depletion, dyspnoea, and measures of pulmonary hypertension in patients with paroxysmal nocturnal haemoglobinuria. Br J Haematol 149:414–425
36. Hill A, Sapsford RJ, Scally A, Kelly R, Richards SJ, Khurisgara G, Sivananthan MU, Hillmen P (2012) Under-recognized complications in patients with paroxysmal nocturnal haemoglobinuria: raised pulmonary pressure and reduced right ventricular function. Br J Haematol 158:409–414
37. Hillmen P, Hall C, Marsh JC, Elebute M, Bombara MP, Petro BE, Cullen MJ, Richards SJ, Rollins SA, Mojcik CF, Rother RP (2004) Effect of eculizumab on hemolysis and transfusion requirements in patients with paroxysmal nocturnal hemoglobinuria. N Engl J Med 350:552–559
38. Hirsch DP, Holloway RH, Tytgat GN, Boeckxstaens GE (1998) Involvement of nitric oxide in human transient lower esophageal sphincter relaxations and esophageal primary peristalsis. Gastroenterology 115:1374–1380
39. Holguin MH, Fredrick LR, Bernshaw NJ, Wilcox LA, Parker CJ (1989) Isolation and characterization of a membrane protein from normal human erythrocytes that inhibits reactive lysis of the erythrocytes of paroxysmal nocturnal hemoglobinuria. J Clin Invest 84:7–17
40. Huang KT, Han TH, Hyduke DR, Vaughn MW, Van HH, Hein TW, Zhang C, Kuo L, Liao JC (2001) Modulation of nitric oxide bioavailability by erythrocytes. Proc Natl Acad Sci U S A 98:11771–11776
41. Ignarro LJ (1989) Heme-dependent activation of soluble guanylate cyclase by nitric oxide: regulation of enzyme activity by porphyrins and metalloporphyrins. Semin Hematol 26:63–76
42. Ignarro LJ, Byrns RE, Buga GM, Wood KS (1987) Mechanisms of endothelium-dependent vascular smooth muscle relaxation elicited by bradykinin and VIP. Am J Physiol 253:H1074–H1082
43. Ignarro LJ, Byrns RE, Buga GM, Wood KS (1987) Endothelium-derived relaxing factor from pulmonary artery and vein possesses pharmacologic and chemical properties identical to those of nitric oxide radical. Circ Res 61:866–879
44. Jison ML, Munson PJ, Barb JJ, Suffredini AF, Talwar S, Logun C, Raghavachari N, Beigel JH, Shelhamer JH, Danner RL, Gladwin MT (2004) Blood mononuclear cell gene expression profiles characterize the oxidant, hemolytic, and inflammatory stress of sickle cell disease. Blood 104:270–280
45. Kato GJ, Gladwin MT, Steinberg MH (2007) Deconstructing sickle cell disease: reappraisal of the role of hemolysis in the development of clinical subphenotypes. Blood Rev 21:37–47
46. Kaul DK, Hebbel RP (2000) Hypoxia/reoxygenation causes inflammatory response in transgenic sickle mice but not in normal mice. J Clin Invest 106:411–420
47. Kaul DK, Liu XD, Chang HY, Nagel RL, Fabry ME (2004) Effect of fetal hemoglobin on microvascular regulation in sickle transgenic-knockout mice. J Clin Invest 114:1136–1145
48. Kaul DK, Liu XD, Fabry ME, Nagel RL (2000) Impaired nitric oxide-mediated vasodilation in transgenic sickle mouse. Am J Physiol Heart Circ Physiol 278:H1799–H1806
49. Kristiansen M, Graversen JH, Jacobsen C, Sonne O, Hoffman HJ, Law SK, Moestrup SK (2001) Identification of the haemoglobin scavenger receptor. Nature 409:198–201

50. LaMuraglia GM, O'Hara PJ, Baker WH, Naslund TC, Norris EJ, Li J, Vandermeersch E (2000) The reduction of the allogenic transfusion requirement in aortic surgery with a hemoglobin-based solution. J Vasc Surg 31:299–308
51. Lamy ML, Daily EK, Brichant JF, Larbuisson RP, Demeyere RH, Vandermeersch EA, Lehot JJ, Parsloe MR, Berridge JC, Sinclair CJ, Baron JF, Przybelski RJ (2000) Randomized trial of diaspirin cross-linked hemoglobin solution as an alternative to blood transfusion after cardiac surgery. The DCLHb Cardiac Surgery Trial Collaborative Group. Anesthesiology 92:646–656
52. Langlois MR, Delanghe JR (1996) Biological and clinical significance of haptoglobin polymorphism in humans. Clin Chem 42:1589–1600
53. Lee R, Neya K, Svizzero TA, Vlahakes GJ (1995) Limitations of the efficacy of hemoglobin-based oxygen-carrying solutions. J Appl Physiol 79:236–242
54. Liao JC, Hein TW, Vaughn MW, Huang KT, Kuo L (1999) Intravascular flow decreases erythrocyte consumption of nitric oxide. Proc Natl Acad Sci U S A 96:8757–8761
55. Liu X, Miller MJ, Joshi MS, Sadowska-Krowicka H, Clark DA, Lancaster JR Jr (1998) Diffusion-limited reaction of free nitric oxide with erythrocytes. J Biol Chem 273:18709–18713
56. Loscalzo J (2001) Genetic clues to the cause of primary pulmonary hypertension. N Engl J Med 345:367–371
57. Mack AK, Kato GJ (2006) Sickle cell disease and nitric oxide: a paradigm shift? Int J Biochem Cell Biol 38:1237–1243
58. Minneci PC, Deans KJ, Zhi H, Yuen PS, Star RA, Banks SM, Schechter AN, Natanson C, Gladwin MT, Solomon SB (2005) Hemolysis-associated endothelial dysfunction mediated by accelerated NO inactivation by decompartmentalized oxyhemoglobin. J Clin Invest 115:3409–3417
59. Moestrup SK, Moller HJ (2004) CD163: a regulated hemoglobin scavenger receptor with a role in the anti-inflammatory response. Ann Med 36:347–354
60. Moncada S, Higgs A (1993) The L-arginine-nitric oxide pathway. N Engl J Med 329:2002–2012
61. Moraes D, Loscalzo J (1997) Pulmonary hypertension: newer concepts in diagnosis and management. Clin Cardiol 20:676–682
62. Morris CR (2006) New strategies for the treatment of pulmonary hypertension in sickle cell disease: the rationale for arginine therapy. Treat Respir Med 5:31–45
63. Morris CR, Kato GJ, Poljakovic M, Wang X, Blackwelder WC, Sachdev V, Hazen SL, Vichinsky EP, Morris SM Jr, Gladwin MT (2005) Dysregulated arginine metabolism, hemolysis-associated pulmonary hypertension, and mortality in sickle cell disease. JAMA 294:81–90
64. Morris CR, Kuypers FA, Kato GJ, Lavrisha L, Larkin S, Singer T, Vichinsky EP (2005) Hemolysis-associated pulmonary hypertension in thalassemia. Ann N Y Acad Sci 1054:481–485
65. Morris CR, Kuypers FA, Larkin S, Vichinsky EP, Styles LA (2000) Patterns of arginine and nitric oxide in patients with sickle cell disease with vaso-occlusive crisis and acute chest syndrome. J Pediatr Hematol Oncol 22:515–520
66. Morris CR, Morris SM Jr, Hagar W, Van Warmerdam J, Claster S, Kepka-Lenhart D, Machado L, Kuypers FA, Vichinsky EP (2003) Arginine therapy: a new treatment for pulmonary hypertension in sickle cell disease? Am J Respir Crit Care Med 168:63–69
67. Morris CR, Poljakovic M, Lavrisha L, Machado L, Kuypers FA, Morris SM Jr (2004) Decreased arginine bioavailability and increased serum arginase activity in asthma. Am J Respir Crit Care Med 170:148–153
68. Morris CR, Singer ST, Walters MC (2006) Clinical hemoglobinopathies: iron, lungs and new blood. Curr Opin Hematol 13:407–418
69. Motoyama N, Okada N, Yamashina M, Okada H (1992) Paroxysmal nocturnal hemoglobinuria due to hereditary nucleotide deletion in the HRF20 (CD59) gene. Eur J Immunol 22:2669–2673

70. Moyo VM, Mukhina GL, Garrett ES, Brodsky RA (2004) Natural history of paroxysmal nocturnal haemoglobinuria using modern diagnostic assays. Br J Haematol 126:133–138
71. Murray JA, Ledlow A, Launspach J, Evans D, Loveday M, Conklin JL (1995) The effects of recombinant human hemoglobin on esophageal motor functions in humans. Gastroenterology 109:1241–1248
72. Nagel RL, Gibson QH (1971) The binding of hemoglobin to haptoglobin and its relation to subunit dissociation of hemoglobin. J Biol Chem 246:69–73
73. Nath KA, Shah V, Haggard JJ, Croatt AJ, Smith LA, Hebbel RP, Katusic ZS (2000) Mechanisms of vascular instability in a transgenic mouse model of sickle cell disease. Am J Physiol Regul Integr Comp Physiol 279:R1949–R1955
74. Naumann HN, Diggs LW, Barreras L, Williams BJ (1971) Plasma hemoglobin and hemoglobin fractions in sickle cell crisis. Am J Clin Pathol 56:137–147
75. Nielsen MJ, Petersen SV, Jacobsen C, Oxvig C, Rees D, Moller HJ, Moestrup SK (2006) Haptoglobin-related protein is a high-affinity hemoglobin-binding plasma protein. Blood 108:2846–2849
76. Olsen SB, Tang DB, Jackson MR, Gomez ER, Ayala B, Alving BM (1996) Enhancement of platelet deposition by cross-linked hemoglobin in a rat carotid endarterectomy model. Circulation 93:327–332
77. Olson JS, Foley EW, Rogge C, Tsai AL, Doyle MP, Lemon DD (2004) No scavenging and the hypertensive effect of hemoglobin-based blood substitutes. Free Radic Biol Med 36:685–697
78. Otterbein LE, Zuckerbraun BS, Haga M, Liu F, Song R, Usheva A, Stachulak C, Bodyak N, Smith RN, Csizmadia E, Tyagi S, Akamatsu Y, Flavell RJ, Billiar TR, Tzeng E, Bach FH, Choi AM, Soares MP (2003) Carbon monoxide suppresses arteriosclerotic lesions associated with chronic graft rejection and with balloon injury. Nat Med 9:183–190
79. Palmer RM, Ferrige AG, Moncada S (1987) Nitric oxide release accounts for the biological activity of endothelium-derived relaxing factor. Nature 327:524–526
80. Peng HB, Spiecker M, Liao JK (1998) Inducible nitric oxide: an autoregulatory feedback inhibitor of vascular inflammation. J Immunol 161:1970–1976
81. Philippidis P, Mason JC, Evans BJ, Nadra I, Taylor KM, Haskard DO, Landis RC (2004) Hemoglobin scavenger receptor CD163 mediates interleukin-10 release and heme oxygenase-1 synthesis: antiinflammatory monocyte-macrophage responses in vitro, in resolving skin blisters in vivo, and after cardiopulmonary bypass surgery. Circ Res 94:119–126
82. Piatti G, Allegra L, Fasano V, Gambardella C, Bisaccia M, Cappellini MD (2006) Lung function in beta-thalassemia patients: a longitudinal study. Acta Haematol 116:25–29
83. Prestera T, Talalay P, Alam J, Ahn YI, Lee PJ, Choi AM (1995) Parallel induction of heme oxygenase-1 and chemoprotective phase 2 enzymes by electrophiles and antioxidants: regulation by upstream antioxidant-responsive elements (ARE). Mol Med 1:827–837
84. Przybelski RJ, Daily EK, Kisicki JC, Mattia-Goldberg C, Bounds MJ, Colburn WA (1996) Phase I study of the safety and pharmacologic effects of diaspirin cross-linked hemoglobin solution. Crit Care Med 24:1993–2000
85. Radomski MW, Palmer RM, Moncada S (1987) Endogenous nitric oxide inhibits human platelet adhesion to vascular endothelium. Lancet 2:1057–1058
86. Reiter CD, Gladwin MT (2003) An emerging role for nitric oxide in sickle cell disease vascular homeostasis and therapy. Curr Opin Hematol 10:99–107
87. Reiter CD, Wang X, Tanus-Santos JE, Hogg N, Cannon RO III, Schechter AN, Gladwin MT (2002) Cell-free hemoglobin limits nitric oxide bioavailability in sickle-cell disease. Nat Med 8:1383–1389
88. Reynolds J, Follette JH, Valentine WN (1957) The arginase activity of erythrocytes and leukocytes with particular reference to pernicious anemia and thalassemia major. J Lab Clin Med 50:78–92
89. Rosse WF (2000) Paroxysmal nocturnal hemoglobinuria. In: Hoffman R (ed), Churchill Livingstone, New York, pp 331–342

90. Rother RP, Bell L, Hillmen P, Gladwin MT (2005) The clinical sequelae of intravascular hemolysis and extracellular plasma hemoglobin: a novel mechanism of human disease. JAMA 293:1653–1662
91. Ryter SW, Otterbein LE, Morse D, Choi AM (2002) Heme oxygenase/carbon monoxide signaling pathways: regulation and functional significance. Mol Cell Biochem 234–235:249–263
92. Savitsky JP, Doczi J, Black J, Arnold JD (1978) A clinical safety trial of stroma-free hemoglobin. Clin Pharmacol Ther 23:73–80
93. Saxena R, Wijnhoud AD, Carton H, Hacke W, Kaste M, Przybelski RJ, Stern KN, Koudstaal PJ (1999) Controlled safety study of a hemoglobin-based oxygen carrier, DCLHb, in acute ischemic stroke. Stroke 30:993–996
94. Schafer A, Wiesmann F, Neubauer S, Eigenthaler M, Bauersachs J, Channon KM (2004) Rapid regulation of platelet activation in vivo by nitric oxide. Circulation 109:1819–1822
95. Schechter AN, Gladwin MT (2003) Hemoglobin and the paracrine and endocrine functions of nitric oxide. N Engl J Med 348:1483–1485
96. Schnog JJ, Jager EH, van der Dijs FP, Duits AJ, Moshage H, Muskiet FD, Muskiet FA (2004) Evidence for a metabolic shift of arginine metabolism in sickle cell disease. Ann Hematol 83:371–375
97. Sears DA (1970) Disposal of plasma heme in normal man and patients with intravascular hemolysis. J Clin Invest 49:5–14
98. Sedlak TW, Snyder SH (2004) Bilirubin benefits: cellular protection by a biliverdin reductase antioxidant cycle. Pediatrics 113:1776–1782
99. Semenza GL (2005) Involvement of hypoxia-inducible factor 1 in pulmonary pathophysiology. Chest 128:592S–594S
100. Singer ST, Kuypers FA, Styles L, Vichinsky EP, Foote D, Rosenfeld H (2006) Pulmonary hypertension in thalassemia: association with platelet activation and hypercoagulable state. Am J Hematol 81:670–675
101. Sloan EP, Koenigsberg M, Gens D, Cipolle M, Runge J, Mallory MN, Rodman G Jr (1999) Diaspirin cross-linked hemoglobin (DCLHb) in the treatment of severe traumatic hemorrhagic shock: a randomized controlled efficacy trial. JAMA 282:1857–1864
102. Tabbara IA (1992) Hemolytic anemias. Diagnosis and management. Med Clin North Am 76:649–668
103. Ulatowski JA, Nishikawa T, Matheson-Urbaitis B, Bucci E, Traystman RJ, Koehler RC (1996) Regional blood flow alterations after bovine fumaryl beta beta-crosslinked hemoglobin transfusion and nitric oxide synthase inhibition. Crit Care Med 24:558–565
104. Valla D, Dhumeaux D, Babany G, Hillon P, Rueff B, Rochant H, Benhamou JP (1987) Hepatic vein thrombosis in paroxysmal nocturnal hemoglobinuria. A spectrum from asymptomatic occlusion of hepatic venules to fatal Budd-Chiari syndrome. Gastroenterology 93:569–575
105. Van Lente F, Marchand A, Galen RS (1981) Diagnosis of hemolytic disease by electrophoresis of erythrocyte lactate dehydrogenase isoenzymes on cellulose acetate or Agarose. Clin Chem 27:1453–1455
106. Vaughn MW, Huang KT, Kuo L, Liao JC (2000) Erythrocytes possess an intrinsic barrier to nitric oxide consumption. J Biol Chem 275:2342–2348
107. Vaughn MW, Kuo L, Liao JC (1998) Effective diffusion distance of nitric oxide in the microcirculation. Am J Physiol 274:H1705–H1714
108. Viele MK, Weiskopf RB, Fisher D (1997) Recombinant human hemoglobin does not affect renal function in humans: analysis of safety and pharmacokinetics. Anesthesiology 86:848–858
109. Voetsch B, Jin RC, Loscalzo J (2004) Nitric oxide insufficiency and atherothrombosis. Histochem Cell Biol 122:353–367
110. Vogel WM, Dennis RC, Cassidy G, Apstein CS, Valeri CR (1986) Coronary constrictor effect of stroma-free hemoglobin solutions. Am J Physiol 251:H413–H420

111. Wagener FA, Eggert A, Boerman OC, Oyen WJ, Verhofstad A, Abraham NG, Adema G, van Kooyk Y, de Witte T, Figdor CG (2001) Heme is a potent inducer of inflammation in mice and is counteracted by heme oxygenase. Blood 98:1802–1811
112. Wang J, Weigand L, Lu W, Sylvester JT, Semenza GL, Shimoda LA (2006) Hypoxia inducible factor 1 mediates hypoxia-induced TRPC expression and elevated intracellular Ca2+ in pulmonary arterial smooth muscle cells. Circ Res 98:1528–1537
113. Wink DA, Mitchell JB (1998) Chemical biology of nitric oxide: insights into regulatory, cytotoxic, and cytoprotective mechanisms of nitric oxide. Free Radic Biol Med 25:434–456
114. Wood KC, Hebbel RP, Granger DN (2005) Endothelial cell NADPH oxidase mediates the cerebral microvascular dysfunction in sickle cell transgenic mice. FASEB J 19:989–991
115. Wu G, Morris SM Jr (1998) Arginine metabolism: nitric oxide and beyond. Biochem J 336(Pt 1):1–17
116. Yamashina M, Ueda E, Kinoshita T, Takami T, Ojima A, Ono H, Tanaka H, Kondo N, Orii T, Okada N (1990) Inherited complete deficiency of 20-kilodalton homologous restriction factor (CD59) as a cause of paroxysmal nocturnal hemoglobinuria. N Engl J Med 323:1184–1189
117. Zakynthinos E, Vassilakopoulos T, Kaltsas P, Malagari E, Daniil Z, Roussos C, Zakynthinos SG (2001) Pulmonary hypertension, interstitial lung fibrosis, and lung iron deposition in thalassaemia major. Thorax 56:737–739

Chapter 8
Bone Marrow Failure in PNH

Britta Höchsmann and Hubert Schrezenmeier

Abstract Bone marrow failure is a relevant aspect in PNH, as PNH frequently arises in association with bone marrow failure syndromes, particularly aplastic anemia. There is increasing evidence that autoimmune mechanisms support PNH clones to selectively survive in the injured bone marrow of bone marrow failure syndromes, leading to clinical manifestations characteristic for PNH.

This article comments on PNH in context of bone marrow failure syndromes contributing to pathophysiology and diagnostic and therapeutic approaches with respect to the new treatment option by complement inhibition. It elucidates the highly variable presentation and course of these disorders which are often characterized by overlap syndromes. Current options to distinguish the various bone marrow failure syndromes will be discussed. Furthermore, the challenges and management of the treatment in such overlap syndromes will be focused.

Based on an improved overall survival of PNH patients with a sufficient complement inhibition, it could be speculated that in context with the natural history of the disease, the number of combined PNH-bone marrow failure cases will increase in the coming years. Thus, the optimizing of diagnostic and therapeutic approaches in PNH-BMF syndromes might be an important task and a key for a further elongation of life expectancy in PNH patients.

Keywords Bone marrow failure syndrome • Paroxysmal nocturnal hemoglobinuria • Aplastic anemia • Hypoplastic MDS

B. Höchsmann, M.D. (✉) • H. Schrezenmeier, M.D.
Institute of Transfusion Medicine, University of Ulm,
Helmholtzstraße 10, 89081 Ulm, Germany

Institute of Clinical Transfusion Medicine and Immunogenetics Ulm, German Red Cross Blood Transfusion Service Baden-Württemberg – Hessen and University Hospital Ulm,
Helmholtzstraße 10, 89081 Ulm, Germany
e-mail: b.hoechsmann@blutspende.de

Y. Kanakura et al. (eds.), *Paroxysmal Nocturnal Hemoglobinuria*,
DOI 10.1007/978-4-431-56003-6_8

8.1 Introduction

Hemolysis and cytopenia are like the two sides of the same coin and the most important causes for a reduced life expectancy in PNH patients [1–6]. The pathophysiology and risk resulting from complement-mediated hemolysis were already described in the previous chapter.

Subsequently, we will elucidate the topic "bone marrow failure (BMF) in PNH" as well as the issue "PNH in BMF," because both are inseparably connected [7, 8].

The bone marrow failure (BMF) syndromes themselves are a heterogeneous group of clinical and pathophysiological distinct but often overlapping disorders associated with cytopenias and failure of normal hematopoiesis [9–11]. Additionally, the natural history of PNH itself is highly variable [1–6]. Therefore, the combination of both is leading to a large variety of subgroups with different characteristics: PNH can arise de novo in the absence of, or in association with, other bone marrow disorders (BMDs). Additionally, PNH may develop secondary to BMDs such as aplastic anemia (AA) or myelodysplastic syndrome. Finally, PNH may present as subclinical PNH in context of bone marrow failure syndromes [1, 3, 5, 12–17]. Due to the large spectrum of manifestations, the coexistence of PNH and bone marrow failure syndromes might be without relevance for the patient or can complicate diagnosis as well as treatment with the risk of a higher mortality due to the associated complications.

8.2 Bone Marrow Failure Syndromes

Over the last two decades, the knowledge about the bone marrow failure syndromes expanded tremendously. This is true not only for the aspects which the distinct bone marrow failure disorders share, especially in context of the frequent overlapping syndromes, but also for the characteristics which distinguish between the several entities.

The etiology of bone marrow failure syndromes includes the following mechanisms: (A) a decrease or damage of the hematopoietic stem cells and their microenvironment, (B) maturation defects, and (C) differentiation defects [9–11, 18, 19].

Thus, the elucidation of the causes of bone marrow failure syndromes increases the understanding of the healthy hematopoiesis itself. The identification of gene mutations in inherited bone marrow failure syndromes (IBMFS), for example, gave a valuable clue in defining the precise functions of the corresponding proteins in normal cells [18, 20, 21].

In general bone marrow failure syndromes may manifest as single-lineage cytopenia (e.g., erythroid, myeloid, or megakaryocytic) or as bi- or pancytopenia. They can be either inherited or acquired. The group of bone marrow failure syndromes includes a huge spectrum of different disorders like the myelodysplastic syndromes (MDS), especially hypoplastic MDS (hMDS), aplastic anemia (AA), pure red cell aplasia (PRCA), amegakaryocytic thrombocytopenia, myeloproliferative neoplasms (MPN), and the large field of inherited bone marrow failure syndromes (like Fanconi anemia (FA), dyskeratosis congenita (DC), congenital neutropenia, Diamond-Blackfan anemia (DBA), Shwachman-Diamond syndrome, congenital amegakaryocytic thrombocytopenia (CAMT), thrombocytopenia-absent radii (TAR) syndrome). Finally, paroxysmal nocturnal hemoglobinuria (PNH) is often associated with bone marrow failure [3, 9, 17–20, 22, 23].

Nevertheless, it has to be discussed whether the PNH itself is a bone marrow failure syndrome too or if it is just accompanying other bone marrow failure syndromes as a consequence of the underlying pathomechanisms.

As GPI-deficient cells occur also in healthy individuals, the two-hit model is the common hypothesis regarding the development of a clinically significant PNH. This thesis postulates as first step a primary *PIG-A* mutation creating GPI-deficient cells followed by a second step (e.g., immune mechanism, second mutation) leading to the expansion of the GPI-deficient clone. Therefore, the GPI-deficient cells might just develop a relative growth advantage over normal hematopoietic cells in the setting of bone marrow failure syndromes. Additional mechanisms like a resistance against apoptosis might further support this growth advantage. Thus, a relative advantage of *PIG-A*-mutated mono- or oligoclonal hematopoiesis versus non-*PIG-A*-mutated polyclonal hematopoiesis could explain the concomitant presentation of bone marrow failure together with the expansion of GPI-deficient clones [7, 8, 12, 14, 15, 17, 24–28].

8.3 Diagnostic Approaches in Bone Marrow Failure Syndromes

In spite of the improved diagnostic tools, like the identification of molecular abnormalities, the accurate diagnosis sometimes remains unclear. This is especially true in overlap syndromes and in the early stages of disease.

The first steps during diagnosis of a bone marrow failure syndrome are:

1. To separate these disorders from malignant disorders as well as from reactive cytopenias [10, 29–33]
2. To rule out spontaneously reversible causes [9]
3. To distinguish between acquired and inherited bone marrow failure [18, 20, 21, 34]

The basic diagnostic methods for these issues are a detailed patient and family history regarding the duration, clinical symptoms, and potential causes (e.g., drugs, infections) of cytopenia as well as a complete physical examination with respect to signs of bleeding, infections, and anemia as well as hints for an inherited etiology like abnormalities in height, facial morphology, limb, urogenital tract, mucosa, skin, or nail. As bone marrow failure syndromes are often accompanied with PNH,

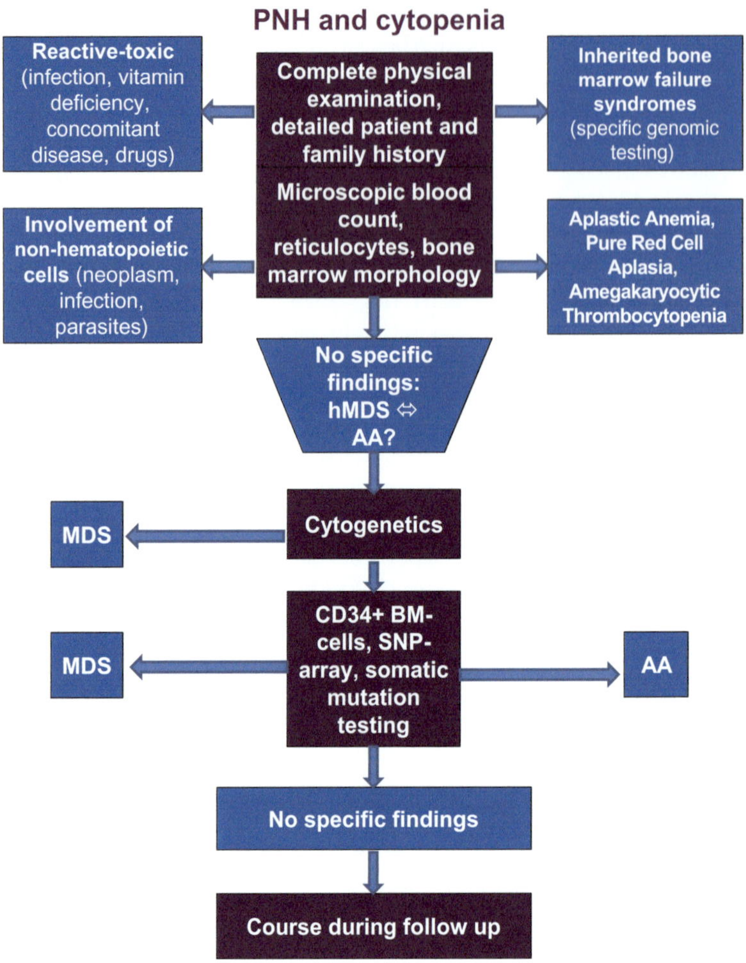

Fig. 8.1 Diagnostic algorithm in BMF-PNH syndromes

history and physical examination should especially address signs of hemolysis (Fig. 8.1).

The most important laboratory diagnostic tools are a complete blood count including microscopic differential, reticulocyte counts and morphologic studies of the bone marrow by assessment of marrow cellularity, fibrosis, and dysplasia (Fig. 8.1). It should be mentioned that bone marrow aspirate and trephine biopsy must be taken, and especially in bone marrow failure syndromes, the quality of the bone marrow sample (e.g., length of trephine biopsy) is essential.

Further laboratory tests are often indispensable to determine the subgroup and the prognosis of the bone marrow failure syndrome and include chemistries, virus serology, flow cytometry, chromosome breakage tests, telomere length and mutational analysis, SNP array, FISH, cytogenetics, and colony-forming assays [1, 10, 11, 16, 18, 19, 21, 25, 28, 30–33, 35–42].

The most difficult diagnostic cases present usually as hypoplastic bone marrow, normal karyotype, and nonspecific types of dysplasia leading to the question whether this is the presentation of a hypoplastic MDS or aplastic anemia (Fig. 8.1) [32].

Aplastic anemia is defined as at least bicytopenia and hypocellular bone marrow without previous chemotherapy or radiation and without the presence of abnormal cells or marrow fibrosis [23, 43]. Depending on the severity of cytopenia, aplastic anemia is classified as non-severe, severe, and very severe aplastic anemia [35].

In contrast, myelodysplastic syndromes (MDS) are clonal hematopoietic stem cell disorders with ineffective hematopoiesis and morphologic abnormalities like dysplasia, ring sideroblasts, myeloblasts, pseudo Pelger-Huet cells, and/or fibrosis. Cytogenetic analyses can identify pathognomonic mutations for MDS or acute myeloid leukemia (Fig. 8.1), like del 5q, monosomy 7, or inversion 3 [30, 32, 37]. However, the cytogenetic abnormalities considered to be specific for MDS occur only in about 50 % of the cases aggravated by the fact that cytogenetic analyses may be less valid in hypocellular bone marrow. This is the case in 5–20 % of the patients although the majority of MDS patients presents with normal to increased bone marrow cellularity [10, 19, 31, 32]. Furthermore, some of the morphologic abnormalities which were found in context of bone marrow failure are not specific for MDS. For example, findings like megaloblastic erythroid maturation or megakaryocytic atypias are not uncommon in aplastic anemia, especially in context of an additional PNH and the increased proliferation which is associated with hemolysis and the influence of vitamin B12 and folic acid consumption.

Also the measurement of GPI-deficient populations is not sufficient to discriminate between hypoplastic MDS and aplastic anemia, as they can occur in both disorders [14, 15, 24].

The most helpful tool, especially in these hypoplastic cases, might be CD34 measurement by immunohistochemistry or by flow cytometry of bone marrow cells. The method bases on the central role of CD34 + progenitor cells in the pathogenesis of AA and MDS. The portion of CD34+ cells in normal bone marrow ranges from 0.5 to 5 %. They are the target for the autoimmune attack in context of AA and therefore are decreased in this context. In contrast, CD34 expression increases during neoplastic clonal expansion and is therefore associated with the presence of a MDS (Fig. 8.1) [40].

Nevertheless, the discrimination between hypoplastic MDS with normal karyotype and AA often remains a challenge. Sometimes a final diagnosis, which is important due to its clinical relevance, is only available during the course of the disease (Fig. 8.1). Therefore, critical reassessment of initial diagnosis during follow-up is necessary, in particular, in case of a lack of response to treatment.

Thus, there is a need for methods addressing this question to improve diagnosis in these cases. New diagnostics, for example, the genome-wide genotyping technology, seem to be a promising approach to answer such questions [33].

8.4 Frequency and Course of GPI Deficiency in Bone Marrow Failure Syndromes

Close ties are not only between hypoplastic MDS and AA. There are numerous other interferences in the field of bone marrow failure syndromes. Another important subgroup in this aspect is the combination of bone marrow failure syndromes with clinical or subclinical PNH. Notable in this context is the large variability of the clinical presentation of these overlap syndromes at initial diagnosis and during the time course [7, 8, 13–17, 24, 25, 28, 39, 44].

In order to study the dynamics of GPI-AP-deficient cell populations over time, serial monitoring was analyzed during a median follow-up of 1039 days in 155 patients by our group. During follow-up in 9 %, a new PNH diagnosis and, in 28 %, a significant change of size or lineage involvement were demonstrated [16].

There are several possible settings (Fig. 8.2). A subgroup of the patients present with significant GPI-deficient populations at time of initial diagnosis of the bone marrow failure syndrome. These cases could be classified as PNH in the setting of another specified bone marrow disorder or as subclinical PNH (PNH-sc) [1, 3, 5]. A recent analysis of the international PNH patient registry data showed that 50 % of the 1550 evaluable PNH patients had another bone marrow disorder in the patient history and the majority of 45 % had an AA, respectively [6].

The patients of the subgroup PNH in the setting of another specified bone marrow disorder have clinical and laboratory evidence of hemolysis and have or had a defined bone marrow disorder (like AA, MDS, or CMPS).

The subcategory subclinical PNH (PNH-sc) is characterized by the missing of a clinical or laboratory evidence of hemolysis, in spite of significant GPI-AP-deficient populations, and is particularly observed in bone marrow failure syndromes [1, 3, 5].

If the underlying bone marrow disorder is successfully treated with a non-transplant approach, both conditions could change into a pure PNH (Fig. 8.2).

A development vice versa from a BMF-PNH syndrome in an isolated BMF syndrome is possible (Fig. 8.2), and sporadically spontaneous remissions have been reported but seem to be disputable in most cases or very rare [3]. Allogeneic stem cell transplantation is the only curative intervention up to now. In case of a successful allogeneic stem cell transplantation, both PNH and the BMF syndrome should be cured [26]. We and others have observed disappearance of GPI-deficient populations in patients with AA-PNH syndrome. However, this was associated with improvement of hematopoiesis and non-isolated disappearance of the PNH clone [16, 27].

Thus, the development from a BMF-PNH syndrome in an isolated BMF syndrome seems unlikely.

Another subgroup will present initially as classic PNH. These patients have evidence of intravascular hemolysis in the absence of another defined bone marrow abnormality [1]. During follow-up, about 20–30 % of the patients with classic PNH

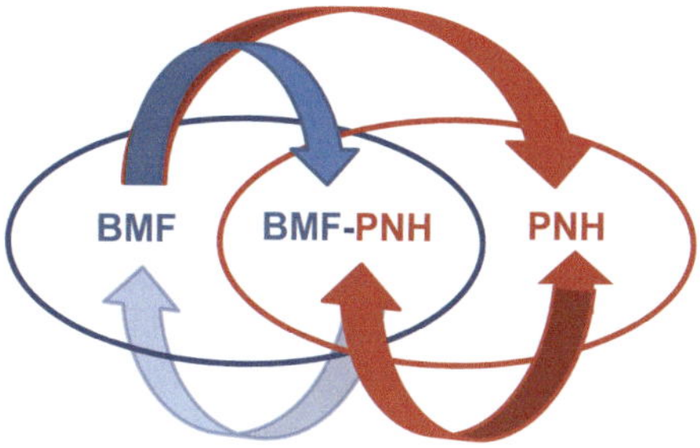

Fig. 8.2 Relationship between bone marrow failure (BMF) and paroxysmal nocturnal hemoglobinuria (PNH)

subsequently developed pancytopenia, which was associated with worse outcomes (Fig. 8.2) [4, 5].

Finally, even 15–20 % of patients, initially diagnosed with a bone marrow failure syndrome without GPI-deficient populations, could develop subclinically or clinically relevant GPI-deficient populations during the follow-up independent of the status of the bone marrow failure syndrome (Fig. 8.2) [14, 23, 43].

8.4.1 GPI-Deficient Populations and PIG-A Mutations in AA

As a proof of the close pathophysiological link between PNH and acquired aplastic anemia, the coincidence of significant GPI-deficient populations is a common event in these patients. Thus, up to 70 % of patients with acquired aplastic anemia demonstrate PNH clones [8, 13–15, 24]. At diagnosis the majority of these patients present GPI-deficient granulocyte populations less than 20 % [1]. Therefore, screening for PNH in patients with aplastic anemia, even in the absence of clinical evidence of hemolysis, is recommended at diagnosis and during follow-up.

The value of GPI deficiency testing is beyond the diagnosis of a symptomatic PNH as several studies suggest a clinical significance of small GPI-deficient populations as prognostic markers in response to immunosuppressive therapy. Sugimori et al. reported data on 122 AA patients showing that 91 % of patients with a significant number of GPI-deficient cells responded to antithymocyte globulin (ATG) + cyclosporine (CsA) therapy, whereas only 48 % without GPI deficiency did. Failure-free survival rates were significantly higher (64 %) among patients with GPI-deficient populations than among patients without GPI deficiency (12 %) at 5 years, although overall survival rates were comparable between the groups. These data suggest that the GPI-deficient cells are sensitive to immunosuppressive therapy and represent therefore a valuable prognostic marker for a positive treatment response [15]. Further analyses confirmed *PIG-A* mutations in the GPI-deficient cells of AA patients by DNA [17, 25]. More than 100 somatic *PIG-A* gene mutations have been reported distributed throughout the *PIG-A* sequence. A 5-bp GTACT deletion in exon 2 at nt. 662–666 was suspected as mutational hot spot in aplastic anemia patients. The large majority of AA/PNH patients have multiple *PIG-A* mutations suggesting a process of hypermutation in the *PIG-A* gene in AA stem cells [28].

Interestingly, a recent study negates such a connection of GPI deficiency with inherited bone marrow failure syndromes, because none of the analyzed patients with an inherited bone marrow syndrome showed PNH clones [44]. However, Dacie et al. reported in 1944 a case with a combined presentation of Fanconi anemia with PNH, which could not be proofed by GPI-AP flow cytometry at those times [34]. If the negative correlation of GPI deficiency with inherited bone marrow failure syndromes will be confirmed in a larger patient group, the existence of significant GPI-deficient populations might be a useful diagnostic tool to exclude the diagnosis of an inherited bone marrow syndrome and focus the workup and treatment on an acquired form of marrow failure.

8.4.2 GPI-Deficient Populations and PIG-A Mutations in MDS

There are several studies reporting significant GPI-deficient populations even for MDS patients. Wang et al. showed small but significant GPI-deficient populations in 12 % of MDS patients with a number of blasts lower than 5 % [24]. The characteristics of the MDS patients with significant GPI-deficient populations tend to be refractory anemia with a hypocellular marrow, HLA-DR15 positivity, normal cytogenetics, moderate to severe thrombocytopenia, and a high likelihood of response to immunosuppressive therapy [14, 15, 24]. Therefore, it has to be discussed if these patient groups have more likely a moderate aplastic anemia rather than MDS. As mentioned earlier, distinguishing hypoplastic MDS from aplastic anemia is often difficult [40].

Routine screening of patients with subcategories of MDS other than refractory anemia or with other clonal myelopathies (e.g., myelofibrosis) who have no clinical or biochemical evidence of hemolysis is not recommended.

It has to be notified that in many of the MDS studies, *PIG-A* mutational analysis to establish clonality has not been performed in many of these studies [17].

8.5 Treatment of BMF-PNH Syndromes

8.5.1 Treatment Decision in BMF-PNH Syndromes

As discussed earlier the presentation of BMF-PNH is manifold, and the treatment has to be adapted to the current situation of the individual patient.

The first important step in this context is to become aware of the patients leading clinical presentation (Fig. 8.3).

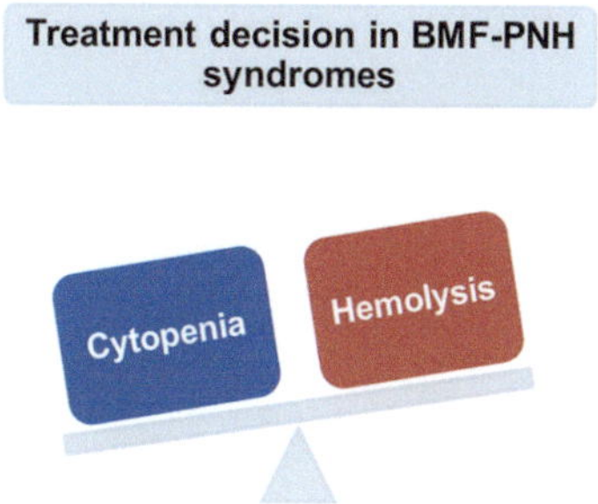

Fig. 8.3 Treatment decision in BMF-PNH syndromes should be triggered by the clinical presentation in the individual patient

The aplastic component of the disorder has to be treated first in BMF-PNH syndromes with symptoms predominately caused by cytopenias [22, 23, 31, 43]. It has to be considered that there are possible effects of those treatment procedures to the PNH as well. A successful stem cell transplantation of an AA or a MDS will also cure the PNH [26, 45, 46]. Furthermore, GPI-deficient populations can increase or decrease clinically relevant in consequence of an immunosuppressive treatment [12, 15, 16, 47, 48].

In case of a clinically significant hemolysis, especially in case of thromboembolism, renal insufficiency, and pulmonal hypertension, the PNH has to be treated [1, 2, 49–52].

If there is a need to treat cytopenic as well as hemolytic symptoms, both conditions should be addressed by the treatment regime [53].

In patients with BMF-PNH syndromes without clinically relevant symptoms by hemolysis and cytopenia, a watch-and-wait strategy flanked by a sufficient supportive therapy should be followed [22, 30, 51].

8.5.2 Treatment Options in BMF-PNH Syndromes

For an overview of the treatment options, see Fig. 8.4.

1. Treatment in aplastic MDS cases without relevant hemolysis should be based on the valid guidelines and adapted to the patient's risk profile and comorbidities and ranges from watch-and-wait strategies to transfusion therapy, iron chelation treatment, growth factors, ATG, administration of lenalidomide and 5-azacitidine, or allogeneic transplantation [30, 31, 37].
2. Treatment in AA cases without relevant hemolysis should be performed according to the valid guidelines adjusted to the severity of the disease, age, and availability of HLA-identical stem cell donor. An additional PNH clone on its own is neither a contraindication of an immunosuppressive therapy nor an indication for stem cell transplantation. The treatment approaches range from watch-and-wait strategies to transfusion therapy, iron chelation treatment, cyclosporine, ATG, alemtuzumab, eltrombopag, androgens, or allogeneic transplantation [22, 23, 43, 47, 48].

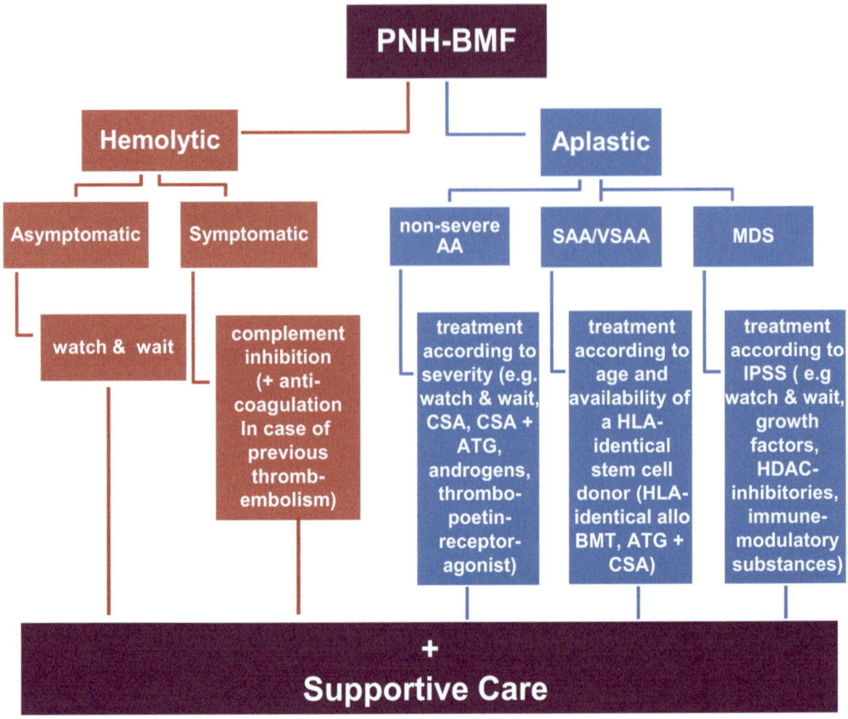

Fig. 8.4 Treatment algorithm in BMF-PNH syndromes based on the main clinical symptoms – hemolysis and cytopenia

3. In case of hemolytic symptomatic PNH, the primary therapeutic strategy is the inhibition of the terminal complement system. The approved humanized monoclonal antibody eculizumab binds to complement factor C5, preventing its cleavage into the fragments C5a and C5b, and thus blocks the subsequent formation of the terminal complement complex C5b-9. Therapy with eculizumab usually is a long-term treatment, as the underlying cellular defect is not influenced by the administration of the antibody. The drug should be administered particularly in case of complications such as transfusion-requiring anemia, previous thromboembolic events, PNH-associated renal failure, crises of abdominal pain, or other serious PNH-related symptoms. In the combined BMF-PNH syndromes, it is sometimes difficult to distinguish in which case hemolysis, respectively aplasia is the leading cause for the clinical symptoms, especially for a reduced quality of life. Patients with a symptomatic PNH can benefit from a long-term therapy with eculizumab as it reduces the symptoms and complications associated with the disease, while survival has also been significantly improved as compared to that of a historical control group [1, 2, 4, 49–52].
4. In patients with the need for an immunosuppression and terminal complement inhibition, IST and eculizumab can be given together. A post hoc review of the PNH clinical trial database (N = 195) demonstrated that eculizumab appears

well tolerated in patients (n = 17) receiving concomitant IST for their marrow failure [53]. A larger analysis of the international PNH patient registry database which is addressing this question is in process.

5. A secondary bone marrow disorder (e.g., SAA/VSAA, MDS, or transformation into an acute leukemia) as well as recurrent life-threatening complications in spite of sufficient complement inhibition might present potential situations from which an indication for allogeneic stem cell therapy might ensue [22, 23, 31, 43, 45, 46, 51].

In vitro and in vivo studies have shown that PNH cells can be eradicated following SCT [26]. But a recent analysis of 211 patients transplanted for PNH confirmed a considerable transplantation-associated morbidity and mortality due to high rates of transplant rejections and GVHD. The 5-year overall survival rate was 68 ± 3 % in all transplanted patients, 54 ± 7 % in the case of additional thromboembolism, 69 ± 5 % in the case of additional AA without thromboembolism, and 86 ± 6 % in the case of recurrent hemolytic anemia without thromboembolism or AA. Matched-pair analysis with non-transplanted PNH patients confirmed a worse overall survival for transplanted PNH patients with thromboembolic events ($p = 0.007$) and no significant differences for the patient group with additional AA ($p = 0.06$). Thus, allogeneic stem cell transplantation could not be used as standard of care option in PNH. Especially, it is not the treatment of first choice for life-threatening thromboembolism in paroxysmal nocturnal hemoglobinuria. Nevertheless, the allogeneic stem cell transplantation is still a sufficient treatment option in AA-PNH syndromes if it is performed analogous to the SAA/VSAA treatment guidelines [22, 46].

A new aspect is the use of eculizumab during the peri-transplant period to reduce the risk of complications during stem cell transplantation of PNH patients. Due to preliminary data, this seems to be a successful approach especially in preventing thromboembolism and further toxicity (e.g., renal insufficiency) associated with stem cell transplantation. Larger studies and uniform strategies are needed to evaluate the optimal use of anticomplement therapy for SAA/PNH patients undergoing HSCT [54, 55].

8.6 Conclusion

PNH and BMF syndromes present a lot of overlapping subgroups. A proper diagnosis is important to estimate prognosis and to choose the best treatment for the individual patient.

If standard criteria do not lead to a distinct diagnosis, more experienced diagnostic tools like CD34 measurement of bone marrow cells might be useful.

For an appropriate treatment of these cases, the individual clinical characteristics of the disease have to be considered.

PNH as well as BMF syndromes are not steady states. The treating physician has to be aware of the possible changes of the disorders during the follow-up. Especially, due to current longer overall survival of PNH patients by sufficient complement inhibition, a transformation to aplastic anemia, myelodysplastic syndromes, or even leukemias might be seen more often in the future.

Financial Disclosure/Acknowledgments H.S. and B.H. received research grants from Genzyme, now Sanofi Aventis, GlaxoSmithKline, and Alexion for research projects. H.S. received honoraria for presentations in Genzyme-sponsored symposia. H.S. and B. H. received honoraria for presentations in Alexion-sponsored symposia. B.H. received honoraria for presentations in GSK-sponsored symposia. H.S. and B.H were members in advisory boards for Alexion.

No writing assistance was utilized in the production of this manuscript.

References

1. Parker C, Omine M, Richards S, Nishimura J, Bessler M, Ware R et al (2005) Diagnosis and management of paroxysmal nocturnal hemoglobinuria. Blood 106(12):3699–3709.
2. Kelly RJ, Hill A, Arnold LM, Brooksbank GL, Richards SJ, Cullen M et al (2011) Long-term treatment with eculizumab in paroxysmal nocturnal hemoglobinuria: sustained efficacy and improved survival. Blood 117(25):6786–6792
3. Hillmen P, Lewis SM, Bessler M, Luzzatto L, Dacie JV (1995) Natural history of paroxysmal nocturnal hemoglobinuria. N Engl J Med 333(19):1253–1258
4. Socié G, Mary JY, de Gramont A, Rio B, Leporrier M, Rose C et al (1996) Paroxysmal nocturnal haemoglobinuria: long-term follow-up and prognostic factors. French Soc Haematol Lancet 348(9027):573–577
5. de Latour RP, Mary JY, Salanoubat C, Terriou L, Etienne G, Mohty M et al (2008) Paroxysmal nocturnal hemoglobinuria: natural history of disease subcategories. Blood 112(8):3099–3106
6. Schrezenmeier H, Muus P, Socié G, Szer J, Urbano-Ispizua A, Maciejewsk JP et al (2014) Baseline characteristics and disease burden in patients in the International Paroxysmal Nocturnal Hemoglobinuria Registry. Haematologica 99(5):922–929
7. Ware RE, Pickens CV, DeCastro CM, Howard TA (2001) Circulating PIG-A mutant T lymphocytes in healthy adults and patients with bone marrow failure syndromes. Exp Hematol 29:1403–1409
8. Schrezenmeier H, Hertenstein B, Wagner B, Raghavachar A, Heimpel H (1995) A pathogenetic link between aplastic anemia and paroxysmal nocturnal hemoglobinuria is suggested by a high frequency of aplastic anemia patients with a deficiency of phosphatidylinositol glycan anchored proteins. Exp Hematol 23:81–87
9. Jain A, Naniwadekar M (2013) An etiological reappraisal of pancytopenia – largest series reported to date from a single tertiary care teaching hospital. BMC Hematol 13:10. doi:10.1186/2052-1839-13-10
10. Barrett J, Sauntharajah Y, Molidrem J (2000) Myelodysplastic syndromes and aplastic anemia: distinct entities or disease linked by common pathophysiology? Semin Hematol 37:15–29
11. DeZern AE, Sekeres MA (2014) The challenging world of cytopenias: distinguishing myelodysplastic syndromes from other disorders of marrow failure. Oncologist 19(7):735–745, Epub 2014 Jun 4
12. Pu JJ, Mukhina G, Wang H, Savage WJ, Brodsky RA (2011) Natural history of paroxysmal nocturnal hemoglobinuria clones in patients presenting as aplastic anemia. Eur J Haematol 87(1):37–45

13. Mukhina GL, Buckley JT, Barber JP, Jones RJ, Brodsky RA (2001) Multilineage glycosylphosphatidylinositol anchor deficient hematopoiesis in untreated aplastic anemia. Br J Haematol 115:476–482
14. Dunn DE, Tanawattanacharoen P, Boccuni P et al (1999) Paroxysmal nocturnal hemoglobinuria cells in patients with bone marrow failure syndromes. Ann Intern Med 131:401–408
15. Sugimori C, Chuhjo T, Feng X et al (2006) Minor population of CD55–CD59- blood cells predicts response to immunosuppressive therapy and prognosis in patients with aplastic anemia. Blood 107:1308–1314
16. Höchsmann B, Rojewski M, Schrezenmeier H (2011) Paroxysmal nocturnal hemoglobinuria (PNH): higher sensitivity and validity in diagnosis and serial monitoring by flow cytometric analysis of reticulocytes. Ann Hematol. doi:10.1007/s00277-011-1177-4
17. Young NS (2009) Paroxysmal nocturnal hemoglobinuria and myelodysplastic syndromes: clonal expansion of PIG-A-mutant hematopoietic cells in bone marrow failure. Haematologica 94(1):3
18. Alter BP (2007) Diagnosis, genetics and management of inherited bone marrow failure syndromes. Hematol Am Soc Hematol Educ Program 2007:29–39
19. Trefferi A, VArdiman JW (2009) Myelodsyplastic syndromes. N Engl J Med 361:1872–1885
20. Shimamura A, Alter BP (2010) Pathophysiology and management of inherited bone marrow failure syndromes. Blood Rev 24:101–122
21. Tsangaris E, Klaassen R, Fernandez CV et al (2011) Genetic analysis of inherited bone marrow failure syndromes from one prospective, comprehensive and population-based cohort and identification of novel mutations. J Med Genet 48:618–628
22. Schrezenmeier H, Brümmendorf T, Linkesch W, Schubert J, Röth A, Höchsmann B, Deeg HJ (2012) Guidline for the diagnostic and treatment of Aplastic Anemia of the German society of hematology and oncology, version 2012. https://www.onkopedia-guidelines.info/en/onkopedia/guidelines/aplastic-anemia-diagnostics-and-therapy-of/index_html
23. Young NS, Calado RT, Phillip S (2006) Current concepts in the pathophysiology and treatment of aplastic anemia. Hematol Am Soc Hematol Educ Program 108:2509–2519
24. Wang H, Chuhjo T, Yasue S, Omine M, Nakao S (2002) Clinical significance of a minor population of paroxysmal nocturnal hemoglobinuria-type cells in bone marrow failure syndrome. Blood 100:3897–3902
25. Nagarajan S, Brodsky RA, Young NS, Medof ME (1995) Genetic defects underlying paroxysmal nocturnal hemoglobinuria that arises out of aplastic anemia. Blood 86:4656–4661
26. Takahashi Y, McCoy JP Jr, Carvallo C, Rivera C, Igarashi T, Srinivasan R et al (2004) In vitro and in vivo evidence of PNH cell sensitivity to immune attack after nonmyeloablative allogeneic hematopoietic cell transplantation. Blood 103(4):1383–1390
27. Schrezenmeier H, Hildebrand A, Rojewski M, Hacker H, Heimpel H, Raghavachar A (2000) Paroxysmal nocturnal haemoglobinuria: a replacement of haematopoietic tissue? Acta Haematol 103:41–48
28. Mortazavi Y, Merk B, McIntosh J, Marsh JC, Schrezenmeier H, Rutherford TR, BIOMED II Pathophysiology and Treatment of Aplastic Anaemia Study Group (2003) The spectrum of PIG-A gene mutations in aplastic anemia/paroxysmal nocturnal hemoglobinuria (AA/PNH): a high incidence of multiple mutations and evidence of a mutational hot spot. Blood 101(7):2833–2841, Epub 2002 Nov 7
29. Swerdlow SH, Campo E, Harris NL (2008) WHO classification of tumours of the haematopoietic and lymphoid tissues. International Agency for Research on Cancer, Lyon
30. Haase D, Germing U, Schanz J et al (2007) New insights into the prognostic impact of the karyotype in MDS and correlation with subtypes: evidence from a core data set of 2124 patients. Blood 110:4385–4395
31. Germing U, Kobbe G, Haas R (2013) Gattermann N Myelodysplastic syndromes: diagnosis, prognosis and treatment. Dtsch Arztebl Int 110(46):783–790

32. Bennett JM, Orazi A (2009) Diagnostic criteria to distinguish hypocellular acute myeloid leukemia from hypocellular myelodysplastic syndromes and aplastic anemia: recommendations for a standardized approach. Haematologica 94:264–268
33. Maciejewski JP, Mufti GJ (2008) Whole genome scanning as a cytogenetic tool in hematologic malignancies. Blood 112:965–974
34. Dacie JV, Gilpin A (1944) Refractory anaemia (Fanconi type) and its incidence in three members of one family, with in one case a relationship to chronic haemolytic anaemia with nocturnal haemo-globinuria (Marchiafava-Micheli Disease or 'Nocturnal Haemoglobinuria'). Arch Dis Child 19(100):155–162
35. Camitta BM, Thomas ED, Nathan DG et al (1976) Severe aplastic anemia: a prospective study of the effect of early marrow transplantation on acute mortality. Blood 48:63–70
36. Moyo VM, Mukhina GL, Garrett ES, Brodsky RA (2004) Natural history of paroxysmal nocturnal haemoglobinuria using modern diagnostic assays. Br J Haematol 126(1):133–138
37. Schanz J, Steidl C, Fonatsch C et al (2011) Coalesced multicentric analysis of 2351 patients with myelodysplastic syndromes indicates an underestimation of poor-risk cytogenetics of myelodysplastic syndromes in the International Prognostic Scoring System. J Clin Oncol 29:1963–1970
38. Lee JW, Jang JH, Kim JS, Yoon S-S, Lee JH, Kim Y-K et al (2013) Clinical signs and symptoms associated with increased risk for thrombosis in patients with paroxysmal nocturnal hemoglobinuria from a Korean Registry. Int J Hematol 97(6):749–757
39. Nishimura J, Kanakura Y, Ware RE, Shichishima T, Nakakuma H, Ninomiya H et al (2004) Clinical course and flow cytometric analysis of paroxysmal nocturnal hemoglobinuria in the United States and Japan. Medicine 83(3):193–207
40. Matsui WH, Brodsky RA, Smith BD, Borowitz MJ, Jones RJ (2006) Quantitative analysis of bone marrow CD34 cells in aplastic anemia and hypoplastic myelodysplastic syndromes. Leukemia 20:458–462
41. Brummendorf TH, Maciejewski JP, Mak J, Young NS, Lansdorp PM (2001) Telomere length in leukocyte subpopulations of patients with aplastic anemia. Blood 97(4):895–900
42. Yamaguchi H, Calado RT, Ly H, Kajigaya S, Baerlocher GM, Chanock SJ, Lansdorp PM, Young NS (2005) Mutations in TERT, the gene for telomerase reverse transcriptase, in aplastic anemia. N Engl J Med 352(14):1413–1424
43. EBMT working party Aplastic anemia. Diagnosis and treatment of aplastic anemia. Bone Marrow Transplantation (2013) 48:161, doi:10.1038/bmt.2012.229 (complete issue)
44. DeZern AE, Symons HJ, Resar LS, Borowitz MJ, Armanios MY, Brodsky RA (2014) Detection of paroxysmal nocturnal hemoglobinuria clones to exclude inherited bone marrow failure syndromes. Eur J Haematol 92(6):467–470. doi:10.1111/ejh.12299, Epub 2014 Mar 18
45. Santarone S, Bacigalupo A, Risitano AM, Tagliaferri E, Di Bartolomeo E, Paola Iori A et al (2010) Hematopoietic stem cell transplantation for paroxysmal nocturnal hemoglobinuria: long-term results of a retrospective study on behalf of the Gruppo Italiano Trapianto Midollo Osseo (GITMO). Haematologica 95(6):983–988
46. Peffault de Latour R, Schrezenmeier H, Bacigalupo A, Blaise D, De Souza CA, Vigouroux S et al (2012) Allogeneic stem cell transplantation in paroxysmal nocturnal hemoglobinuria. Haematologica 97(11):1666–1673
47. Tichelli A, Schrezenmeier H, Socie G, Marsh J, Bacigalupo A, Duhrsen U, Franzke A, Hallek M, Thiel E, Wilhelm M, Hochsmann B, Barrois A, Champion K, Passweg JR (2011) A randomized controlled study in patients with newly diagnosed severe aplastic anemia receiving antithymocyte globulin (ATG), cyclosporine, with or without G-CSF: a study of the SAA Working Party of the European Group for Blood and Marrow Transplantation. Blood 117(17):4434–4441
48. Marsh JC, Bacigalupo A, Schrezenmeier H, Tichelli A, Risitano AM, Passweg JR, Killick SB, Warren AJ, Foukaneli T, Aljurf M, Al-Zahrani HA, Höchsmann B, Schafhausen P, Roth A, Franzke A, Brummendorf TH, Dufour C, Oneto R, Sedgwick P, Barrois A, Kordasti S, Elebute MO, Mufti GJ, Socie G (2012) Prospective study of rabbit antithymocyte globulin and

cyclosporine for aplastic anemia from the EBMT Severe Aplastic Anaemia Working Party. Blood 119(23):5391–5396
49. Hillmen P, Young NS, Schubert J, Brodsky RA, Socié G, Muus P et al (2006) The complement inhibitor eculizumab in paroxysmal nocturnal hemoglobinuria. N Engl J Med 355(12):1233–1243
50. Brodsky RA, Young NS, Antonioli E, Risitano AM, Schrezenmeier H, Schubert J et al (2008) Multicenter phase 3 study of the complement inhibitor eculizumab for the treatment of patients with paroxysmal nocturnal hemoglobinuria. Blood 111(4):1840–1847
51. Schubert J, Röth A, Bettelheim P, Stüssi G, Brümmendorf T, Schrezenmeier H (2012) Guidline for the treatment of Paroxysmal Nocturnal hemoglobinuria of the German society of hematology and oncology, version 2012. https://www.onkopedia-guidelines.info/en/onkopedia/guidelines/paroxysmal-nocturnal-hemoglobinuria-pnh
52. Schrezenmeier H, Höchsmann B (2009) Eculizumab opens a new era of treatment for paroxysmal nocturnal hemoglobinuria. Expert Rev Hematol 2:7–16
53. Schrezenmeier H, Schubert J, Luzzatto L, Muus P, Socie G, Risitano A, Hill A (2009) Hillmen P effects of Eculizumab therapy in patients with Paroxysmal Nocturnal Hemoglobinuria (PNH) receiving concurrent immunosuppressive therapy for bone marrow insufficiency. Blood 114:3012
54. Kulasekararaj AG, Potter VT, Gandhi SA, Benson-Quarm N, Joanna L, Antonio P, Mufti GJ, Judith M (2013) Feasibility and optimal schedule of using Eculizumab in patients with hemolytic Paroxysmal Nocturnal Hemoglobinuria (hPNH) with Severe Aplastic Anemia (SAA) prior to Haemopoietic Stem Cell Transplant (HSCT). Blood 122:2482
55. Michael M, Larisa S, Elena K, Elena B, Alexey L, Yakov M, Vlasta B, Varvara K, Irina K, Dina B, Dmitriy B, Galina N, Alexey M (2013) Graft TCR-alpha/beta depletion and peri-transplant use of Eculizumab in matched unrelated donor transplantation for severe aplastic anemia-paroxysmal nocturnal hemoglobinuria: report of two cases. Blood 122:4870

Chapter 9
Thrombophilia in PNH

Haruhiko Ninomiya and Anita Hill

Abstract Thromboembolic event is the most important complication of paroxysmal nocturnal hemoglobinuria (PNH) affecting its mortality. The pathophysiological mechanisms underlying thrombosis in PNH have not been fully clarified; multiple factors are likely to be involved. They are likely to be related to the complement activation on/around red blood cells (RBC), white blood cells, and particularly platelets. Intravascular hemolysis also contributes to the mechanisms through the release of free hemoglobin, depletion of nitric oxide (NO), and generation of RBC-derived microparticles (MP). Elevated MP in the plasma which derive from platelets, endothelial cells, and RBC, in total, enhance the prothrombotic states in the circulation. Recent researches have revealed close interactions between coagulation and complement systems, enhancing each other. Continuous activation of complement makes a vicious loop enhancing the coagulation/complement systems interacting with blood cells and endothelial cells in PNH.

Furthermore, the key role of complement activation in the development of thrombosis has been shown also by the effectiveness of eculizumab (humanized monoclonal antihuman C5 antibody) in the prevention of thromboembolic events in PNH. Because thrombotic complications impact mortality and eculizumab exerts a dramatic effect, commencement of eculizumab is recommended for patients with PNH who have had thromboembolic episodes. If eculizumab is not available or is ineffective, prophylactic anticoagulation is required in those with larger proportion of PNH white cells. It should be noted that cases with smaller proportions of PNH cells also have a higher risk of thrombosis than normal individuals.

Keywords PNH • Thrombosis • Complement • NO • Microparticle

H. Ninomiya, M.D., Ph.D. (✉)
Faculty of Medicine, University of Tsukuba,
1-1-1 Tennodai, Tsukuba, Ibaraki 305-8575, Japan
e-mail: ninomiya.haruhiko.ft@u.tsukuba.ac.jp

A. Hill, MBChB (Hons), Ph.D.
Department of Haematology, St. James' University Hospital,
Beckett Street, Leeds, West Yorkshire LS9 7TF, UK

Y. Kanakura et al. (eds.), *Paroxysmal Nocturnal Hemoglobinuria*,
DOI 10.1007/978-4-431-56003-6_9

9.1 Introduction

The clinical manifestations of paroxysmal nocturnal hemoglobinuria (PNH) include hemolytic anemia, thrombosis, bone marrow failure, and progression to myelodysplastic syndrome or acute leukemia, which are primarily related to the abnormal hematopoiesis in PNH [1]. The hematopoietic abnormalities in PNH are caused by a somatic mutation in the *PIG-A* gene, which encodes the glycosyl phosphatidylinositol (GPI)-anchor synthesis [2]. Whereas the pathogenesis of intravascular hemolysis has been thoroughly understood by the deficiency of two GPI-anchored proteins with complement regulatory activities, CD55 and CD59, in PNH-affected RBC, the pathophysiology underlying thrombosis in PNH has remained to be clarified.

A retrospective study of 220 patients, published in 1996 [3], found that the 8-year incidence rates of thrombosis was 28 %. A further publication from this group, published in 2008 [4], covered a total of 460 patients, indicated a 10-year incidence rates of thrombosis 30.7 %; evolution to thrombosis affected the survivals (hazard ratio (HR) 7.8 in classic PNH; HR 33.0 in aplastic anemia-PNH). Hillmen et al. reported one or more episodes of venous thrombosis during the course of PNH in 31 of 80 (39 %) patients with PNH referred to Hammersmith Hospital between 1940 and 1970 [5]. Intra-abdominal veins are the commonly affected sites of thrombosis; cerebral vein and superficial dermal vein also appear to be affected by thrombosis disproportionately. Fatal thrombosis usually involves the hepatic vein, portal system, or the cerebral veins [5].

The risk of thrombosis appears to be significantly related to the size of PNH clone [6, 7]. In two series, almost all patients who developed thrombosis had >50 % [6] or >61 % [7] PNH clone size (of PNH-affected granulocytes).

Thromboembolic events occur principally in relation to the intravascular hemolysis and platelet activation, which further enhance the interactions between complement and coagulation system. Real integration between the coagulation and complement systems with many complexities has been demonstrated [8–11].

9.2 Incidence and Sites of Thrombosis

9.2.1 Incidence

Thromboembolism is the most common cause of mortality in patients with PNH and accounts for approximately 40–67 % of deaths of which the cause is known. Poor survival was associated with the occurrence of thrombosis as a complication in PNH (relative risk 10.2) by a report from French Society of Haematology [3]. A comparative study of the United States and Japan also demonstrated that the relative risk of death was increased five to 15.4-fold by the complication of thrombosis [6]. During the course of the disease, 29–44 % of patients with PNH have been reported to have at least one thromboembolic events, although the reasons of sudden onset of a thrombotic event remain unclear [1, 3–7, 12]. According to the recent report on 1610 patients enrolled in the international PNH registry, 16 % patients had a history of thrombotic events at their enrollment [13].

Thrombosis in PNH may occur at any site. Common sites include the intra-abdominal and cerebral veins. An explanation for the propensity of intra-abdominal thrombosis in PNH is still to be clarified. Multiple sites are involved in more than one-fifth of the cases. Hepatic vein thrombosis (Budd-Chiari syndrome) is recognized as one of the most common sites of thrombosis and affects 7.5–25 % of patients with PNH [14–16] and may lead to hepatic failure and thereby may cause death in PNH [17].

In PNH, recognizing venous thrombosis is difficult, because episodes may be intra-abdominal or intracranial. Severe abdominal pain or an unusual headache with or without neurological deficit must be taken seriously, and appropriate imaging studies should be taken. An increase in the level of serum LDH, alanine aminotransferase (ALT), and aspartate aminotransferase (AST) may be an early clue to the presence of hepatic vein thrombosis. Plasma concentration of direct bilirubin also may increase, but other biochemical tests are of limited value. The incidence rates of thrombosis in PNH appear to be underestimated, because a study using sensitive imaging techniques detected abnormalities suggestive of previous subclinical pulmonary thrombosis in six of ten patients with PNH (without known prior thrombosis), even in patients with recent onset of PNH. There was also evidence that subclinical thrombosis could lead to long-term organ damage as reflected by compromised cardiac function in the majority of these patients [18].

The theory that patients from different ethnic groups may have additional genetic prothrombotic traits was refuted by a study demonstrating no correlation between known inherited thrombophilia (factor V Leiden mutation) and thrombosis in PNH [19]. Dragoni et al. have found a high rate of antiphospholipid antibodies in patients with PNH compared with healthy volunteers and patients with aplastic anemia, and they suggested that it could be a contributory factor to the thrombosis in PNH [20].

9.2.2 *Sites of Thrombosis*

1. Hepatic vein thrombosis

Venous thrombosis occurs frequently in the intra-abdominal veins, particularly the hepatic veins [21, 22]. The onset of hepatic vein thrombosis may be insidious or can occur suddenly, frequently in association with an exaggeration of hemolysis [21]. Hepatic vein thromboses could be detected by magnetic resonance imaging (MRI) [23, 24]. However, even MRI may miss thrombosis of hepatic veins. Flow within the hepatic system can be demonstrated by ultrasound Doppler techniques. Hepatic venography is definitive, but this procedure carries more risk than noninvasive techniques. Once it has occurred, hepatic vein thrombosis tends to recur, ultimately causing cirrhosis and rerouting of the blood from the drainage. The latter

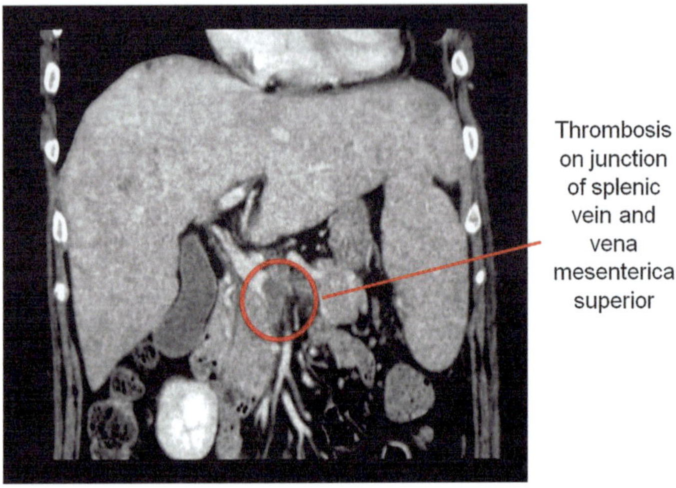

Fig. 9.1 Contrast-enhanced CT scan of the abdomen of a patient with PNH (37-year-old female with 14-year history of PNH). An extensive thrombosis in splenic vein was revealed. This patient was then treated with eculizumab. 14 weeks after the eculizumab administration, splenic vein thrombosis disappeared. (This CT is kindly provided with permission by Dr. Shinya Katsutani, Hiroshima University Hospital, Hiroshima, Japan)

change exaggerated by the portal vein thrombosis, which often occurs in the same patients [24]. The development of Budd-Chiari syndrome is associated with a poor prognosis. Treatment with eculizumab appears to reduce the incidence of Budd-Chiari syndrome and may reverse the disease process [25].

2. Thrombosis of other intra-abdominal veins (Fig. 9.1)

Thrombosis of other intra-abdominal veins, particularly the portal vein, the splenic vein, and the inferior vena cava, is also common in PNH. This may result in splenomegaly or splenic rupture [26]. Infarction of the intestinal tract is also seen with signs and symptoms of ileus. Mesenteric vein thrombosis results in abdominal pain that may be disproportionately exaggerated relative to the physical examination [27]. Thrombosis may affect the small peripheral mesenteric veins and induce transient ischemia of intestines. Abdominal pain, fever, obstruction, and rectal bleeding may be associated. Duodenal venous thrombosis is associated with papillary endothelial hyperplasia, ulceration, and a circumferential mass in the third portion of the duodenum [28]. Large vein thrombosis can be detected by MRI, radiologic CT scanning, or ultrasonography; however, detection of thrombosis in smaller vessels is rarely accomplished even by these imaging techniques. Figure 9.1 is a CT of a patient with PNH complicated with splenic vein thrombosis, which was successfully treated with eculizumab and no recurrence of thrombosis has been observed afterwards (Fig. 9.1 is provided by courtesy of Dr. Shinya Katsutani, Hiroshima University Hospital, Japan) [29].

3. Thrombosis of cerebral veins

Thrombosis of cerebral veins occurs less frequently in PNH than intra-abdominal veins. Cerebral vein thrombosis can occur as a catastrophic event or with an insidious onset [30]. Small-vessel thrombosis may cause severe and refractory headaches or progress to cerebrovascular thrombosis [21]. Major venous sinuses (*e.g.*, superior sagittal, lateral, cavernous, sigmoid) are often involved, but thrombosis may be limited to the veins covering cerebrum, particularly the parietal lobe. The diagnosis of cerebral vein thrombosis is often difficult to establish, even with MRI or other imaging techniques.

4. Thrombosis of other veins

The thrombotic process can affect other veins including those of the legs, kidneys, and skin. Dermal vein thrombosis can present as discrete areas of erythema, swelling, and pain or as a syndrome resembling purpura fulminans [31–33]. Dermal vein thrombosis may result in painful discolored skin lesions. These lesions rarely ulcerate, but a separate condition resembling purpura fulminans can develop, affecting larger areas of skin with necrosis [32]. It may occur in areas of trauma or in sites of previous inflammation or allergy. Deep vein thrombosis of the lower limbs occurs more frequently in patients with PNH than in the general population and has been reported in approximately one-third of patients [5, 34]. Thrombosis in the pulmonary artery is also recognized but not always in the form of emboli related to the deep vein thrombosis in the lower limb.

5. Arterial thrombosis

Arterial thrombosis (*e.g.*, cerebral, coronary arteries) has been described in patients with PNH, but much less commonly than venous thrombosis [35, 36], accounting for approximately 8 % of thrombosis. However, arterial thrombosis may not be rare, according to a South Korean National PNH Registry reporting the incidence rates of arterial vs venous thrombosis, at 31.5 % vs 68.5 %, respectively [37]. The sites of arterial thrombosis in PNH are not particular, although they occur at a younger age than expected in the overall population.

9.3 Proposed Mechanisms of Thrombosis in PNH

In contrast to our thorough understanding on the mechanisms of hemolysis, much less is known about the mechanisms underlying the thrombophilia of PNH. Because the hematopoietic cells are abnormal in PNH, it has been suggested that these defects are somehow responsible also for the thrombosis. Intrinsic relationships between the coagulation and complement systems [8, 9, 11] are likely to amplify the developmental process of thrombosis in PNH.

Complement-mediated platelet activation, complement-mediated hemolysis, impaired NO bioavailability, impaired fibrinolytic system, and inflammatory mediators are all responsible for the increased thrombotic risk in PNH. These multiple factors are likely to contribute to any one thrombotic event.

9.3.1 Platelet Activation

Platelet activation by the action of complement is likely to be the main factor contributing to the thrombosis in PNH [38–40]. Furthermore, many mechanisms are thought to induce platelet activation in patients with PNH, as summarized by Hill et al. [11]. The deficiency of CD59 renders PNH-affected platelets susceptible to the formation of membrane attack complex of complement (MAC, *i.e.*, C5b-9 complex) on their surface. Although complement activation on platelets may result in the lysis or removal of platelets from the circulation and thereby induce thrombocytopenia in some extent, the survival of platelets in PNH patients has been demonstrated to be normal [41].

The formation of C5b-9 complex leads to an increased expression of activation-dependent proteins, and platelet stimulation is accompanied by the loss of membrane phospholipid asymmetry [40, 42, 43]. Platelet-derived microparticles (MP), with highly procoagulant activity, are present at significantly elevated levels in the plasma of patients with PNH. The externalized phosphatidylserine (PS) on the MP acts as a high-affinity binding site for prothrombinase [44] and factor Xase complexes [45]. Therefore, deficiency of CD59 in platelets probably leads to thrombin generation, an increased sensitivity to platelet aggregation by thrombin and thereby increases the thrombotic risk, both venous and arterial [40, 46]. Activation of complement on the surface of platelets stimulates removal of complement complexes by vesiculation; then highly prothrombotic, PS-exposed, MP are released to the circulation [47]. Figure 9.2 shows that PS-exposed MP are released from PNH platelets as well as RBC upon complement activation in vitro. Thrombin, generated on the surface of PS-exposed MP, further reacts with the thrombin receptor on platelets, leading to platelet activation and aggregation, possibly initiating the clot formation [48].

The PS externalization and MP production are recognized in apoptotic cells. PS becomes a marker for phagocyte recognition of senescent or apoptotic cells to be removed [23] and may contribute to the thrombocytopenia in some extent, whereas bone marrow failure is the main cause of thrombocytopenia in PNH. Administration of eculizumab for PNH did not raise the platelet counts significantly in a clinical study [49], suggesting complement-induced platelet activation do not induce thrombocytopenia in PNH in vivo, at least under a static condition.

Activated platelets also interact with neutrophils and can promote thrombus formation by the release of neutrophil serine proteases (elastase and cathepsin G) and nucleosomes, synergistically activating factor X further thus triggering blood coagulation primarily through the extrinsic coagulation pathway [50].

The platelet activation may also in itself perpetuate or exacerbate prothrombotic process in patients through continuous activation of the alternative pathway of com-

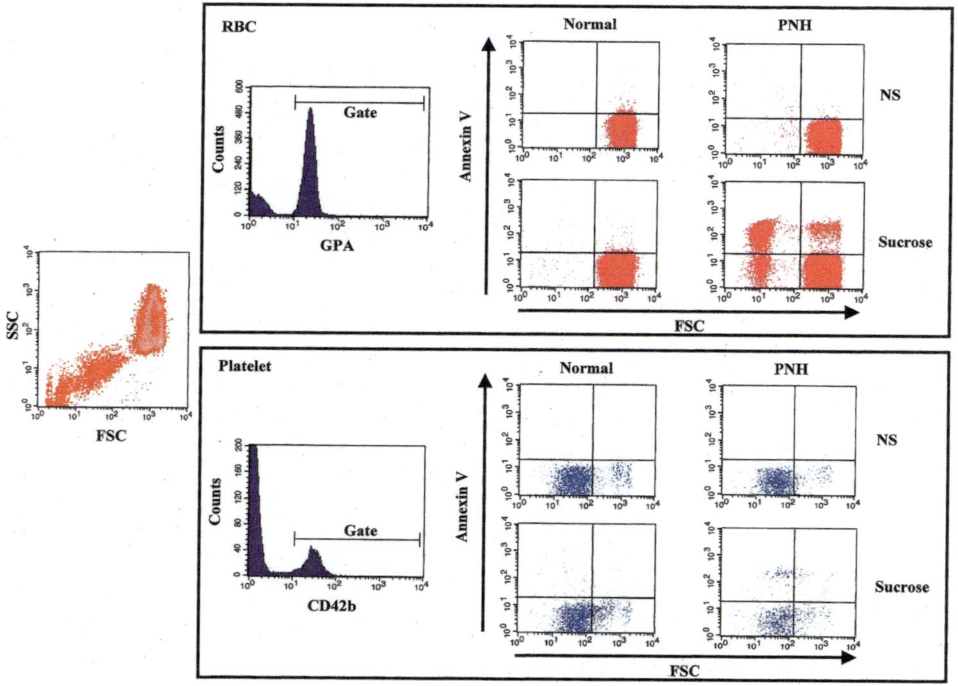

Fig. 9.2 MP released from RBC and platelets upon complement activation in PNH. Whole blood anticoagulated with sodium citrate was incubated in normal saline (NS) or sucrose buffer containing calcium and magnesium ions, and then aliquots were stained with RBC- or platelet-specific markers, glycophorin A (GPA) or CD42b, respectively, and FITC-labeled annexin V. MP determined according to the FSC and the annexin V-binding flow cytometry. CD42b-positive and GPA-positive MP are released from platelets and RBC, respectively, upon complement activation in vitro. (These data were obtained in cooperation with Yukinori Kozuma, University of Tsukuba, Tsukuba, Japan)

plement (through P-selectin (CD62P) expression on activated platelets) [51] and by initiating activation of the classical pathway of complement by platelet-derived chondroitin sulfate [52].

Further mechanisms of platelet activation in PNH are due to depletion of nitric oxide (NO), direct toxicity of free hemoglobin, increased reactive oxygen species (ROS) causing oxidative stress, generation of thrombin, and as a consequence of endothelial dysfunction.

One study demonstrated that the platelets in PNH were hyporeactive and they concluded that this may be due to chronic stimulation of platelets by continual complement activation [53]. Activation of platelets assessed by the surface expression of P-selectin, fibrinogen, von Willebrand factor (vWF), thrombospondin, and lysosomal protein was demonstrated in vivo in PNH patients; they suggested a relation of platelet activation with the grade of hemolysis [39].

Although the complement activation does not appear to cause significant thrombocytopenia in PNH patients at least under a static condition, it is also recognized clinically that an unexpected drop in a patient's platelet count may be an indicator of a complication of thrombosis. Lower resting platelet counts in PNH may be a consequence of an increased sensitivity of megakaryocyte progenitors PNH to complement [54] additionally to the bone marrow failure.

9.3.2 Intravascular Hemolysis: NO Depletion, Toxicity of Free Hemoglobin, and RBC-Derived MP

Thrombotic events have been coincided with increased hemolysis [36], and intravascular hemolysis is also likely to be one of the principle contributors to thromboembolism in an animal model [55]. Multiple mechanisms by which intravascular hemolysis may contribute to thrombosis is summarized by Hill et al. [11].

Hemolysis, through several factors such as toxicity of free hemoglobin and NO depletion, has been implicated in the initiation of platelet activation and aggregation [56]. The role of free hemoglobin has been demonstrated by the infusion of cross-linked hemoglobin in rats, which increase platelet aggregation and adhesion in vivo on prothrombotic surfaces such as injured vessel wall [57]. Further, administration of heme in healthy volunteers causes thrombophlebitis, demonstrating that heme can cause vascular inflammation followed by vascular obstruction in vivo [58]. The addition of free hemoglobin (>2 g/L) to human serum causes inhibition of metalloprotease ADAMTS-13, an enzyme critical in limiting platelet thrombus formation [59]. Further, disintegration of heme releases toxic species of iron, which participates in biochemical reactions that generate free radicals and thus catalyze the formation of ROS and result in loss of membrane lipid organization [60]. PS-exposed RBC are more likely to adhere to endothelium as well as provide basis for the factor

Xase and prothrombinase complexes. ROS were higher and reduced glutathione lower in CD55-/CD59-negative cells than CD55-/CD59-positive cells or cells of normal control, suggesting the PNH cells were under oxidative stress [61].

NO, a free radical, binds avidly to soluble guanylate cyclase resulting in increased intracellular cyclic guanosine monophosphate (cGMP) [62]. cGMP activates cGMP-dependent kinase that decreases intracellular calcium concentration in smooth muscle, producing relaxation, vasodilatation, and increased regional blood flow, primarily suppressing platelet aggregation, expression of cell adhesion molecules on endothelial cells, and secretion of procoagulant proteins [56, 63]. NO also inhibits platelet aggregation and ischemia-reperfusion injury [64], modulates endothelial proliferation [65], and has anti-inflammatory properties [66]. Conversely, NO depletion is associated with platelet activation and an increase in soluble P-selectin expression [67], which in itself can further activate the complement system [51].

NO also interacts with components of the coagulation cascade to downregulate the clot formation. For example, NO has been shown to chemically modify and inhibit factor XIII, suggesting that NO depletion would enhance clot stability [68]. Further, NO depletion causes increase in fibrin degradation products (FDP) and thrombin-antithrombin (TAT) complexes, leading to significant fibrin deposition and thrombus formation in an animal model [69]. Reduced NO production in L-arginine deficiency in lysinuric protein intolerance has been associated with increased TAT and FDP, whereas reversal of NO deficiency with L-arginine causes a reduction in intravascular coagulopathy [70].

The reaction of NO with oxyhemoglobin is fast and irreversible [71]. The chronic nature of the hemolysis in PNH is such that even at baseline, there is sufficient release of free hemoglobin to saturate biochemical systems in place to remove it, resulting in NO depletion. The rate of NO depletion correlates with the severity of intravascular hemolysis of which LDH is a sensitive marker [72]. In addition to NO scavenging by free hemoglobin, intravascular hemolysis also releases RBC arginase, an enzyme that converts L-arginine, the substrate for NO synthesis, to ornithine, thereby further reducing the systemic availability of NO [73].

Circulating procoagulant MP are elevated in the plasma of patients with PNH, whereas those derived from RBC were reported to be relatively low [46, 74]. The procoagulant MP derived from endothelial cell, platelets, and RBC, in total, could provide disseminated prothrombotic seats in the circulation [46]. Figure 9.2 shows that complement activation induces a release of procoagulant, PS-exposed MP from RBC [75] as well as platelets in vitro in PNH (Fig. 9.2). Complement-induced hemolytic attack may increase the risk of thrombosis through the accumulation of procoagulant MP in the plasma by addition of RBC-derived MP as well as platelet- or endothelial cell-derived MP.

9.3.3 Deficiency of Other GPI-Linked (or Associated) Proteins: uPAR (CD87), TFPI

Urokinase-type plasminogen activator receptor (uPAR: CD87) is a GPI-anchored protein that is therefore deficient in PNH monocytes and granulocytes. Pro-urokinase (uPA) bound to CD87 on the cell surface converts plasminogen to plasmin and results in degradation of fibrin. It is possible that the deficiency of CD87 in the surface of PNH cells results in an increased tendency to thrombosis as a result of impaired fibrinolysis and reduced clot dissolution [76]. Because of a lack of anchorage of CD87 to the cell membrane, increased soluble CD87 in the plasma is thought to also contribute to the increased risk of venous thrombosis by competing with membrane-bound CD87 [77, 78]. It may potentiate thrombosis but is unlikely to be a sole cause of thrombosis in PNH.

Tissue factor pathway inhibitor (TFPI) is predominantly released by the endothelium (but is also present on the surface of monocytes, within platelets, and in the plasma) and is anchored, most likely indirectly, through the GPI anchor [79]. It is a potent anticoagulant protein that abrogates blood coagulation by inhibiting both factor Xa and tissue factor (TF)-factor VIIa catalytic complex, making it the only physiologically active inhibitor of the initiation of the extrinsic coagulation pathway. It has been suggested that defective expression or reduced activity of TFPI (as TFPI is downregulated by inflammatory cytokines) potentially contributes to both arterial and venous thrombosis in PNH [79]. The localization of the clot to the vessel wall may occur because complement activation and the generation of MAC on the defective blood cells stimulate the expression of TF on endothelial cells [80]. Such a site would provide a localized area for aggregated platelets, particularly in the areas where the blood flow is sufficiently slow to allow stimulation of the endothelium to occur and aggregated platelets to adhere. Deficiency of the GPI-linked protein, TFPI, is a likely contributor to abnormality of this procoagulant pathway [79], whereas it has not been studied on the problem whether endothelial cells are deficient in the expression of GPI-anchored proteins in PNH similarly to the case of PNH-affected blood cells.

9.3.4 Endothelial Dysfunction

Endothelial dysfunction occurs during any thrombotic event. TF which is originally expressed in subendothelial mural cells and adventitial fibroblasts in the vessel wall is linked to the coagulation and complement cascade by its exposure on endothelial cells. The endothelium has also been implicated in the pathogenesis of thrombosis in hemolytic states [81], *i.e.*, free hemoglobin directly impairs endothelial function. Free hemoglobin and its breakdown oxidative product heme can directly activate endothelial cells and further promote inflammation and coagulation as well as increase TF production and release of high molecular weight vWF. In particular, the activation of C5 as an inflammatory response can cause an increased expression of functionally active TF in leukocytes [82]. In addition, C5a [83] and the cytolytically inactive MAC [84] can induce TF expression on human endothelial cells.

MP elevated in the plasma of PNH express endothelial markers: ICAM-1 (CD54), sVCAM-1, vWF, CD144 (VE-cadherin), and CD105 (endoglin), indicating chronic endothelial activation in PNH. CD144, similar to CD105, is derived from a subpopulation of endothelial cell junctions. It has a very short half-life in the circulation; therefore its presence in the plasma in PNH indicates persistent endothelial damage associated with the chronic hemolysis of PNH [74, 85]. A similar association has been described in sickle-cell disease [65].

9.3.5 Other Complement-Mediated Procoagulant Mechanisms (Independent of Hemolysis)

Complement activation plays a major role in vascular inflammation. C5a may result in proinflammatory and prothrombotic processes through the generation of inflammatory cytokines such as IL-6, IL-8, and TNF-α. These will further activate the endothelium with the production of endothelial MP, potentially self-perpetuating the problem. Complement activation on the surface of neutrophils and monocytes is also followed by the MAC formation. On these cells, MAC formation induces cell activation and also proliferation [86]. Both the MAC formation and C5a may induce the expression of TF as well as PAI-1 by these leukocytes. One study demonstrated that complement activation and downstream signaling via C5a receptor in neutrophils lead to the induction of TF [87]. Markedly elevated plasma levels of leukocyte-derived TF in PNH are referred to this mechanism [88]. IL-6 may additionally deregulate the immune system and inhibit ADAMTS-13 (vWF-cleaving protease) activity [89]. Preliminary data suggest that low-grade in vivo activation of clotting is common in PNH, an abnormality that is enhanced with increased activation of complement and decreased when PNH is treated with eculizumab [47].

Infection triggers the coincidence of increased hemolysis and thrombotic complication in PNH. In addition to the intravascular hemolysis-related mechanisms contributing to the thrombosis as described above, there are also hemolysis-independent thrombogenic mechanisms. The invading pathogens are recognized by antigen-presenting cells, neutrophils, monocytes, macrophages, endothelial cells, and platelets, resulting in the TF expression that is sustained by cytokine and chemokines. The pathogens also further induce complement activation, promoting generation of more C5a and MAC. C5a feeds back to promote expression of TF [9].

The pathway turns full circle with the knowledge that a fourth pathway (separate from the classic, lectin, and alternative) has been described to activate the complement system in which thrombin itself cleaves and activates C3 and C5 (independent of C3) [90]. Subsequent investigation has revealed that both C3 and C5 can be proteolytically activated by several components of coagulation cascade in addition to thrombin [91]. Therefore, thrombosis activates complement, perhaps leading to further thrombosis in PNH and then a vicious circle ensues. This might explain the observation that once a patient has their first thrombosis, this often heralds further thrombotic complications spiraling out of control, despite anticoagulation, until the patient eventually succumbs [11].

Although studies have reported a strong correlation between a larger PNH neutrophil clone and the occurrence of thrombosis [4, 7, 92], thrombosis appears to also occur frequently in patients with smaller PNH clones, as low as 10 %, when compared with the normal population [92, 93]. In addition, Hugel et al. found no correlation between circulating platelet-derived MP level and PNH clone size [46], which partly explains the unpredictability of thrombosis in PNH.

9.4 Management of Thrombosis in PNH

A definitive guideline for the management of thrombosis in PNH has not been established yet in the era of eculizumab. There are several personal views, by PNH experts, on the management of PNH including thrombosis management published [11, 94, 95]. Because PNH is a rare disorder, prospective studies on the management are difficult to design. We have to further accumulate the clinical experiences to reach a consensus on the management of PNH.

9.4.1 Acute Treatment

Anticoagulation is required for the treatment of thrombosis associated with PNH, and the commencement of eculizumab therapy is recommended in the acute setting. Mild to moderate thrombocytopenia (platelets $50–100 \times 10^9$/L) is not a contraindication to anticoagulation; however, platelet transfusion may be required for patients with platelet counts $<50 \times 10^9$/L. If there is evidence of thrombosis in a patient who is not on anticoagulation prophylaxis, this should be instituted immediately; but it is important to notice that venous thrombosis can develop in a patient with PNH who is fully anticoagulated.

Occasional episodes of hemolysis coincident with the administration of heparin have been reported [96], and the phenomenon has been attributed to activation of the alternative pathway of complement by heparin. However, concern for exacerbation of hemolysis by heparin should not deter in its use in standard pharmacologic doses in situations where anticoagulation is warranted. Once adequately anticoagulated with heparin, warfarin therapy should be initiated with a target INR of 2.5. Although data on recurrence rates have not been demonstrated, patients with PNH who experience a thromboembolic episode probably warrant life-long anticoagulation.

Thrombolytic therapy has previously been advocated for extensive, acute, or life-threatening hepatic vein thrombosis if the clot is less than 3–4 days old and in whom there are no contraindications but experience is limited [12, 14, 95, 97]. Even with heparin therapy, extensive vein thrombosis is associated with a poor prognosis [14, 21]. If there is no resolution of thrombosis within 2–3 days, and especially if the patient reports with signs and symptoms of thrombosis going back several days, serious consideration should be given to thrombolytic therapy with tissue-type plasminogen activator (t-PA). The use of this appears to have reduced with quick commencement of eculizumab. Fibrinolytic therapy may be dangerous in those with cerebral vein thrombosis, since it may convert thrombotic stroke into hemorrhagic one. A recent review of nine patients receiving intravenous t-PA on 15 occasions reported serious complications in three, so thrombolysis must be considered a high-risk intervention [98]. The use of eculizumab during the initial treatment of acute thrombosis has also been recommended [11]. The increasing use of eculizumab in the management of acute thrombosis in patients with PNH is providing effective and positive experience in a number of cases including acute Budd-Chiari syndrome [99, 100]. Development of any thrombosis in a patient with PNH is now considered one of the primary indications for eculizumab therapy, and this should be done without delay.

Patients with recurrent episodes are managed as other patients with a clinically manifested hypercoagulable state, using warfarin for an identified period in addition to eculizumab. In the absence of concomitant treatment with eculizumab, antithrombotic therapy alone has not been effective in preventing further episodes of thrombosis in PNH.

9.4.2 *Prophylaxis*

In the study of Socie et al. [3], 30 % of French patients experienced an episode of thrombosis within 8 years of the diagnosis of PNH, and approximately 50 % of patients were predicted to have this complication within 15 years. Because of the relatively high incidence of thrombosis and its associated morbidity and mortality, an argument can be made for prophylactic anticoagulation in patients without contraindications such as severe thrombocytopenia and who are not receiving eculizumab therapy [5, 92]. A nonrandomized study with a relatively short follow-up period suggested a significant reduction in the thrombotic events when PNH patients with >50 % PNH clones received prophylactic anticoagulation with Coumadin [92]. A second retrospective study supports the use of prophylactic anticoagulation for patients with large PNH clones (>50–60 %) [7]. The benefits of prophylactic anticoagulation, however, must be weighed against potential adverse effects of long-term anticoagulation.

Eculizumab appears to reduce the risk of thromboembolic complications [34]. For patients being treated with eculizumab who have no prior history of thromboembolic complications, prophylactic anticoagulation may be unnecessary [49]. Recently, Hillmen et al. analyzed long-term safety and efficacy of eculizumab in 195 patients over 66 months: the administration of eculizumab reduced the thromboembolic incidence rate from 11.13 events per 100 patient-years to 2.14 events per 100 patient-years, a relative reduction of 81.8 % [101]. Administration of eculizumab decreases markers of thrombin generation and inflammation in patients with PNH, indicating the central role of complement activation in the pathogenesis of thrombosis in PNH [102]. Successful discontinuation of anticoagulation following eculizumab administration has been reported in three PNH patients with severe thrombotic history [103]. However, others recommend continuing anticoagulation even with eculizumab therapy when there has been a prior thrombosis in PNH patients if no contraindication [11, 49, 104]. Accumulation of the long-term management with eculizumab alone in the prevention of thrombosis may change the standard protocol against thrombosis in PNH.

Anticoagulation when not clinically contraindicated for patients for whom eculizumab is not available for any reason: If a patient has had one or more episodes of thrombosis, whether witnessed or presumed from the history, anticoagulation is required. Long-term anticoagulation with a target INR of 2.5 for patients with large proportion of PNH cells (PNH granulocytes or monocytes >50 %) and a platelet count greater than 100×10^9/L is recommended; anticoagulation can also be considered for patients with smaller proportion of PNH cells and platelet counts less than 100×10^9/L dependent on additional factors for thrombosis and bleeding [105].

Prophylaxis with heparin (7,500–10,000 units twice a day) or LMW heparin should be instituted in any perioperative period, during immobilization, or when an indwelling intravenous catheter is used. Such prophylaxis should also be started in the first trimester of pregnancy and continued until 6 weeks postpartum. The role of eculizumab in these settings is discussed in Chap. 21 by Dr. Miyasaka.

9.5 Conclusion

Thrombotic complication is the leading cause of death in PNH. Prevention of thrombosis and effective treatment of thrombosis at early stage improve its prognosis. Although multiple factors are likely to be involved in the development of thrombosis in PNH and all of them are contributing in some extent, complement activation plays a central role in the pathophysiology. Intercommunication between the two major host protection systems, the coagulation and complement cascades, obviously makes a vicious circle potentiating the thrombotic mechanisms in PNH. The key role of complement activation in the development of thrombosis is clinically demonstrated by the effectiveness of the administration of eculizumab in the prevention of thrombosis in PNH. Management of thrombosis in PNH should be designed according to the understanding of the pathophysiology underlying the thrombosis in PNH, with appropriate usage of eculizumab in combination with thrombolytic and anticoagulation strategies.

Acknowledgment We thank Dr. Shinya Katsutani, Hiroshima University Hospital, for his provision of a CT of splenic vein thrombosis in a patient with PNH. We also thank Dr. Yukinori Kozuma, University of Tsukuba, for his cooperation with HN at flow cytometric analysis of complement-mediated activation of platelets in PNH.

References

1. Parker C, Omine M, Richards S et al (2005) International PNH International Interest Group. Diagnosis and management of paroxysmal nocturnal hemoglobinuria. Blood 106:3699–3709
2. Takeda J, Miyata T, Kawagoe K et al (1993) Deficiency of the GPI anchor caused by a somatic mutation of the PIG-A gene in paroxysmal nocturnal hemoglobinuria. Cell 73:703–711
3. Socie G, Mary JY, de Gramont A et al (1996) Paroxysmal nocturnal haemoglobinuria: long-term follow-up and prognostic factors. Lancet 348:573–577
4. de Latour RP, Mary JY, Salanoubat C et al (2008) Paroxysmal nocturnal hemoglobinuria: natural history of disease subcategories. Blood 112:3099–3106
5. Hillmen P, Lewis SM, Bessler M et al (1995) Natural history of paroxysmal nocturnal hemoglobinuria. N Engl J Med 333:1253–1258
6. Nishimura J, Kanakura Y, Ware RE et al (2004) Clinical course and flow cytometric analysis of paroxysmal nocturnal hemoglobinuria in the United States and Japan. Medicine 83:193–207
7. Moyo VM, Mukhina GL, Garrett ES et al (2004) Natural history of paroxysmal nocturnal haemoglobinuria using modern diagnostic assays. Br J Haematol 126:133–138
8. Markiewski MM, Nilsson B, Ekdahl KN et al (2007) Complement and coagulation: stranger or partners in crime? Trends Immunol 28:184–192
9. Delvaeye M, Conway EM (2009) Coagulation and innate immune responses: can we view them separately? Blood 114:2367–2374
10. Oikonopoulou K, Ricklin D, Ward PA et al (2012) Interaction between coagulation and complement – their role in inflammation. Semin Immunopathol 34:151–165
11. Hill A, Kelly RJ, Hillmen P (2013) Thrombosis in paroxysmal nocturnal hemoglobinuria. Blood 121:4985–4996
12. Araten DJ, Thaler HT, Luzzatto L (2005) High incidence of thrombosis in African-American and Latin-American patients with paroxysmal nocturnal haemoglobinuria. Thromb Haemost 93:88–91
13. Schrezenmeier H, Muus P, Socie et al (2014) Baseline characteristics and disease burden in patients in the international paroxysmal nocturnal hemoglobinuria registry. Haematologica 99:922–929
14. McMullin MF, Hillmen P, Jackson J et al (1994) Tissue plasminogen activator for hepatic vein thrombosis in paroxysmal nocturnal haemoglobinuria. J Intern Med 235:85–89
15. Ziakas PD, Poulou LS, Rokas GI et al (2007) Thrombosis in paroxysmal nocturnal hemoglobinuria: sites, risks, outcome. An overview. J Thromb Haemost 5:642–645
16. Hoekstra J, Leebeek FW, Plessier A et al (2009) European network for vascular disorders of the liver. Paroxysmal nocturnal hemoglobinuria in Budd-Chiari syndrome: findings from a cohort study. J Hepatol 51:696–706
17. Singer AL, Locke JE, Stewart ZA et al (2009) Successful liver transplantation for Budd-Chiari syndrome in a patient with paroxysmal nocturnal hemoglobinuria treated with the anti-complement antibody eculizumab. Liver Transpl 15:540–543

18. Hill A, Sapsford RJ, Scally A et al (2012) Under-recognized complications in patients with paroxysmal nocturnal haemoglobinuria: raised pulmonary pressure and reduced right ventricular function. Br J Haematol 158:409–414
19. Nafa K, Bessler M, Mason P et al (1996) Factor V Leiden mutation investigated by amplification created restriction enzyme site (ACRES) in PNH patients with and without thrombosis. Haematologica 81:540–542
20. Dragoni F, Iori AP, Pignoloni et al (2010) Thrombophilic screening in patients with paroxysmal nocturnal haemoglobinuria: a pilot study. Br J Haematol 150:492–494
21. Peytremann R, Rhodes RS, Hartmann RC (1972) Thrombosis in paroxysmal nocturnal hemoglobinuria (PNH) with particular reference to progressive, diffuse hepatic venous thrombosis. Ser Hematol 5:115–136
22. Valla D, Dhumeaux D, Babany G et al (1987) Hepatic vein thrombosis in paroxysmal nocturnal hemoglobinuria. A spectrum from asymptomatic occlusion of hepatic venules to fatal Budd-Chiari syndrome. Gatroenterology 93:569–575
23. Allen TM, Williamson P, Schiegel RA (1988) Phosphatidylserine as a determinant of reticuloendothelial recognition of liposome models of the erythrocyte surface. Proc Natl Acad Sci U S A 85:8067–8071
24. Mathieu D, Rahmouni A, Villeneuve P et al (1995) Impact of magnetic resonance imaging on the diagnosis of abdominal complications of paroxysmal nocturnal hemoglobinuria. Blood 85:3283–3288
25. Haughton J et al (2012) Improved outcome of Budd-Chiari syndrome in paroxysmal nocturnal hemoglobinuria with eculizumab therapy. Blood (ASH Annual Meeting Abstracts) 120(21):abstract 3478
26. Zimmerman D, Bell WR (1980) Venous thrombosis and splenic rupture in paroxysmal nocturnal hemoglobinuria. Am J Med 68:275–279
27. Poulou LS, Xila V, Rokas GI et al (2008) Temporal trends in mortality rates from visceral vein thrombosis in paroxysmal nocturnal haemoglobinuria: an optimal view. Thromb Haemost 99:642–645
28. Ziakas PD, Poulou LS, Pomoni A (2008) Thrombosis in paroxysmal nocturnal hemoglobinuria at a glance: a clinical review. Curr Vasc Pharmacol 6:347–353
29. Katsutani S, Ichinohe T (2014) Experience of eculizumab in a case of PNH with recurrent acute renal failure and thrombosis. PNH Front 1:50–53 (Japanese)
30. Donhowe SP, Lazaro RP (1984) Dural sinus thrombosis in paroxysmal nocturnal hemoglobinuria. Clin Neurol Neurosurg 86:149–152
31. Rietschel RL, Lewis CW, Simmons RA et al (1978) Skin lesions in paroxysmal nocturnal hemoglobinuria. Arch Dermatol 114:560–563
32. Watt SG, Winhoven S, Hay CR et al (2007) Purpura fulminans in paroxysmal nocturnal haemoglobinuria. Br J Haematol 137:271
33. Zhao H, Shattil S (2013) Cutaneous thrombosis in PNH. Blood 122:3249
34. Hillmen P, Muus P, Duhrsen U et al (2007) Effect of the complement inhibitor eculizumab on thromboembolism in patients with paroxysmal nocturnal hemoglobinuria. Blood 110:4123–4128
35. von Stuckrad-Barre S, Berkefeld J, Steckel D et al (2003) Cerebral arterial thrombosis in paroxysmal nocturnal hemoglobinuria. J Neurol 250:756–757
36. Audebert HJ, Planck J, Eisenburg M et al (2005) Cerebral ischemic infarction in paroxysmal nocturnal hemoglobinuria report of 2 cases and updated review of 7 previously published patients. J Neurol 252:1379–1386
37. Lee JW, Jang JH, Kim JS et al (2013) Clinical signs and symptoms associated with increased risk for thrombosis in patients with paroxysmal nocturnal hemoglobinuria from a Korean Registry. Int J Hematol 97:749–757
38. Dixon RH, Rosse WF (1977) Mechanism of complement-mediated activation of human blood platelets in vitro. J Clin Invest 59:360–368
39. Gralnick HR, Vail M, McKeown LP et al (1995) Activated platelets in paroxysmal nocturnal haemoglobinuria. Br J Haematol 91:697–702

40. Wiedmer T, Hall SE, Ortel TL et al (1993) Complement-induced vesiculation and exposure of membrane prothrombinase sites in platelets of paroxysmal nocturnal hemoglobinuria. Blood 82:1192–1196
41. Devine DV, Siegel RS, Rosse WF (1987) Interaction of the platelets in paroxysmal nocturnal hemoglobinuria with complement. Relationship to defects in the regulation of complement and to platelet survival in vivo. J Clin Invest 79:131–137
42. Wiedmer T, Esmon CT, Sims PJ (1986) Complement proteins C5b-9 stimulate procoagulant activity through platelet prothrombinase. Blood 68:875–880
43. Shattil SJ, Cunningham M, Wiedmer T et al (1992) Regulation of glycoprotein IIb-IIIa receptor function studied with platelets permeabilized by the pore-forming complement proteins C5b-9. J Biol Chem 267:18424–18431
44. Sims PJ, Fainoni EM, Wiedmer T et al (1988) Complement proteins C5b-9 cause release of membrane vesicles from the platelet surface that are enriched in the membrane receptor factor Va and express prothrombinase activity. J Biol Chem 263:18205–18212
45. Gilbert GE, Sims PJ, Wiedmer T et al (1991) Platelet-derived microparticles express high affinity receptors for factor VIII. J Biol Chem 266:17261–17268
46. Hugel B, Socie G, Vu T et al (1999) Elevated levels of circulating procoagulant microparticles in patients with paroxysmal nocturnal hemoglobinuria and aplastic anemia. Blood 93:3451–3456
47. van Bijnen ST, van Heede WL, Muus P (2012) Mechanisms and clinical implications of thrombosis in paroxysmal nocturnal hemoglobinuria. J Thromb Haemost 10:1–10
48. Harmon JT, Jamieson GA (1986) Activation of platelets by alpha-thrombin is a receptor-mediated event. D-phenylalanyl-L-prolyl-L-arginine chloromethyl ketone-thrombin, but not N alpha-tosyl-L-lysine chloromethyl ketone-thrombin, binds to the high affinity thrombin receptor. J Biol Chem 261:15928–15933
49. Kelly RJ, Hill A, Arnold LM et al (2011) Long-term treatment with eculizumab in paroxysmal nocturnal hemoglobinuria: sustained efficacy and improved survival. Blood 117:6786–6792
50. Massberg S, Grahl L, von Bruehl ML et al (2010) Reciprocal coupling of coagulation and innate immunity via neutrophil serine proteases. Nat Med 16:887–896
51. del Conde I, Cruz MA, Zhang et al (2005) Platelet activation leads to activation and propagation of the complement system. J Exp Med 201:871–879
52. Hamad OA, Ekdahl KN, Nilsson PH et al (2008) Complement activation triggered by chondroitin sulfate released by thrombin receptor-activated platelets. J Thromb Haemost 6:1413–1421
53. Grunewald M, Grunewald A, Schmid A et al (2004) The platelet function defect of paroxysmal nocturnal haemoglobinuria. Platelets 15:145–154
54. Dessypris EN, Gleaton JH, Clark DA (1988) Increased sensitivity to complement of megakaryocyte progenitors in paroxysmal nocturnal haemoglobinuria. Br J Haematol 69:305–309
55. Lewis DA, Nyska A, Potti A et al (2006) Hemostatic activation in a chemically induced rat model of severe hemolysis and thrombosis. Thromb Res 118:747–753
56. Rother RP, Bell L, Hillmen et al (2005) The clinical sequelae of intravascular hemolysis and extracellular plasma hemoglobin: a novel mechanism of human disease. JAMA 293:1653–1662
57. Olsen SB, Tang DB, Jackson MR et al (1996) Enhancement of platelet deposition by cross-linked hemoglobin in a rat carotid endarterectomy model. Circulation 93:327–332
58. Simionatto OS, Cabal R, Jones RL et al (1988) Thrombophlebitis and disturbed hemostasis following administration of intravenous hematin in normal volunteers. Am J Med 85:538–540
59. Studt JD, Kremer Hovinga JA, Antoine G et al (2005) Fatal congenital thrombotic thrombocytopenia purpura with apparent ADAMTS13 inhibitor: in vitro inhibition of ADAMTS13 activity by hemoglobin. Blood 105:542–544

60. Ataga KI, Cappellini MD, Rachmilewitz EA (2007) β-thalassaemia and sickle cell anaemia as paradigms of hypercoagulability. Br J Haematol 139:3–13
61. Amer J, Zelig O, Fibach E (2008) Oxidative status of red blood cells, neutrophils, and platelets in paroxysmal nocturnal hemoglobinuria. Exp Hematol 36:369–377
62. Ignarro LJ, Buga GM, Wood KS et al (1987) Endothelium-derived relaxing factor produced and released from artery and vein is nitric oxide. Proc Natl Acad Sci U S A 84:9265–9269
63. Arnold WP, Mittal CK, Katsuki S et al (1977) Nitric oxide activate guanylate cyclase and increases guanosine 3':5'-cyclic monophosphate levels in various tissue preparations. Proc Natl Acad Sci U S A 74:3203–3207
64. Kaul DK, Hebbel RP (2000) Hypoxia/reoxygenation causes inflammatory response in transgenic sickle mice but not in normal mice. J Clin Invest 106:411–420
65. Hebbel RP, Osarogiagbon R, Kaul D (2004) The endothelial biology of sickle cell disease: inflammation and a chronic vasculopathy. Microcirculation 11:129–151
66. Peng HB, Spiecker M, Liao JK (1998) Inducible nitric oxide: an autoregulatory feedback inhibitor of vascular inflammation. J Immunol 161:1970–1976
67. Hu W, Jin R, Zhang J et al (2010) The critical roles of platelet activation and reduced NO bioavailability in fatal pulmonary arterial hypertension in a murine hemolysis model. Blood 116:1613–1622
68. Catani MV, Bernassola F, Rossi A et al (1998) Inhibition of clotting factor XIII activity by nitric oxide. Biochem Biophys Res Commun 249:275–278
69. Shao J, Miyata T, Yamada K et al (2001) Protective role of nitric oxide in a model of thrombotic microangiopathy in rats. J Am Soc Nephrol 12:2088–2097
70. Kayanoki Y, Kawata S, Yamasaki E et al (1999) Reduced nitric oxide production by L-arginine deficiency in lysinuric protein intolerance exacerbates intravascular coagulation. Metabolism 48:1136–1140
71. Schechter AN, Gladwin MT (2003) Hemoglobin and the paracrine and endocrine of nitric oxide. N Engl J Med 348:1483–1485
72. Hill A, Rother RP, Wang X et al (2010) Effect of eculizumab on haemolysis-associated nitric oxide depletion, dyspnoea, and measures of pulmonary hypertension in patients with paroxysmal nocturnal haemoglobinuria. Br J Haematol 149:411–425
73. Morris CR, Kuypers FA, Larkin S et al (2000) Patterns of arginine and nitric oxide in patients with sickle cell disease with vasoocclusive crisis and acute chest syndrome. J Pediatr Hematol Oncol 22:515–520
74. Simak J, Holada K, Risitano AM et al (2004) Elevated circulating endothelial membrane microparticles in paroxysmal nocturnal haemoglobinuria. Br J Haematol 125:804–813
75. Kozuma Y, Sawahata Y, Takei Y et al (2011) Procoagulant properties of microparticles released from red blood cells in paroxysmal nocturnal haemoglobinuria. Br J Haematol 152:631–639
76. Ploug M, Plesner T, Ronne E et al (1992) The receptor for urokinase-type plasminogen activator is deficient on peripheral blood leukocytes in patients with paroxysmal nocturnal hemoglobinuria. Blood 79:1447–1455
77. Ronne E, Papott H, Grondahl-Hansen J et al (1995) The receptor for urokinase plasminogen activator is present in plasma from healthy donors and elevated in patients with paroxysmal nocturnal haemoglobinuria. Br J Haematol 89:576–581
78. Ninomiya H, Hasegawa Y, Nagasawa T et al (1997) Excess soluble urokinase-type plasminogen activator receptor in the plasma of patients with paroxysmal nocturnal hemoglobinuria inhibits cell-associated fibrinolytic activity. Int J Hematol 65:285–291
79. Maroney SA, Cunningham AC, Ferrel J et al (2006) A GPI-anchored co-receptor for tissue factor pathway inhibitor controls its intracellular trafficking and cell-surface expression. J Thromb Haemost 4:1114–1124

80. Saadi S, Holzknecht RA, Patte CP et al (1995) Complement-mediated regulation of tissue factor activity in endothelium. J Exp Med 182:1807–1814
81. Koshkaryev A, Barshtein G, Nyska A et al (2003) 2-butoxyethanol enhance the adherence of red blood cells. Arch Toxicol 77:465–469
82. Muhlfelder TW, Niemetz J, Kreutzer D et al (1979) C5 chemotactic fragment induces leukocyte production of tissue factor activity: a link between complement and coagulation. J Clin Invest 63:147–150
83. Ikeda K, Nagasawa K, Horiuchi T et al (1997) C5a induces tissue factor activity on endothelial cells. Throm Haemost 77:394–398
84. Tedesco F, Pausa M, Nardon E et al (1997) The cytolytically inactive terminal complement complex activates endothelial cells to express adhesion molecules and tissue factor procoagulant activity. J Exp Med 185:1619–1627
85. Helley D, de Latour RP, Porcher R et al (2010) Evaluation of hemostasis and endothelial function in patients with paroxysmal nocturnal hemoglobinuria receiving eculizumab. Haematologica 95:574–584
86. Cole DS, Morgan BP (2003) Beyond lysis: how complement influences cell surface. Clin Sci 104:455–466
87. Ritis K, Doumas M, Mastellos D et al (2006) A novel C5a receptor-tissue factor cross-talk in neutrophils links innate immunity to coagulation pathways. J Immunol 177:4794–4802
88. Lieben HA, Feinstein (2003) Thrombosis in patients with paroxysmal nocturnal hemoglobinuria is associated with markedly elevated plasma levels of leukocyte-derived tissue factor. Thromb Res 111:235–238
89. Mouzner K, DiNardo A, Goldstein K (2007) Thrombotic thrombocytopenic purpura during immune reconstruction. AIDS 21:2559–2560
90. Huber-Lang M, Sarma JV, Zetoune FS et al (2006) Generation of C5a in the absence of C3: a new complement activation pathway. Nat Med 12:682–687
91. Amara U, Flierl MA, Rittirsch D et al (2010) Molecular intercommunication between the complement and coagulation systems. J Immunol 185:5628–5636
92. Hall C, Richards S, Hillmen P (2003) Primary prophylaxis with warfarin prevents thrombosis in paroxysmal nocturnal hemoglobinuria (PNH). Blood 102:3587–3591
93. Fowkes FJ, Price JF, Fowkes FG (2003) Incidence of diagnosed deep vein thrombosis in the general population: systematic review. Eur J Vasc Endovasc Surg 25:1–5
94. Brodsky RA (2009) How I treat paroxysmal nocturnal hemoglobinuria. Blood 113:6522–6527
95. Luzzatto L, Gianfaldoni G, Notaro R (2011) Management of paroxysmal nocturnal haemoglobinuria: a personal view. Br J Haematol 153:709–720
96. Rosse WF (1982) Treatment of paroxysmal nocturnal hemoglobinuria. Blood 55:20–23
97. Sholar PW, Bell WR (1985) Thrombolytic therapy for inferior vena cava thrombosis in paroxysmal nocturnal hemoglobinuria. Ann Intern Med 103:539–541
98. Araten DJ, Notaro R, Thaler HT et al (2012) Thrombolytic therapy is effective in paroxysmal nocturnal hemoglobinuria: a series of nine patients and a review of the literature. Haematologica 97:344–352
99. Brodsky A, Mazzocchi O, Sanchez G et al (2012) Eculizumab in paroxysmal nocturnal hemoglobinuria with Budd-Chiari syndrome progressing despite anticoagulation. Exp Hematol Oncol 1:26
100. Mandala E, Lafaras C, Tsioni K et al (2013) Treatment of a patient with classical paroxysmal nocturnal hemoglobinuria and Budd-Chiari syndrome, with complement inhibitor eculizumab: case report. Hippokralia 147:81–84
101. Hillmen P, Muus P, Roth A et al (2013) Long-term safety and efficacy of sustained eculizumab treatment in patients with paroxysmal nocturnal haemoglobinuria. Br J Haematol 162:62–73

102. Weitz IC, Razavi P, Rochanda L et al (2012) Eculizumab therapy results in rapid and sustained decreases in markers of thrombin generation and inflammation in patients with PNH independent of its effects on hemolysis and microparticle formation. Thromb Res 130:361–368
103. Emadi A, Brodsky RA (2009) Successful discontinuation of anticoagulation following eculizumab administration in paroxysmal nocturnal hemoglobinuria. Am J Hematol 84:699–701
104. Parker CJ (2011) Management of paroxysmal nocturnal hemoglobinuria in the era of complement inhibitory therapy. Hematol Am Soc Hematol Educ Program 2011:21–29
105. Baglin TP, Keeling DM, Watson HG, British Committee for Standards in Haematology (2005) Guidelines on oral anticoagulation (warfarin): third edition-2005 update. Br J Haematol 132:277–285

Chapter 10
Diagnosis and Classification of PNH

Hideki Nakakuma, Tsutomu Shichishima, and Jun-ichi Nishimura

Abstract PNH is an acquired stem cell disorder of a clonal nature characterized by complement-mediated intravascular hemolysis negative for the direct antiglobulin test (DAT, Coombs test), a thrombotic tendency, bone marrow dysfunction, and infrequent development of leukemia. Hemolysis and thrombosis are currently accepted as ascribable to deficiency of a series of glycosylphosphatidylinositol (GPI)-linked membrane proteins including decay-accelerating factor (DAF, CD55) and CD59 with complement-regulatory activity on blood cells. The deficiency is due to a synthetic defect of GPI caused by mutations of genes (virtually *PIGA*) involved in the steps of GPI biosynthesis. It has been suggested that PNH bone marrow failure is closely associated with acquired aplastic anemia, and it is considered to be immune mediated. For the diagnosis of PNH, identification of the three major clinical manifestations of hemolysis, thrombosis, and bone marrow dysfunction, as well as the detection of a simultaneous lack of multiple GPI-linked membrane proteins in individual blood cell lineages, reflecting the defect of GPI and mutations of GPI biosynthesis genes like *PIGA* in hematopoietic stem cells, is needed. Flow cytometry detects all blood cells lacking any GPI proteins, while conventional hemolytic tests such as the Ham's acidified serum test (the Ham test) and the sugar-water test detect only PNH erythrocytes susceptible to autologous complement. The evaluation of hemolysis, thrombosis, and underlying bone marrow disorder virtually defines PNH classification and disease severity.

Keywords Hemolysis • Complement-regulatory protein • Flow cytometry • Ham test • Thrombosis • Bone marrow failure

---

H. Nakakuma (✉)
Kagoshima-Tokushukai Hospital, 3-8-1 Shimo-Arata, Kagoshima 890-0056, Japan
e-mail: hideki.nakakuma@tokushukai.jp

T. Shichishima, M.D., Ph.D.
Department of Hematology and Oncology, Fukushima Medical University,
1 Hikariga-oka, Fukushima 960-1295, Japan

Fukushima Research Institute of Environment and Medicine,
16-6 Mito-uchi Houkida-aza, Fukushima 960-8560, Japan

J.-i. Nishimura
Department of Hematology and Oncology, Osaka University Graduate School of Medicine,
2-2 Yamadaoka, Suita 565-0871, Osaka, Japan

Y. Kanakura et al. (eds.), *Paroxysmal Nocturnal Hemoglobinuria*,
DOI 10.1007/978-4-431-56003-6_10

10.1 Definition and Diagnostic Criteria for PNH [1, 2]

For clinical manifestations characteristic of PNH, one or more affected stem cells with mutation of the glycosylphosphatidylinositol (GPI) synthesis gene (virtually *PIGA*) clonally expand. Affected stem cells generate progeny deficient in several GPI-linked membrane proteins (Table 10.1). Typical PNH hemolysis is intravascular and caused by the deficiency of complement-regulatory membrane proteins, such as decay-accelerating factor (DAF, CD55) and CD59 on erythrocytes. Thrombophilia is also dependent on GPI deficiency and a major cause of death in Europe and the United States of America compared to Asia and Japan (Table 10.2) [3, 4]. PNH often develops in the context of bone marrow failure syndromes and is closely associated with aplastic anemia [5]. Marrow failure is more marked in patients in Asia than in Europe and North America. The median age at diagnosis of PNH of 176 Duke University patients and 209 Japanese patients was 30 years (ranging from 4 to 80) and 45 years (ranging from 10 to 86 years), respectively [4]. In short, PNH is virtually diagnosed on the basis of an acquired Coombs-negative intravascular hemolysis of GPI-negative erythrocytes susceptible to autologous complement, hemolysis-associated thrombosis, and underlying bone marrow failure.

Table 10.1 GPI-linked membrane proteins missing from PNH blood cells [29]

Complement-regulatory proteins DAF (CD55), CD59	
Enzymes	Neutrophil alkaline phosphatase
	Erythrocyte acetylcholinesterase, BST-1 (CD157)
	Ecto-5′ nucleotidase (CD73)
Receptors	CD14, CD16b (FcγRIII), folate receptor,
	Urokinase-type plasminogen activator receptor (CD87)
Adhesion molecules	
Others	Blast-1 (CD48), LFA-3 (CD58), GPI-80, CD66e (CEA),
	CD66b, CD66c, JMH blood group antigen (CD108),
	CD24, CD52, CD109, CLBgran/5, Thy-1 (CD90),
	NB-1(CD177), cellular prion protein,
	Eosinophil-derived neurotoxin (EDN)

Table 10.2 Clinical and laboratory features at PNH diagnosis [4]

	Duke University 176 patients	Japan 209 patients
Preceding disorder		
Aplastic anemia	51 (29 %)	79 (38 %)
MDS	9 (5 %)	10 (5 %)
Signs and symptoms		
Hemoglobinuria	88 (50 %)	70 (33 %)
Anemia	155 (88 %)	197 (94 %)
Leukocytopenia	80 (45 %)	151 (72 %)
Thrombocytopenia	92 (52 %)	132 (63 %)
Thrombosis	34 (19 %)	13 (6 %)
Laboratory tests (Mean)		
Leukocytes (10^6/L)	4948	3475
Hemoglobin (g/dL)	9.7	8.2
Platelets (10^9/L)	140	96
LDH (U/L)	2337	1572

Table 10.3 Minimal essential diagnostic criteria

A.	Collecting evidence for hemolysis
	Decrease of serum haptoglobin, increase of serum lactate dehydrogenase, increase of unconjugated bilirubin, jaundice, relative reticulocytosis, hemoglobinuria, hemosiderinuria
B.	Detection of blood cells deficient in GPI-anchored membrane proteins
	Detection of PNH type III erythrocytes more than 1 % is recommended in the peripheral blood

10.2 Collecting Evidence Supporting PNH [1, 2, 4]

10.2.1 Hemolysis

Hemolysis is indicated by a decreased serum haptoglobin level, increased serum lactate dehydrogenase (LDH) activity, increased unconjugated bilirubin, jaundice, and relative reticulocytosis (Table 10.3). In contrast with autoimmune hemolytic anemias, hemolysis of PNH erythrocytes that are susceptible to complement does not deplete serum complement (i.e., CH50 level is not low), despite complement-mediated hemolysis. The hemolysis is antibody independent, i.e., negative for Coombs' test (direct antiglobulin test, DAT). Typical PNH hemolysis is intravascular and then manifests hemoglobinuria and hemosiderinuria (Fig. 10.1). The findings of hemolysis are markedly exacerbated in hemolytic precipitation induced by various infections [6].

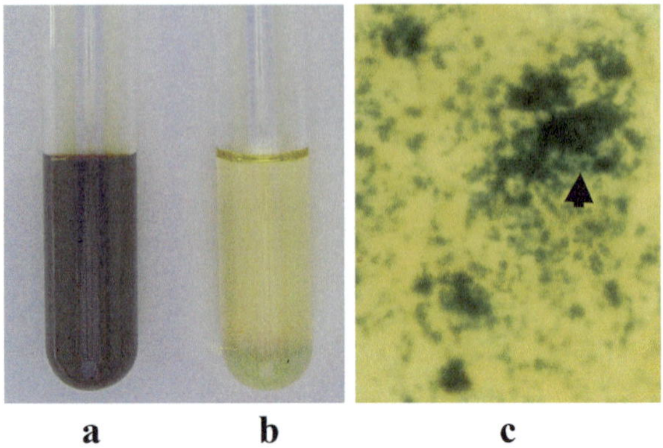

Fig. 10.1 Intravascular hemolysis characteristic of PNH. (**a**) and (**c**), hemoglobinuria (*dark* urine) and hemosiderinuria (the *arrow* indicates hemosiderin), respectively, of a patient with PNH; (**b**) urine of a healthy volunteer

10.2.2 Anemia

Anemia in patients with PNH is ascribable to hemolysis with relative reticulocytosis, iron deficiency associated with intravascular hemolysis, and marrow failure. Depending on each cause, the mean corpuscular volume (MCV) of erythrocytes of PNH patients shows macro-, micro-, and normocytic, respectively.

10.2.3 In Vitro Hemolysis Tests

PNH erythrocytes, which lack GPI-linked complement-regulatory membrane proteins such as DAF (CD55) and CD59, are susceptible to autologous complement. The existence of PNH erythrocytes in peripheral blood is demonstrable by in vitro hemolysis tests such as the Ham test [7] (Fig. 10.2) and sugar-water test. [8] In the Ham test (acidified serum lysis test), the alternative pathway of complement is activated by adjusting the serum pH to around 6.5 with weak acid. In the sugar-water test, complements are activated under low-electrolyte conditions and normal osmolarity maintained by supplying serum with sugar water. Positive results in the hemolysis tests need more than 10 % hemolysis. However, the hemolysis tests require experienced technicians, without whom the results are not always reliable.

10.2.4 Synthetic Defect of GPI in Hematopoietic Stem Cells

The distinct characters of PNH are the blood cell-restricted deficiency of GPI-linked membrane proteins in every blood cell lineage and the coexistence of both blood cells that are positive and negative for GPI-inked membrane proteins.

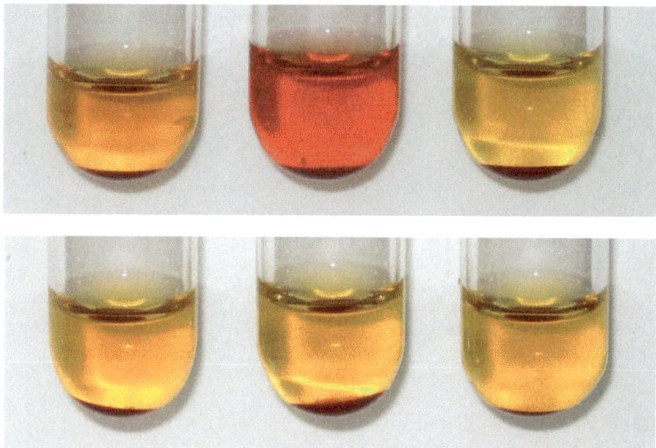

Fig. 10.2 Ham test for the detection of PNH erythrocytes. Affected erythrocytes susceptible to autologous complement of a patient with PNH undergo in vitro hemolysis in complement-activated serum treated with acid. In contrast, affected erythrocytes survive in the pretreatment serum and in the heat-inactivated serum. Erythrocytes of a healthy donor are intact in each serum

The expression of GPI-linked proteins on blood cells is analyzed by labeling with antibodies to GPI-linked proteins and subsequent flow cytometry (Fig. 10.3) [9, 10]. For the diagnosis of PNH, flow cytometry is the most reliable test to detect and quantify affected cells among erythrocytes, leukocytes, and platelets in peripheral blood as well as bone marrow cells [11], in contrast with the hemolysis tests such as the Ham test and sugar-water test that detect only PNH erythrocytes. To ensure PNH diagnosis, demonstration of the deficiency of a series of GPI-linked membrane proteins on two or more blood cell lineages is preferable. Instead of antibodies to GPI-linked proteins, aerolysin (FLAER), a fluorescence-conjugated bateriotoxin, which binds directly to membrane GPI, is used to discriminate PNH cells [12]. However, FLAER is not suitable for the analysis of erythrocytes and platelets because the toxin injures the glycophorin-expressing blood cells. For PNH diagnosis, it is recommended to show that the proportion of affected erythrocytes is above 1 % in peripheral blood (Table 10.3). In general, the proportion of PNH granulocytes is higher than PNH erythrocytes and preferable for the early detection of PNH cells, because PNH granulocytes are not always susceptible to autologous complement. It is known that PNH granulocytes lack DAF and CD59 but express non-GPI-linked complement-regulatory proteins such as membrane cofactor protein (MCP). The proportions of PNH granulocytes and reticulocytes are then useful to evaluate the PNH clone size [13]. Flow cytometry is convenient to discriminate PNH from HEMPAS (hereditary erythroblastic multinuclearity associated with a positive acidified serum test) which is positive with the Ham test.

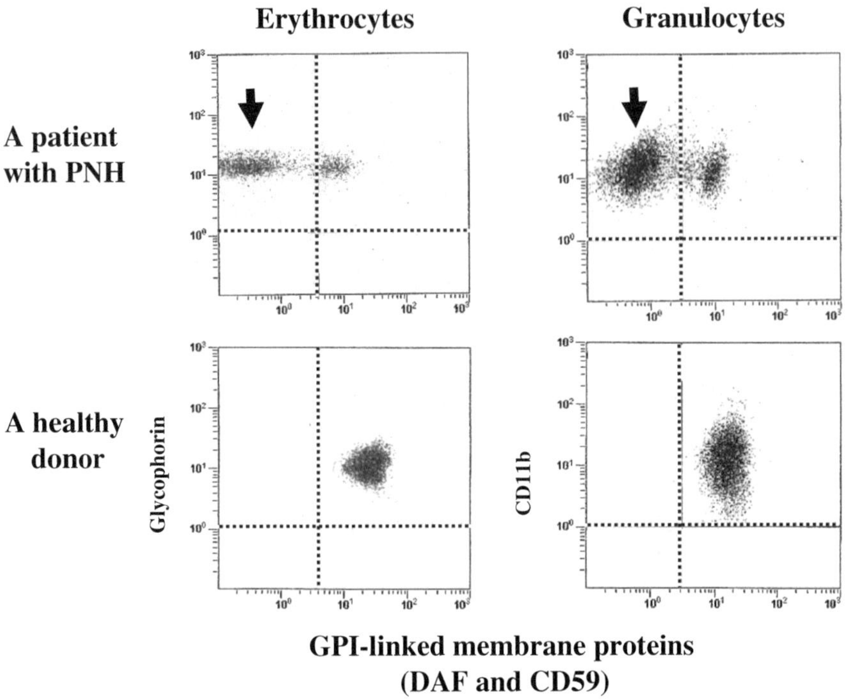

Fig. 10.3 Flow cytometric detection of PNH blood cells. Arrows indicate PNH cells that are negative for GPI-linked membrane proteins such as DAF (CD55) and CD59 of a patient with PNH. Coexistence of blood cells positive and negative for the proteins in a single patient is of note. None of the blood cells of a healthy donor are negative for DAF and CD59

10.2.5 PIGA *Mutations*

An acquired somatic null mutation of *PIGA* causes both the synthetic defect of GPI and deficiency of GPI-linked membrane proteins of blood cells (Fig. 10.4), leading to clinical manifestations characteristic of PNH. Germ line null mutations of *PIGA* have been suggested to be lethal [14, 15]. PNH hemolysis is not demonstrable in hypomorphic inherited germ line mutations of *PIGA* [16]. Although the detection of *PIGA* mutation confirms the PNH diagnosis, technical problems limit its routine clinical application for the diagnosis. It has been reported that, in a single patient with PNH, multiple affected clones with individual *PIGA* mutations are often detected, indicating that PNH is oligoclonal rather than clonal [17]. In support of this, PNH cells are often not phenotypically homogenous but rather mosaic. For example, a single patient with PNH has blood cells both completely negative (type III) and partially positive (type II) for DAF and CD59 [1]. Of note, instead of

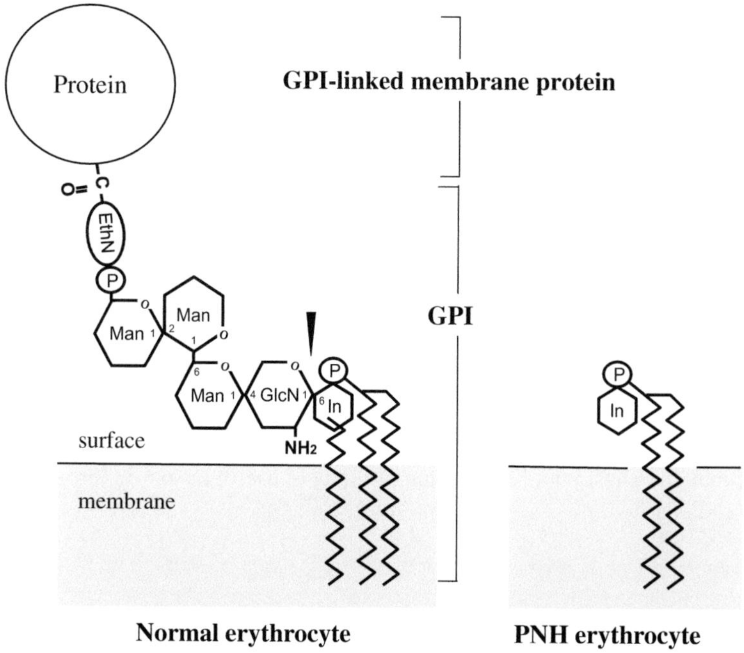

Fig. 10.4 Synthetic defect of GPI in PNH blood cells [29]. In the normal erythrocyte (*left panel*), GPI is composed of phosphatidylinositol (InP), N-acetylglucosamine (GlcN), 3 mannoses (Man), and ethanolamine phosphate (EthN-P). Proteins are covalently attached to EthN-P of GPI. In contrast, in the PNH erythrocyte (*right panel*), both the carbohydrate chain of GPI and protein are missing

somatic mutations in X-linked *PIGA*, the current report shows an exceptional PNH case with both a heterozygous germ line mutation and a somatic mutation in autosomal *PIGT*, which is important for attachment of the preassembled GPI anchor to proteins [18].

10.2.6 Acquired Bone Marrow Failure

The bone marrow of patients with PNH shows various degrees of hypoplasia, which is compatible with differential peripheral cytopenia [5]. There are no PNH-specific morphological features in the bone marrow cells of PNH patients. Nonrandom karyotypic abnormalities associated with PNH have not been identified yet, although karyotypic abnormalities such as trisomy 8 are infrequently detected in PNH, especially in the setting of other specific bone marrow disorders such as MDS [19].

Table 10.4 Classification of PNH [1]

A.	Classic PNH
B.	PNH in the setting of another specified bone marrow disorder (e.g., PNH/aplastic anemia or PNH/refractory anemia-MDS)
C.	PNH-subclinical (PNH-sc) in the setting of another specified bone marrow disorder (e.g., PNH-sc/aplastic anemia)

10.2.7 Thrombotic Tendency

Thrombosis of unknown origin must be present to screen for PNH, i.e., Budd-Chiari syndrome, and thrombosis of veins (e.g., hepatic vein, portal vein, vena cava, mesenteric, central nervous system vein, pulmonary vein) and thrombosis of coronary and cerebral arteries. Arterial thrombosis is infrequent. Common symptoms are abdominal and chest pain [20]. Serum D-dimer is useful to survey thrombotic tendency in PNH.

10.3 PNH Classification [1]

Based on the current proposal by the members of the International PNH Interest Group, patients with PNH are classified into three subcategories: classic PNH, PNH in the setting of another specified bone marrow failure, and subclinical PNH (Table 10.4) [11, 21].

10.3.1 Classic PNH

Patients in this subcategory manifest clinically evident intravascular hemolysis (macroscopic hemoglobinuria is frequent or persistent), but do not show apparent bone marrow failure or myelodysplasia. Bone marrow shows erythroid hyperplasia and morphologically normal hematopoiesis. Eculizumab, a humanized monoclonal antibody, is effective for the florid hemolysis, because the antibody inhibits the terminal complement activation pathway by binding to complement C5 when injected intravenously [22–24].

PNH in the setting of another specified bone marrow failure. Patients in this subcategory manifest mild to moderate intravascular hemolysis (macroscopic hemoglobinuria is intermittent or absent) and also show preceding or concomitant underlying bone marrow failure mostly associated with aplastic anemia and refractory anemia/myelodysplastic syndrome [5, 11, 25]. PNH with preceding aplastic anemia is termed aplastic anemia-PNH syndrome. Approximately 30 % of PNH patients had preceding aplastic anemia. Flow cytometry showed that an average of 25 % (range, 13–52 %) of 517 patients with aplastic anemia in 7 reports had a proportion (1 % or higher) of blood cells with the PNH phenotype. PNH-type blood cells were also detected in 10–23 % of patients with myelodysplastic syndromes [25–27].

10.3.2 Subclinical PNH

Patients in this subcategory show no clinical or laboratory evidence of intravascular hemolysis, but do show evidence of concomitant bone marrow failure syndromes, such as aplastic anemia and refractory anemia/myelodysplastic syndrome [5, 11, 21, 25–27]. There is no benefit of eculizumab for PNH patients in this category [23].

10.4 Clinical Stages of PNH

PNH clones develop in hematopoietic bone marrow cells and expand to generate differentiated blood cells, including affected erythrocytes susceptible to autologous complement, leading to clinical manifestations such as intravascular hemolysis and thrombosis. Overt PNH infrequently results in spontaneous or therapy-related remission [3, 21, 28]. To assess the entire course of PNH, a staging system has been proposed: stage I, latent PNH with affected cells in bone marrow alone; stage II, smoldering PNH with affected cells in both bone marrow and peripheral leukocytes but not in erythrocytes; stage III, overt PNH which satisfies the conventional diagnostic criteria; and stage IV, dormant PNH with clinical remission [21]. However, the clinical relevance of the staging has yet to be evaluated.

10.5 Clinical Severity

The distinct character of PNH involves its complex pathophysiology and various clinical manifestations, such as intravascular hemolysis, thrombosis, and bone marrow failure. The disease severity is then dependent on the major clinical manifestations. However, it appears difficult to propose a globally applicable grading system of the disease severity that matches with the prognosis of individual patients with PNH all over the world. It is partly because major causes of death vary among races, i.e., between patients in Japan and in the United States of America [4]. Furthermore, the molecular relationships among the manifestations are not yet fully clear.

References

1. Parker CJ, Omine M, Richard S et al (2005) Diagnosis and management of paroxysmal nocturnal hemoglobinuria. Blood 106:3699–3709
2. Parker CJ (2008) Ask the hematologist: how do I diagnose and treat PNH? Hematol ASH News Rep 5:4–5
3. Hillmen P, Lewis SM, Bessler M, Luzzatto L, Dacie JV (1995) Natural history of paroxysmal nocturnal hemoglobinuria. N Engl J Med 333:1253–1258
4. Nishimura J, Kanakura Y, Ware RE et al (2004) Clinical and flow cytometric analysis of paroxysmal nocturnal hemoglobinuria in the United States and Japan. Medicine 83:193–207
5. Young NS (2000) Acquired aplastic anemia. In: Young NS (ed) Bone marrow failure syndromes. WB Saunders, Philadelphia, pp 1–46
6. Nakakuma H, Hidaka M, Nagakura S et al (1995) Expression of cryptantigen Th on paroxysmal nocturnal hemoglobinuria erythrocytes in association with a hemolytic exacerbation. J Clin Invest 96:201–206
7. Ham TH, Dingle JH (1939) Studies on destruction of red blood cells. II. Chronic hemolytic anemia with paroxysmal nocturnal hemoglobinuria: certain immunological aspects of the hemolytic mechanism with special reference to serum complement. J Clin Invest 18:657–672
8. Hartmann RC, Jenkins DE Jr (1966) The sugar-water test for paroxysmal nocturnal hemoglobinuria. N Engl J Med 275:155–157
9. van der Schoot CE, Huizinga TW, van't Veer-Korthof ET, Wijimans R, Pinkster J, von dem Borne AE (1990) Deficiency of glycosyl-phosphatidylinositol-linked membrane glycoproteins of leukocytes in paroxysmal nocturnal hemoglobinuria, description of a new diagnostic cytofluorometric assay. Blood 76:1853–1859
10. Shichishima T, Terasawa T, Saitoh Y, Hashimoto C, Ohto H, Maruyama Y (1993) Diagnosis of paroxysmal nocturnal haemoglobinuria by phenotypic analysis of erythrocytes using two-colour flow cytometry with monoclonal antibodies to DAF and CD59/MACIF. Br J Haematol 85:378–386
11. Nakakuma H, Nagakura S, Iwamoto N et al (1995) Paroxysmal nocturnal hemoglobinuria clone in bone marrow of patients with pancytopenia. Blood 85:1371–1376
12. Brodsky RA, Muhhina GL, Li S et al (2000) Improved detection and characterization of paroxysmal nocturnal hemoglobinuria using fluorescent aerolysin. Am J Clin Pathol 114:459–466
13. Iwamoto N, Kawaguchi T, Nagakura S et al (1995) Markedly high population of affected reticulocytes negative for decay-accelerating factor and CD59 in paroxysmal nocturnal hemoglobinuria. Blood 85:2228–2232
14. Keller P, Tremml G, Rosti V, Bessler M (1999) X inactivation and somatic cell selection rescue female mice carrying a Piga-null mutation. Proc Natl Acad Sci U S A 96:7479–7483
15. Chen G, Ye Z, Yu X, Zou J, Mali P, Brodsky RA, Cheng L (2008) Trophoblast differentiation defect in human embryonic stem cells lacking PIG-A and GPI-anchored cell-surface proteins. Cell Stem Cell 2:345–355
16. Johnston JJ, Gropman AL, Sapp JC et al (2012) The phenotype of a germline mutation in PIGA: the gene somatically mutated in paroxysmal nocturnal hemoglobinuria. Am J Hum Genet 90:295–300
17. Endo M, Ware RE, Vreeke TM et al (1996) Molecular basis of the heterogeneity of expression of glycosyl phosphatidylinositol anchored proteins in paroxysmal nocturnal hemoglobinuria. Blood 87:2546–2557
18. Krawitz PM, Hochsmann B, Murakami Y et al (2013) A case of paroxysmal nocturnal hemoglobinuria caused by a germline mutation and a somatic mutation in *PIGT*. Blood 122:1312–1315
19. Araten DJ, Swirsky D, Karadimitris A et al (2001) Cytogenetic and morphological abnormalities in paroxysmal nocturnal haemoglobinuria. Br J Haematol 115:360–368

20. Schrezenmeier H, Muus P, Socie G et al (2014) Baseline characteristics and disease burden in patients in the international paroxysmal nocturnal haemoglobinuria registry. Haematologica 99:922–929
21. Nakakuma H, Kawaguchi T, Horikawa K et al (1995) Proposal for a classification of the clinical stages of paroxysmal nocturnal hemoglobinuria. Blood 86:2051–2052
22. Hillmen P, Hall C, Marsh JC et al (2004) Effect of eculizumab on hemolysis and transfusion requirements in patients with paroxysmal nocturnal hemoglobinuria. N Engl J Med 350:552–559
23. Parker CJ (2009) Eculizumab for paroxysmal nocturnal hemoglobinuria. Lancet 373:759–767
24. Kanakura Y, Ohyashiki K, Shichishima T et al (2011) Safety and efficacy of the terminal complement inhibitor eculizumab in Japanese patients with paroxysmal nocturnal hemoglobinuria: the AEGIS clinical trial. Int J Hematol 93:36–46
25. Iwanaga M, Furukawa K, Amenomori T et al (1998) Paroxysmal nocturnal haemoglobinuria clones in patients with myelodysplastic syndromes. Br J Haematol 102:465–474
26. Dunn DE, Tanawattanacharoen P, Boccuni P et al (1999) Paroxysmal nocturnal hemoglobinuria cells in patients with bone marrow failure syndromes. Ann Intern Med 131:401–408
27. Kawaguchi T, Nakakuma H (2007) New insight into molecular pathogenesis of bone marrow failure in paroxysmal nocturnal hemoglobinuria. Int J Hematol 86:27–32
28. Nakakuma H, Nagakura S, Kawaguchi T et al (1994) Persistence of affected T-lymphocytes in long-term clinical remission in paroxysmal nocturnal hemoglobinuria. Blood 84:3925–3928
29. Nakakuma H, Kawaguchi T (1996) Paroxysmal nocturnal hemoglobinuria (PNH): mechanism of intravascular hemolysis. Crit Rev Oncol/Hematol 24:213–229

Chapter 11
Clinical Significance of a Small Population of Glycosylphosphatidylinositol-Anchored Membrane Proteins (GPI-APs)-Deficient Cells in the Management of Bone Marrow Failure

Shinji Nakao

Abstract Althoughan increased blood cell deficiency of glycosylphosphatidylinositol-anchored membrane proteins (GPI-APs) has often been detected in patients with aplastic anemia (AA) and myelodysplastic syndrome (MDS), the clinical significance of such GPI-APs$^-$ cells remains to be elucidated. We established a sensitive flow cytometric assay capable of precisely detecting less than 0.01 % GPI-APs$^-$ blood cells and have examined a large number of patients with bone marrow (BM) failure. The assay failed to detect a significant increase in GPI-APs$^-$ cells in the peripheral blood (PB) of 190 of 192 healthy individuals, while noting significant increases in two individuals. On the other hand, an increase in the percentage of GPI-APs$^-$ cells was detectable in approximately 50 % of all AA patients and in 20 % of all refractory anemia (RA)-MDS patients, while it was undetectable in any patients with RA with ringed sideroblasts (RARS) or an excess of blasts (RAEB) or in those with hematological malignancies, including acute myelogenous leukemia and multiple myeloma. Several recent studies have shown that the presence of an increased number of GPI-APs$^-$ cells predicted a good response to immunosuppressive therapy and a favorable prognosis among patients with AA and RA. A sensitive flow cytometric analysis that can detect a small population of GPI-APs$^-$ cells in the PB is therefore an important examination that can guide the management of BM failure.

Keywords GPI-APs$^-$ blood cells • PNH-sc • Bone marrow failure • Immunosuppressive therapy

S. Nakao, M.D., Ph.D. (✉)
Department of Hematology, Faculty of Medicine, Institute of Medical, Pharmaceutical and Health, Kanazawa University, 13-1 Takaramachi, Kanazawa, Ishikawa 920-8640, Japan
e-mail: snakao8205@staff.kanazawa-u.ac.jp

Y. Kanakura et al. (eds.), *Paroxysmal Nocturnal Hemoglobinuria*,
DOI 10.1007/978-4-431-56003-6_11

11.1 Introduction

Paroxysmal nocturnal hemoglobinuria (PNH) is an acquired hemolytic anemia characterized by an increased number of glycosylphosphatidylinositol (GPI)-anchored membrane proteins (GPI-APs$^-$)-deficient cells derived from hematopoietic stem cells (HSCs) with a *PIGA* gene mutation [10]. A small population of GPI-APs$^-$ blood cells are often detected in bone marrow (BM) failure patients who do not show either clinical or laboratory signs of hemolysis. This type of BM failure was defined as subclinical PNH (PNH-sc) by the International PNH Interest Group [12]. Several studies have attempted to clarify the clinical significance of such GPI-APs$^-$ cells in BM failure patients [1, 5, 17, 21, 22]. Some studies have revealed that the presence of GPI-APs$^-$ cells in patients with myelodysplastic syndrome (MDS) and aplastic anemia (AA) predicts a good response to immunosuppressive therapy (IST) [5, 17, 21], while others failed to confirm the predictive value of GPI-APs$^-$ cells [4, 13, 15, 19, 23]. This discrepancy may be due to differences in the sensitivity and specificity of the flow cytometric assays which were used to detect GPI-APs$^-$ cells in the previous studies.

We have been detecting GPI-APs$^-$ cells in the peripheral blood (PB) of patients with various types of BM failure using a high-sensitivity flow cytometric assay and postulated the significance of an increase in the percentage of GPI-APs$^-$ cells as a marker for the immune pathophysiology of AA and refractory anemia (RA)-MDS according to the FAB classification [17, 21]. In this review article, I summarize our experience regarding the detection of GPI-APs$^-$ cells in patients with various hematological diseases and also discuss the current results of a nationwide multicenter prospective observational study (OPTIMA) while emphasizing the importance of using a high-sensitivity flow cytometric assay to detect small populations of GPI-APs$^-$ cells in the management of BM failure.

11.2 High-Sensitivity Flow Cytometry Assay

Conventional flow cytometric assays using a single color fluorescence-labeled antibodies specific to GPI-APs have defined the presence of GPI-APs$^-$ cells by more than 1 % of the total cells as a significant increase in the GPI-APs$^-$ cells. The cutoff value was set based on the fact that damaged or immature GPI-APs$^+$ cells are mistakenly identified to be GPI-APs$^-$ due to the poor binding of specific antibodies or fluorescence-labeled antibodies or fluorescent-labeled inactive toxin aerolysin (FLAER) to GPI-APs$^-$ cells [3]. The cutoff value can be reduced to a level of 0.01 % by eliminating SSC^{dim} and CD11b^{dim} granulocytes or glycophorin A^{dim} RBCs, as well as 7-amino-actinomycin D (7-AAD)-positive (damaged) cells [17]. Moreover, the threshold can be further reduced to 0.003 % for granulocytes and 0.005 % for erythrocytes by examining a large number of healthy individuals. In this high-sensitivity assay, the position of the border between GPI-APs$^+$ and GPI-APs$^-$ cells was set so that it did not include any dots in the GPI-AP s$^-$ cell area of the scattergrams obtained from more than 50 different samples from healthy individuals.

11.3 GPI-APs⁻ Cells in Healthy Individuals

Detecting small populations of GPI-APs$^-$ cells may be meaningless in the management of BM failure if they are often detectable in healthy individuals or if there is no clear-cut border in the percentage of GPI-APs$^-$ cells between healthy individuals and BM failure patients. Araten et al. identified 0.0001–0.0051 % CD55$^-$CD59$^-$ CD11b$^+$ granulocytes in the PB of all nine healthy individuals, as well as *PIGA* mutations in sorted CD55$^-$CD59$^-$ CD11b$^+$ granulocytes [2]. They speculated that the *PIGA* mutant HSCs generating GPI-APs$^-$ granulocytes do not persist for very long based on their findings that the same *PIGA* mutations were not detectable in the second samples taken more than 6 months after the first analysis. On the other hand, Hu et al. demonstrated that various *PIGA* mutations were detectable in the progenies of GPI-APs$^+$ colony forming units-granulocytes and macrophages that were cultured in vitro and thereby indicated a possibility that the GPI-APs$^-$ cells detected in vivo are derived from committed progenitor cells that developed *PIGA* mutations as a result of their extensive proliferation [6]. These data were compatible with the finding by Araten et al. that the GPI-APs$^-$ cells with a specific mutation did not persist over 6 months.

We screened the PB of 192 healthy volunteers for the presence of GPI-APs$^-$ cells using the abovementioned high-sensitivity method that was originally designed not to detect more than 0.003 % GPI-APs$^-$ cells in healthy individuals [8]. Notably, two of these patients were found to bear detectable levels of GPI-APs$^-$ cells, and in both of them, GPI-APs$^-$ cells were detected in limited lineages, representing granulocytes (G), monocytes (M), erythrocytes (E, GME), and GE-type cells (Fig. 11.1). The similar percentages and lineage combinations of GPI-APs$^-$ cells persisted more than 3 years in these two individuals, indicating that the GPI-APs$^-$ were derived from HSCs, rather than hematopoietic progenitor cells. Together with previous reports, our findings indicate that GPI-APs$^-$ cells derived from *PIGA* mutant HSCs that are selected by chance to contribute to hematopoiesis in the absence of immune pressures in the BM exist in healthy individuals, but at a very low incidence, and that our assay can clearly distinguish long-lived small populations of GPI-APs$^-$ cells from short-lived GPI-APs$^-$ cells.

11.4 GPI-APs⁻ Cells in Patients with BM Failure

We have examined the PB of a total of more than 9000 patients with BM failure for the presence of GPI-APs$^-$ cells using the highly sensitive flow cytometric assay. Figure 11.2 shows the results of the GPI-APs$^-$ cell detection in the first 1656 patients [18]. A total of 49 % of AA and 17 % of RA patients were positive for increased GPI-APs$^-$ cells, while none of the patients with RA with an excess of blasts (RAEB) or patients with other types of BM failure associated with hematological malignancies and collagen diseases were positive for the increase in GPI-APs$^-$ cells. Notably, more than 80 % of all PNH-sc patients had less than 1 % GPI-APs$^-$ cells, with a median percentage of 0.239 %, which might have been overlooked if they were

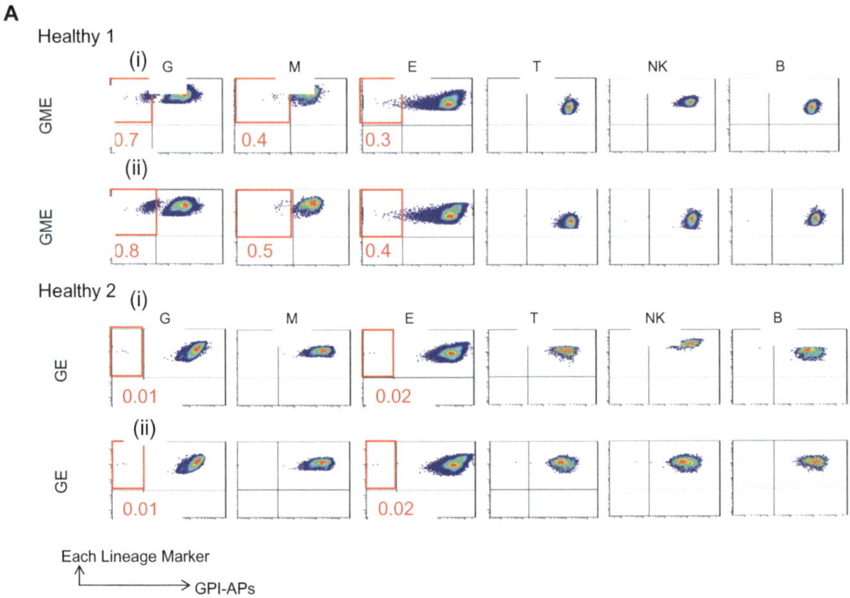

Fig. 11.1 Detection of GPI-APs⁻ cells in different lineages of blood cells from two healthy individuals [8]. The profiles of the peripheral blood cells of two healthy individuals (Healthy 1 and Healthy 2) showing GPI-APs⁻ cells in the GME and GE lineages are shown. They exhibited GPI-APs⁻ cells in the same lineage combination pattern at the first sampling (*i*) and 13 and 7 months after the first sampling (*ii*), respectively

examined with conventional flow cytometry. The prevalence of increased GPI-APs⁻ cells in each subset of patients as of August 2014 remained similar to the findings reported in 2009. Of particular note, increased GPI-APs⁻ cells have not been detected in more than 200 patients with RA with ringed sideroblasts (RARS) or RAEB, except for a few patients whose disease onset times were unclear. Thus, the presence of increased GPI-APs⁻ cells at the onset of BM failure rules out the diagnosis of advanced MDS with definite preleukemic features.

11.5 Response to Immunosuppressive Therapy (IST) in BM Failure Patients Bearing Increased Numbers of GPI-APs⁻ Cells

11.5.1 The Response to Antithymocyte Globulin (ATG)

The impact of the presence of increased GPI-APs⁻ blood cells on the response to IST in patients with BM failure was first demonstrated by Dunn et al. [5]. They showed that patients with MDS bearing GPI-APs⁻ cells that were revealed by a

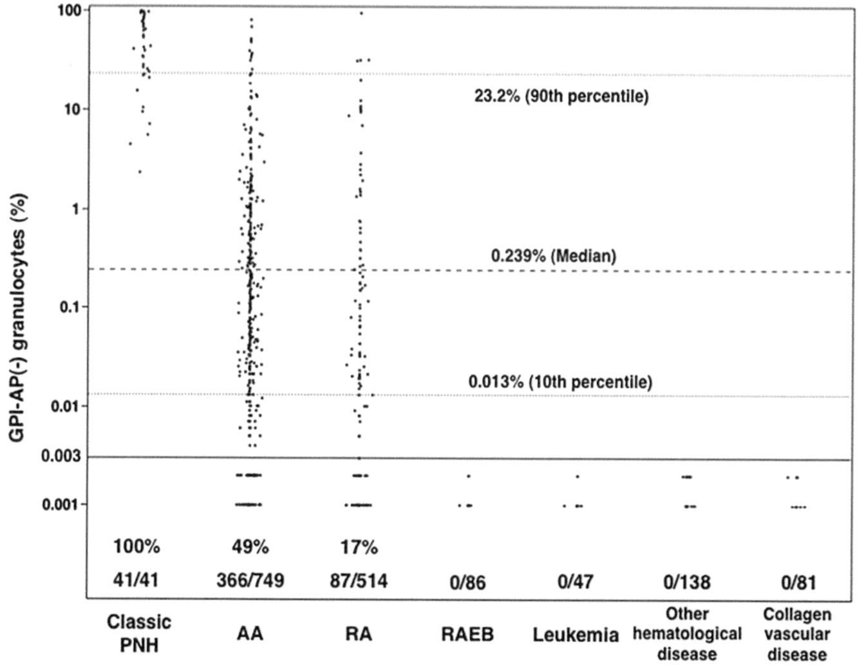

Fig. 11.2 The percentages of GPI-APs⁻ granulocytes in patients with various types of bone marrow failure. The percentages of GPI-APs⁻ granulocytes in each patient group are plotted on a semilogarithmic graph. The numbers above the disease name represent the prevalence of patients bearing a significant increase in the percentage of GPI-APs⁻ granulocytes and the number of patients evaluated

conventional flow cytometry method responded to ATG significantly better than did MDS patients not bearing GPI-APs⁻ cells. However, the NIH group and others failed to observe a difference in the response rate to IST in favor of patients with GPI-APs⁻ cells in AA patients [5, 14, 19, 23].

Our retrospective analysis using the high-sensitivity flow cytometry method demonstrated that the response to IST (91 %) and the probability of surviving failure-free at 5 years (64.2 %) in 83 AA patients bearing an increased percentage of GPI-APs⁻ were significantly higher than those (48 % and 12.3 %) in 39 AA patients without such an increase [17]. As shown in Fig. 11.3, there were no significant differences in the rates of achieving response to IST among different subpopulations of AA patients defined by the percentage of GPI-APs⁻ granulocytes; every subpopulation with increased GPI-APs⁻ cells showed a significantly better response than patients without GPI-APs⁻ cells.

The predictive value of an increased proportion of GPI-APs⁻ for a favorable prognosis in AA was recently confirmed by two prospective studies from Russia [9] (Fig. 11.4) and Canada [20] in which high-sensitivity flow cytometry assays similar

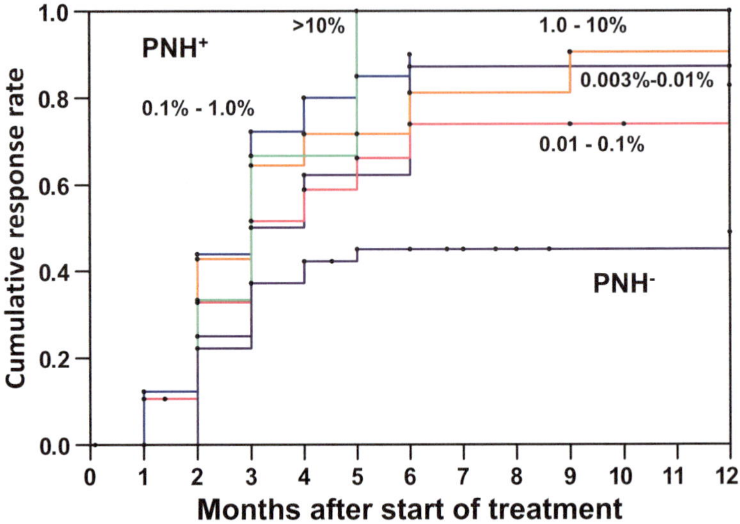

Fig. 11.3 The response to immunosuppressive therapy according to the PNH clone size. The cumulative response rates to antithymocyte globulin (ATG) plus cyclosporine (CsA) therapy in AA patients based on the GPI-APs⁻ cell percentage are shown. Every subpopulation of patients bearing increased GPI-APs⁻ cells (PNH⁺ patients) showed a significantly better response than did the patients not bearing GPI-APs⁻ cells (PNH⁻). The *number* on each line represents the percentage of GPI-APs⁻ cells

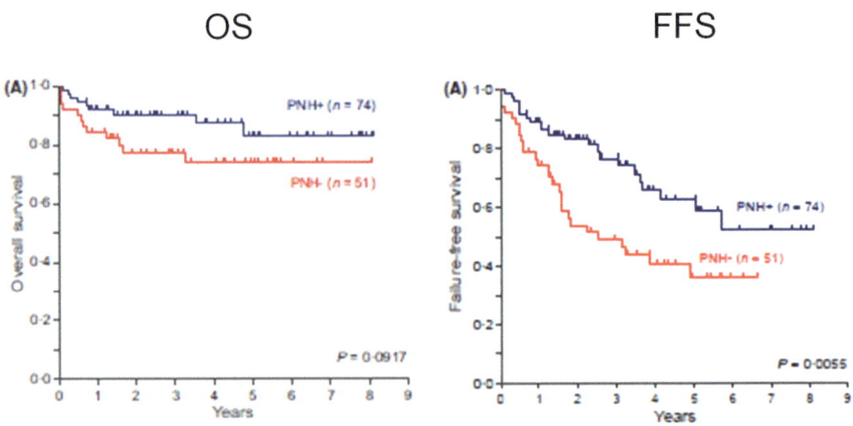

Fig. 11.4 The prognostic values of GPI-APs⁻ cells in patients with AA treated with ATG+CsA [9]. The overall and failure-free survival probabilities according to baseline PNH status are shown

to our method were employed. These results indicate that a minor population of GPI-APs⁻ cells represents a reliable marker of a positive ATG response and a favorable prognosis among patients with AA.

11.5.2 Response to CsA

Our previous retrospective study provided the first evidence of a better response rate to monotherapy with CsA in MDS-RA patients bearing increased GPI-APs$^-$ cells than in patients without GPI-APs$^-$ cells [21]. Thereafter, Ishikawa et al. conducted a prospective study to assess the efficacy of CsA in the treatment of patients with low-risk MDS and analyzed the factors associated with a good response to CsA [7]. A short duration (<4 months) of illness and the presence of GPI-APs$^-$ blood cells were identified as factors significantly associated with a good response to CsA; five (71 %) of seven patients with increased GPI-APs$^-$ cells improved with CsA, whereas only one (10 %) of ten patients without increased GPI-APs$^-$ cells responded to the treatment.

11.6 The Actual Pathophysiology of MDS Patients with Increased GPI-APs$^-$ Cells

Although MDS is defined as a clonal disorder associated with a risk of developing acute myelogenous leukemia (AML), its diagnosis relies on the presence of dysplastic signs in the immature BM cells and normocellular or hypercellular BM, despite the presence of pancytopenia. The discordance in the definition between the disease concept and diagnostic criteria leads to confusion among physicians. The following case represents a typical example of such confusion [11]. A 14-year-old male was found to have mild pancytopenia in 2009. His complete blood count showed a red blood cell count of 3.24×10^{12}/L, hemoglobin level of 11.0 g/dL, and a white blood cell count of 2.85×10^9/L with a differential count of 36 % neutrophils, 58 % lymphocytes, 1 % eosinophils, 1 % basophils, 5 % monocytes, and a platelet count of 26×10^9/L. BM aspiration and biopsy showed hypercellularity with some dysplastic signs and a relative decrease in megakaryocytes with a normal karyotype (Fig. 11.5a). Morphology experts diagnosed this patient to have RAEB or refractory cytopenia of childhood and suggested allogeneic stem cell transplantation from an HLA-identical unrelated donor as a therapeutic option. However, our high-sensitivity flow cytometry assay detected small populations of GPI-APs$^-$ cells in erythrocytes (0.139 %) and granulocytes (0.461 %) in the patient's PB (Fig. 11.5b), suggesting the presence of immune pathophysiology in this patient. Magnetic resonance imaging (MRI) of the thoracolumbar spine showed abundant hematopoietic nests in the bilateral iliac bones, but typical fatty marrow in the thoracoabdominal spines. Although the BM biopsy findings did not meet the criteria for the diagnosis of AA, he was eventually diagnosed to have AA mimicking MDS and was treated with CsA alone. He achieved complete hematological recovery within 1 year without receiving any blood transfusions and has been in remission for 3 years after the cessation of the treatment.

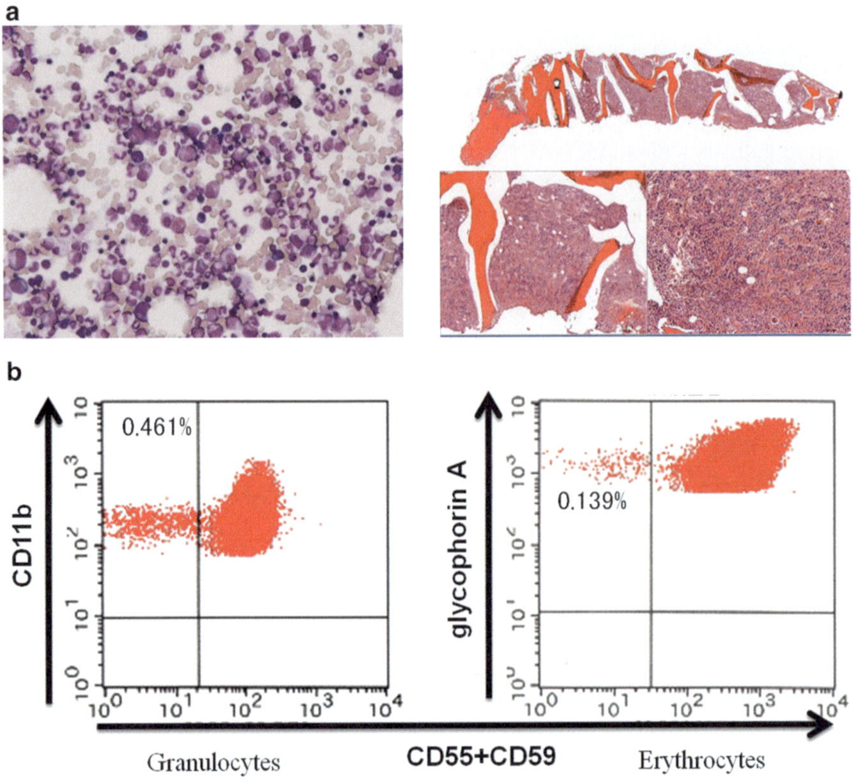

Fig. 11.5 The bone marrow findings and the results of the high-sensitivity flow cytometry assay. (**a**), Bone marrow smear and biopsy specimens showed hypercellularity; (**b**) GPI-APs⁻ cells were revealed in both granulocytes and erythrocytes

We have been following many patients bearing increased GPI-APs⁻ cells who met the morphological criteria for refractory cytopenia with unilineage dysplasia (RCUD) or refractory cytopenia with multilineage dysplasia (RCMD) defined by the WHO 2008 for many years. Some of them progressed to RAEB or AML, but the incidence of these findings was less than 3 %, similar to that observed in patients with typical AA [16]. Thus, the pathophysiology of MDS patients bearing GPI-APs⁻ cells is thought to be essentially the same as that of AA.

11.7 A Nationwide Multicenter Prospective Observational Study: The OPTIMA

The significance of detecting small GPI-APs⁻ cell populations <0.1 % in the management of BM failure has only been documented by a limited number of groups, probably because the sensitive flow cytometric assay has not been popularized due to its very low cutoff values. To verify its clinical significance, the Japanese PNH Study Group started a nationwide multicenter prospective observational study named the OPTIMA (Observation of GPI-anchored protein-deficient (PNH-type) cells In Japanese patients with bone Marrow failure syndrome) in July 2011. Japanese patients with AA, MDS, and BM failure suspected of having PNH were prospectively enrolled in the OPTIMA study. The high-sensitivity flow cytometry technique that was developed at Kanazawa University was transferred to six different university laboratories assigned as regional analysis centers in Japan. PB samples from various types of BM failure patients were sent to these centers for the detection of GPI-APs⁻ granulocytes and erythrocytes. For each patient, the percentage of PNH-type cells was measured using a high-resolution flow cytometry-based method using a liquid FLAER method for granulocytes and a cocktail method with anti-CD55 and anti-CD59 antibodies for erythrocytes, and the relationships among increased GPI-APs⁻ cells, IST, and the prognosis of BM failure were analyzed.

To check the quality of the individual flow cytometry assays, negative (no GPI-APs⁻ cells) and positive (approximately 0.01 % GPI-APs⁻ cells) samples were periodically sent, unannounced, to the six laboratories. The periodic blind validation tests revealed that the interlaboratory differences in the PNH-type cell percentage were always within 0.02 %.

As of July 2013, flow cytometry data on 1210 cases (386 AA, 339 MDS, 55 PNH, and 430 with undiagnosed BM failure) were collected for an interim analysis. A total of 457 (37.8 % and 57 % of the AA, 19.8 % of MDS, and 100 % of PNH) patients were found to be positive for GPI-APs⁻ cells. Among the different subsets of patients with MDS, increased PNH-type cells were detectable in 20 (21.3 %) of the 94 patients with RCUD, 33 (21.7 %) of 152 with RCMD, and five (27 %) of 22 with MDS unclassifiable, but not in any of 14 RARS or 32 RAEB patients, a finding compatible with our previous study.

11.8 Conclusions

The detection of a small population of GPI-APs⁻ cells is the most fundamental examination that can be performed to assess the pathophysiology of BM failure. High-sensitivity flow cytometry can be performed anywhere by following a standard protocol. The predictive value of an increased proportion of PNH-type cells for a favorable prognosis of patients with BM failure will be clarified by the final analyses of the OPTIMA data in a few years.

References

1. Afable MG 2nd, Shaik M, Sugimoto Y, Elson P, Clemente M, Makishima H, Sekeres MA, Lichtin A, Advani A, Kalaycio M, Tiu RV, O'Keefe CL, Maciejewski JP (2011) Efficacy of rabbit anti-thymocyte globulin in severe aplastic anemia. Haematologica 96(9):1269–1275, doi:haematol.2011.042622 [pii] 10.3324/haematol.2011.042622
2. Araten DJ, Nafa K, Pakdeesuwan K, Luzzatto L (1999) Clonal populations of hematopoietic cells with paroxysmal nocturnal hemoglobinuria genotype and phenotype are present in normal individuals. Proc Natl Acad Sci U S A 96(9):5209–5214

3. Brodsky RA, Mukhina GL, Li S, Nelson KL, Chiurazzi PL, Buckley JT, Borowitz MJ (2000) Improved detection and characterization of paroxysmal nocturnal hemoglobinuria using fluorescent aerolysin. Am J Clin Pathol 114(3):459–466
4. De Lord C, Tooze JA, Saso R, Marsh JC, Gordon-Smith EC (1998) Deficiency of glycosylphosphatidyl inositol-anchored proteins in patients with aplastic anaemia does not affect response to immunosuppressive therapy. Br J Haematol 101(1):90–93
5. Dunn DE, Tanawattanacharoen P, Boccuni P, Nagakura S, Green SW, Kirby MR, Kumar MS, Rosenfeld S, Young NS (1999) Paroxysmal nocturnal hemoglobinuria cells in patients with bone marrow failure syndromes. Ann Intern Med 131(6):401–408
6. Hu R, Mukhina GL, Piantadosi S, Barber JP, Jones RJ, Brodsky RA (2005) PIG-A mutations in normal hematopoiesis. Blood 105(10):3848–3854
7. Ishikawa T, Tohyama K, Nakao S, Yoshida Y, Teramura M, Motoji T, Takatoku M, Kurokawa M, Mitani K, Uchiyama T, Omine M (2007) A prospective study of cyclosporine A treatment of patients with low-risk myelodysplastic syndrome: presence of CD55(−)CD59(−) blood cells predicts platelet response. Int J Hematol 86(2):150–157, doi:B825VRU20K835K14 [pii] 10.1532/IJH97.07052
8. Katagiri T, Kawamoto H, Nakakuki T, Ishiyama K, Okada-Hatakeyama M, Ohtake S, Seiki Y, Hosokawa K, Nakao S (2013) Individual hematopoietic stem cells in human bone marrow of patients with aplastic anemia or myelodysplastic syndrome stably give rise to limited cell lineages. Stem Cells 31(3):536–546. doi:10.1002/stem.1301
9. Kulagin A, Lisukov I, Ivanova M, Golubovskaya I, Kruchkova I, Bondarenko S, Vavilov V, Stancheva N, Babenko E, Sipol A, Pronkina N, Kozlov V, Afanasyev B (2014) Prognostic value of paroxysmal nocturnal haemoglobinuria clone presence in aplastic anaemia patients treated with combined immunosuppression: results of two-centre prospective study. Br J Haematol 164(4):546–554. doi:10.1111/bjh.12661
10. Miyata T, Takeda J, Iida Y, Yamada N, Inoue N, Takahashi M, Maeda K, Kitani T, Kinoshita T (1993) The cloning of PIG-A, a component in the early step of GPI-anchor biosynthesis. Science 259(5099):1318–1320
11. Nishimura R, Mase S, Araki R, Fujiki T, Kuroda R, Maeba H, Koizumi S, Yachie A (2014) Massive hyper-reactive hematopoietic nests in bilateral iliac bones in a patient with mild aplastic anemia. Pediatr Blood Cancer 61(10):1903–1904. doi:10.1002/pbc.25140
12. Parker C, Omine M, Richards S, Nishimura J, Bessler M, Ware R, Hillmen P, Luzzatto L, Young N, Kinoshita T, Rosse W, Socie G, International PNHIG (2005) Diagnosis and management of paroxysmal nocturnal hemoglobinuria. Blood 106(12):3699–3709. doi:10.1182/blood-2005-04-1717
13. Sauntharajah Y, Nakamura R, Wesley R, Wang QJ, Barrett AJ (2003) A simple method to predict response to immunosuppressive therapy in patients with myelodysplastic syndrome. Blood 102(8):3025–3027
14. Scheinberg P, Marte M, Nunez O, Young NS (2010) Paroxysmal nocturnal hemoglobinuria clones in severe aplastic anemia patients treated with horse anti-thymocyte globulin plus cyclosporine. Haematologica 95(7):1075–1080. doi:10.3324/haematol.2009.017889
15. Schrezenmeier H, Hertenstein B, Wagner B, Raghavachar A, Heimpel H (1995) A pathogenetic link between aplastic anemia and paroxysmal nocturnal hemoglobinuria is suggested by a high frequency of aplastic anemia patients with a deficiency of phosphatidylinositol glycan anchored proteins. Exp Hematol 23(1):81–87
16. Seiki Y, Sasaki Y, Hosokawa K, Saito C, Sugimori N, Yamazaki H, Takami A, Nakao S (2013) Increased plasma thrombopoietin levels in patients with myelodysplastic syndrome: a reliable marker for a benign subset of bone marrow failure. Haematologica 98(6):901–907. doi:10.3324/haematol.2012.066217
17. Sugimori C, Chuhjo T, Feng X, Yamazaki H, Takami A, Teramura M, Mizoguchi H, Omine M, Nakao S (2006) Minor population of CD55-CD59- blood cells predicts response to immunosuppressive therapy and prognosis in patients with aplastic anemia. Blood 107(4):1308–1314

18. Sugimori C, Mochizuki K, Qi Z, Sugimori N, Ishiyama K, Kondo Y, Yamazaki H, Takami A, Okumura H, Nakao S (2009) Origin and fate of blood cells deficient in glycosylphosphatidylinositol-anchored protein among patients with bone marrow failure. Br J Haematol 147(1):102–112, doi: BJH7822 [pii] 10.1111/j.1365-2141.2009.07822.x
19. Timeus F, Crescenzio N, Longoni D, Doria A, Foglia L, Pagliano S, Vallero S, Decimi V, Svahn J, Palumbo G, Ruggiero A, Martire B, Pillon M, Marra N, Dufour C, Ramenghi U, Saracco P (2014) Paroxysmal nocturnal hemoglobinuria clones in children with acquired aplastic anemia: a multicentre study. PLoS One 9(7):e101948. doi:10.1371/journal.pone.0101948
20. Tutelman PR, Aubert G, Milner RA, Dalal BI, Schultz KR, Deyell RJ (2014) Paroxysmal nocturnal haemoglobinuria phenotype cells and leucocyte subset telomere length in childhood acquired aplastic anaemia. Br J Haematol 164(5):717–721. doi:10.1111/bjh.12656
21. Wang H, Chuhjo T, Yasue S, Omine M, Nakao S (2002) Clinical significance of a minor population of paroxysmal nocturnal hemoglobinuria-type cells in bone marrow failure syndrome. Blood 100(12):3897–3902
22. Wang SA, Pozdnyakova O, Jorgensen JL, Medeiros LJ, Stachurski D, Anderson M, Raza A, Woda BA (2009) Detection of paroxysmal nocturnal hemoglobinuria clones in patients with myelodysplastic syndromes and related bone marrow diseases, with emphasis on diagnostic pitfalls and caveats. Haematologica 94(1):29–37. doi:10.3324/haematol.13601
23. Yoshida N, Yagasaki H, Takahashi Y, Yamamoto T, Liang J, Wang Y, Tanaka M, Hama A, Nishio N, Kobayashi R, Hotta N, Asami K, Kikuta A, Fukushima T, Hirano N, Kojima S (2008) Clinical impact of HLA-DR15, a minor population of paroxysmal nocturnal haemoglobinuria-type cells, and an aplastic anaemia-associated autoantibody in children with acquired aplastic anaemia. Br J Haematol 142(3):427–435. doi:10.1111/j.1365-2141.2008.07182.x

Chapter 12
Clonal Origin and Clonal Selection in PNH

Lucio Luzzatto

Abstract Paroxysmal nocturnal haemoglobinuria (PNH) is a haemolytic anaemia with rather unique features; indeed, (a) it is also associated with features of bone marrow failure; (b) it is acquired but it is due to an intrinsic red cell abnormality; and (c) it is a clonal disorder of haematopoiesis, but it is not a malignancy. Since it has been known that the clone arises through a somatic mutation of the X-linked *PIG-A* gene, and since *PIG-A* mutations are found also in normal people, the key to understanding the pathogenesis of PNH lies in what makes the *PIG-A* mutant clone expand. In order to rationalize the link between (a) and (c), it was suggested since 1989 that the disease develops when a *PIG-A* mutant haematopoietic stem cell (HSC) finds itself in a bone marrow environment that faces an autoimmune attack – as is thought to be the case in idiopathic aplastic anaemia (AA). In this paper, after a brief historical introduction, the evidence in support of this mechanism from in vitro studies, from animal models and from PNH patients is reviewed. We now have evidence for the notion that in PNH patients there are GPI-reactive CD1d-restricted T cells that selectively attack normal (GPI-positive) HSCs but spare the GPI-negative progeny of the *PIG-A* mutant HSCs.

Keywords Haemolytic anaemia • Somatic mutation • Clonal disorder • T cell-mediated autoimmunity • Darwinian selection • Conditional growth advantage • *PIG-A* gene

---

This paper is dedicated to the memory of my dear colleague and friend Bruno Rotoli.

L. Luzzatto, M.D., Ph.D. (✉)
Istituto Toscano Tumori, Department of Haematology, University of Florence, Viale G. Pieraccini, 6, 50139 Florence, Italy

Present address: Department of Haematology and Blood Transfusion, Muhimbili University of Health and Allied Sciences, Dar-Es-Salaam, Tanzania
e-mail: lluzzatto@blood.ac.tz

Y. Kanakura et al. (eds.), *Paroxysmal Nocturnal Hemoglobinuria*,
DOI 10.1007/978-4-431-56003-6_12

12.1 Historical Introduction

The first report of a patient with paroxysmal nocturnal haemoglobinuria (PNH) is usually credited to the German internist Paul Strübing, who published it in 1882 [1], although the medical historian Voswinckel [2] has traced a much earlier clinical description – in 1648, in Latin – to the Dutch physician Johann Schmidt. Strübing's report was important for at least two reasons. First, his article included a detailed diary of the patient's urine samples, documenting that the passing of dark urine was intermittent; second, it was noted that the patient did not have syphilis, a known cause of paroxysmal cold haemoglobinuria (PCH); thus, PNH was identified as a condition different from PCH. In 1911, Marchiafava [3] confirmed that haemoglobinuria was paroxysmal, but he also demonstrated that haemosiderinuria was 'perpetual', thus pinpointing, already one century ago, that haemolysis takes place all the time in PNH and explaining how PNH patients can become iron deficient.

From then on, PNH was investigated as a haemolytic anaemia, a condition of which several forms were already known at that time. A broad classification recognized that inherited or congenital haemolytic anaemias were due to intracorpuscular causes, whereas acquired haemolytic anaemias were due to extracorpuscular causes (a notion that to a large extent still stands today (see Table 12.1). Against that background, the studies of Ham [4] and Dacie [5] brought up something unexpected: in PNH, certainly an acquired disease, there was strong evidence of an intracorpuscular or intrinsic red cell abnormality. This was suggested by in vitro tests that also revealed two most interesting features: (i) haemolysis depended on the presence of serum, which must be fresh and not preheated, implying that haemolysis depended on complement [6], and (ii) of all the patient's red cells, only a proportion – variable from patient to patient – was susceptible to complement-mediated lysis (see Fig. 12.1).

Table 12.1 Classification of haemolytic anaemias

	Intracorpuscular causes	Extracorpuscular causes
Hereditary	Haemoglobinopathies Enzymopathies Membranopathies Other	Familial Haemolytic-uraemic syndrome (HUS)
Acquired	Paroxysmal Nocturnal Haemoglobinuria (PNH)	Malaria Autoimmune Drug-induced Micro-angiopathic Other

It is seen that in most cases hereditary haemolytic anaemias are due to intracorpuscular causes, whereas acquired haemolytic anaemias are due to extracorpuscular causes. The two exceptions are familial HUS (also currently known as atypical HUS) and PNH. Interestingly, both conditions have to do with complement (C): in familial HUS, a C-regulatory plasma protein (usually factor H) is mutated; in PNH there is a somatic mutation of *PIG-A* that prevents the insertion in the cell membrane of the C regulators CD55 and CD59

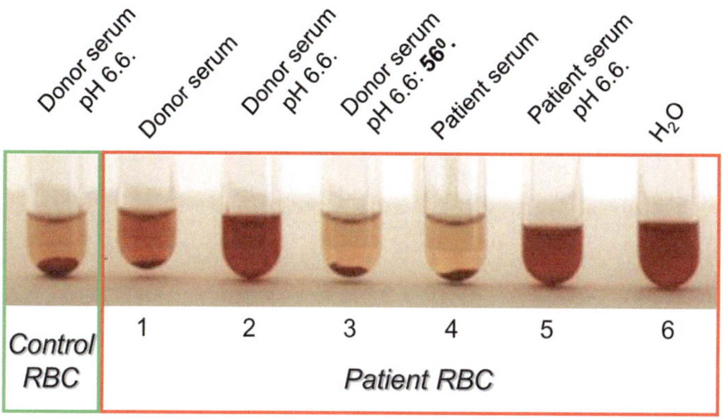

Fig. 12.1 *The acidified serum test demonstrates coexistence of red cells that are susceptible and red cells that are resistant to complement lysis.* In the test tube on the left, red cells from a normal control person have not lysed after incubation for 30 minutes at 37 °C in normal compatible serum acidified with HCl (to pH about 6.6). The 6 test tubes on the *right* all contain red cells from a patient with PNH, and they show in sequence *1*, lysis of a proportion of the red cells in normal compatible serum; *2*, lysis of a larger proportion – *but not all* – of the red cells when the alternative complement pathway is activated by the lower pH; *3*, no lysis if the serum has been pre-heated at 56° (a procedure that denatures some complement proteins); *4*, much less lysis than in tube *1* (the level of some complement proteins may be lower in the patient's serum than in the serum of a normal donor); *5*, once complement is activated by the lower pH the lysis becomes similar to that in tube *2*; and *6*, complete lysis of red cells. By colorimetric quantitation of free haemoglobin in tube *2* or in tube *5*, compared to tube *6*, it is possible to estimate the proportion of PNH red cells in the patient: the proportion is similar to that of PNH III red cells quantitated by flow cytometry

12.2 PNH: A Clonal Disease

If the finding of an intrinsic red cell abnormality in an acquired disease was surprising, the notion that it seemed to affect some red cells but not all of them was utterly baffling. It was John Dacie [7] who, in a landmark address to the Royal Society of Medicine as president of its Pathology Section, first confronted this issue explicitly in 1963, when he noted: 'That two populations *(of red cells)* are present is quite clear both from the laboratory tests and also from the results of red cell survival from a patient with PNH, using ^{51}Cr labeling'. He further noted that it was the patients who had a larger proportion of 'cells that are easily lysed' who had more severe clinical manifestations. The next section in his address was headed the *Somatic Mutation Hypothesis*, which he found attractive but that he judged 'as difficult to prove as to refute'.

To prove that any disease is due to a somatic mutation was indeed a challenge in the pre-DNA sequencing era. Fortunately, the discovery by Mary Lyon [8] in 1961 that female mice were somatic cell mosaics as a result of the X chromosome inactivation phenomenon provided a tool. Ernie Beutler, by using the X-linked gene

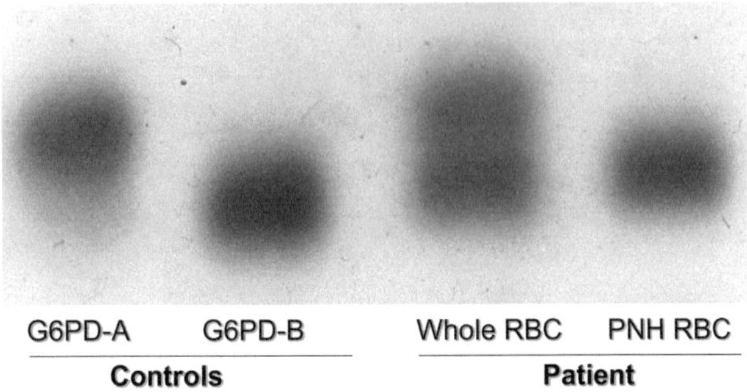

Fig. 12.2 *Clonal origin of PNH red cells based on mono-allelic expression of G6PD in a G6PD*^{A}*/G6PD*^{B} *heterozygous woman*. On the *left*, samples from two normal males who were hemizygous for G6PD A and G6PD B, respectively. On the *right*, samples for one female patient with PNH. It is seen that in the whole red cell population G6PD A and G6PD B are expressed at similar levels; but in the red cells lysed by complement in the acidified serum test only G6PD B is expressed, indicating that they all derive from a single stem cell (From Ref. [12], with permission)

G6PD as a marker, first showed that X-inactivation applied also to human females [9], and Gartler, by an original approach that could be used in females who were heterozygous at the *G6PD* locus, [10] showed that human tumours arose from a single cell within the mosaic. At the time I was working as a haematologist in Nigeria, where the *G6PD* gene is highly polymorphic [11], and nearly 50 % of females are heterozygous. In two women who where *G6PD* heterozygotes, we found that in the red cells that were lysed by complement in vitro, only one *G6PD* allele was expressed [12]. As an internal control, both alleles were expressed in the red cells that were not lysed (see Fig. 12.2). Thus, Dacie's notion was experimentally validated.

From then on, it was accepted that PNH was a clonal disorder: the abnormal clone was referred to as the PNH clone, and gradually its features were characterized. It was already known that acetylcholinesterase was deficient in PNH [13], and several other surface proteins were also found to be deficient, including some, such as the decay-accelerating factor (DAF now CD55) [14] and the membrane inhibitor of reactive lysis (MIRL, now CD59), [15] that bind complement proteins (C3 and C5-8, respectively), thus explaining the exquisite sensitivity to complement of PNH red cells. Deficiencies of these and of numerous other proteins were also discovered on white cells and platelets, supporting the notion that they belonged to the PNH clone and implying that the original lesion must be in a haematopoietic stem cell (HSC). This notion was corroborated by in vitro culture studies; notably when, based on complement sensitivity, two types of erythroid colonies (bursts) were found in the bone marrow of PNH patients, normal and PNH[16], consistent with a somatic mutation upstream of BFU-Es, presumably in an HSC.

It seemed contradictory at first sight that a single somatic mutation could produce multiple abnormalities; however, it emerged that all the proteins involved had something in common [17]: they are surface proteins tethered to the membrane through a glycan phosphatidyl inositol (GPI) molecule. In view of this, it seemed likely that there was an impediment in the biosynthesis of GPI; indeed, biochemical studies pinpointed the metabolic block at the *N*-acetylglucosamine transferase step [18], and by testing somatic cell hybrids, it was found that the gene mutated in PNH cells must be on the X chromosome [19]. At about the same time, Taroh Kinoshita's team, by an elegant expression cloning approach, identified *PIG-A* as the gene defective in a PNH-like cell line [20]: the gene maps indeed to the X chromosome, and it encodes one of the subunits of the *N*-acetyl glucosamine transferase. *PIG-A* was found to have diverse inactivating mutations in peripheral blood cells of PNH patients [21]. Thus, the PNH clone was now defined by a named mutant gene, and its GPI-negative phenotype was explained.

12.3 Features of PNH Clones

In the past, the diagnosis of PNH was based on the acidified serum test [4, 5], which tested the sensitivity to complement of red cells only. Over the past 20 years, flow cytometry analysis [22, 23] has become the standard diagnostic test, and it has made it possible to investigate other blood cells as well. Experience accumulated on large number of patients has established several points:

1. A bimodal distribution, with one population of normal cells and a distinctly separate population of GPI-deficient cells, is seen in all cases [24].
2. The proportion of GPI-deficient cells varies a great deal from patient to patient [25].
3. In each individual patient, the percentage of GPI-deficient cells is much higher in monocytes and in granulocytes compared to erythrocytes; it is much lower in B-lymphocytes and in T-lymphocytes [26].
4. GPI-deficient platelets are also seen [27], but for technical reasons their study is rather difficult.
5. In the erythrocytes, the level of fluorescence of the GPI-deficient population is consistent in most cases with complete deficiency of GPI: these cells are traditionally designated PNH III, but sometimes the level of fluorescence indicates only a partial deficiency of GPI, and these cells are traditionally designated PNH II (the normal cells being designated PNH I) [28].
6. In some patients the distribution of erythrocytes, rather than bimodal, is trimodal, with coexistence of PNH III, PNH II and PNH I cells in the same patient [23, 29, 30].
7. Granulocytes also may show partial or total GPI deficiency: however, the basis for this has niot been worked out and the terms 'PNH II'or 'PNH III' are not applicable to granulocytes.

Some of these features are relevant not just to diagnosis but also to understanding the pathophysiology of PNH. The difference in the proportion of GPI-negative cells in granulocytes versus red cells is explained by the fact that the latter are subject to complement-mediated lysis in vivo: this notion has been confirmed in patients treated with the complement (C5) inhibitor eculizumab, in whom one sees a substantial increase in the proportion of GPI-negative red cells, as they are now protected from complement [31]. Thus, in general, the true size of the PNH clone in an individual patient is larger than the proportion of GPI-negative red cells, and as there is no evidence that monocytes or granulocytes have a decreased life span in PNH in vivo, the size of the clone is reflected rather precisely by the proportion of these cells (rather than of red cells) that are GPI negative. If we find in a PNH patient that 98 % of granulocytes are GPI negative – a not unusual finding – a staggering implication is that the patient's haematopoiesis is supported almost completely by the PNH clone and, therefore, perhaps by a single stem cell.

The finding of PNH II and PNH III type clones has found an explanation at the molecular level. Indeed, there are many different *PIG-A* mutations known [32, 33]. A large number are small indels causing frameshifts that will cause complete loss of function: we presume and in some cases we know that they underlie the PNH III phenotype. Others are missense mutations, where the gene product may retain some enzymatic function: they must underlie the PNH II phenotype. These differences are of considerable clinical significance. Indeed, in first approximation, the severity of haemolysis in PNH correlates, not surprisingly, with clone size but only if we compare patients with PNH III clones. Instead, a patient with a very large PNH II clone may have less haemolysis than a patient with a smaller size PNH III clone.

The functional implications of the GPI-deficient phenotype are different in different types of cells. For mature erythrocytes, the main implication is clearly that they are hyper-susceptible to complement lysis (by virtue of their deficiency of CD55 and CD59), but nucleated erythroid precursors do not seem to be so affected. For platelets, it has been suggested (but never formally proven) that when they are GPI negative, they may be more easily activated by activated complement, and this may be a factor in making PNH a potentially vicious thrombophilic condition. For neutrophils, the phagocytic and bactericidal functions seem unaffected, but trans-endothelial migration is significantly impaired by virtue of the deficiency of CD157 [34]. For lymphocytes, functional abnormalities have not been demonstrated in humans, in keeping with the fact that PNH patients are not immunodeficient (unless they have been or they are on immunosuppressive agents). However, in a mouse model (see below), GPI-deficient T cells have reduced reactivity in tests for delayed-type hypersensitivity [35].

12.4 PNH-Like Clonal Populations Modelled in Mice

Mouse chimaeras obtained by injecting into normal blastocysts embryonic stem cells in which *pig-a* had been knocked out by homologous recombination resulted, depending on the proportion of *pig-a-null* cells that contributed to embryo formation, in either early death of the embryo or in normal mice [36]. In the latter case, interestingly, the proportion of GPI-negative blood cells decreased gradually in late

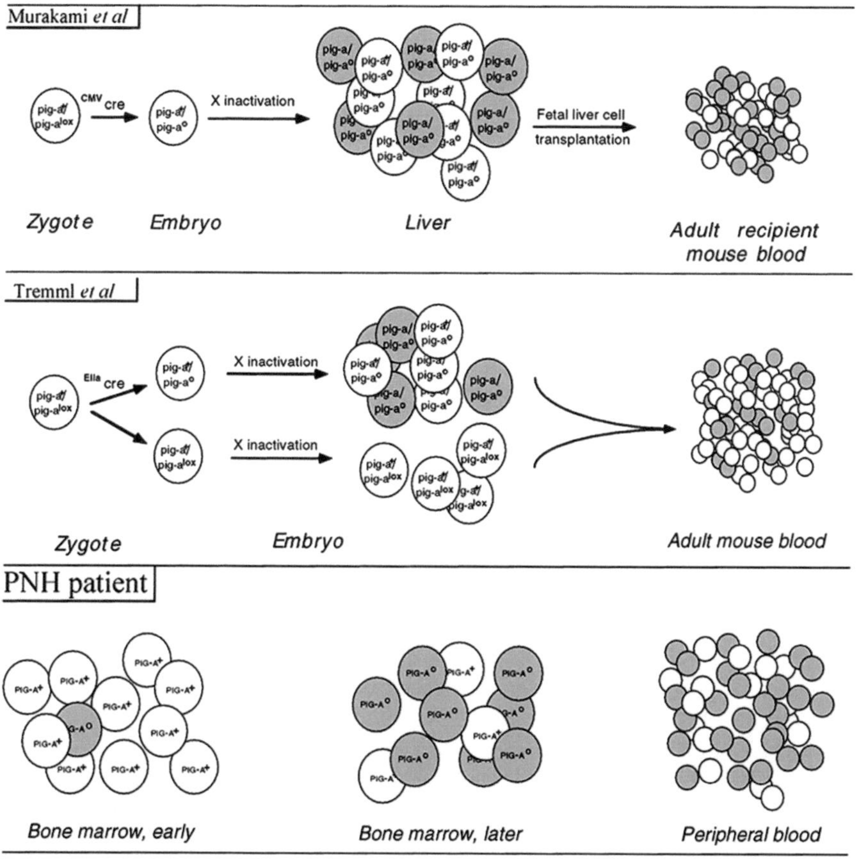

Fig. 12.3 *PNH in mice and humans*. The two *upper panels* represent in cartoon form the mouse models constructed in Refs. [19] and [20], respectively. Although all cells have the same genotype, their phenotype differs depending on which X chromosome has been inactivated: white circles indicate cells in which the X chromosome with the normal *pig-a* gene is active; grey circles indicate cells in which the X chromosome with the inactivated *pig-a* gene (pig-a°) is active. As a result, in the peripheral blood there is a mixture of normal (*white*) and PNH (*grey*) blood cells. In both models, the proportion of PNH cells in the peripheral blood depends on the proportion of cells in which *cre*-mediated recombination has taken place: there is no evidence of selection thereafter. The *bottom panel* represents in cartoon form what happens in the human disease, PNH. Here, unlike in the mice, the entire PNH population arises usually from a single stem cell in which a somatic mutation has taken place (see also Fig. 12.1); therefore, selection must take place at the level of stem cells in order for a large proportion of the blood cells to have the PNH phenotype (From Ref. [39], with permission)

foetal life and virtually disappeared after birth. In order to further investigate how *pig-a* inactivation affects haematopoiesis, two different conditional knockout approaches were used successfully [37, 38] (see Fig. 12.3): the blood phenotype of PNH patients was mimicked, but again there was no increase in GPI negative with time. These findings in mice clearly indicate that a GPI-negative status does not confer a growth advantage onto haematopoietic cells [39]. On the other hand, in an immunological assay designed to test reactivity of normal mouse T cells, these were more reactive against GPI+ than against GPI-negative target cells [40].

12.5 GPI-Negative Clones Outside PNH

As part of our intense efforts to understand the significance of *PIG-A* mutations, we wondered whether GPI-negative blood cells could be found in normal people, and in order to answer this question, we took advantage of three distinct features of this gene. (1) Since the gene maps to the X chromosome and since in somatic cells only one X chromosome is active, a *PIG-A* mutation will yield a phenotype without interference by another allele. (2) Since the gene encodes a protein essential for GPI biosynthesis, with an inactivating mutation, not one but all GPI-linked proteins will be affected. (3) GPI-linked proteins are on the cell surface and therefore conveniently accessible by antibodies suitable for flow cytometry. The combination of these features makes for high sensitivity, provided sufficient numbers of events are accumulated and analysed: when we tested one million (or more) granulocytes (see Fig. 12.4) from normal subjects, we regularly found some that were GPI deficient [41, 42].

This finding was subsequently confirmed by several other investigators [43, 44] (indeed, the 'PIG-A test' is now widely used for testing mutagens [45], PIG-A mutagenesis [46, 47]), and it helped to shift the focus from discovering that a mutant clone exists to understanding what makes a mutant clone expand (see next section). The same finding was also a stimulus to investigating GPI-negative (PNH-like) clones in other conditions, and very small PNH clones (usually well below 1 %) appear to be relatively common in patients with aplastic anaemia (AA), [48] as well as in patients who have been diagnosed with a myelodysplastic syndrome (MDS) [49]. The findings in AA are particularly intriguing, because a close relationship between PNH and AA was identified since 1963 [7], and the term PNH-aplastic anaemia (PNH-AA) syndrome was then coined [50]. Already at the time, it was noted that not infrequently bone marrow failure (BMF) manifesting in AA precedes PNH [7], and this is probably the rule rather than the exception.

12.6 Expansion of PNH Clones

It was precisely in trying to understand the association of PNH and AA that we were confronted with a paradox. At first sight, a haemolytic anaemia such as PNH, with erythroid hyperplasia in the bone marrow, is almost antithetic to bone marrow failure (BMF) as seen in AA: how could they coexist, or why should they follow one another? In addition, PNH and AA are both such rare diseases that it seemed unconceivable that their association could be coincidental. In 1989, together with Bruno

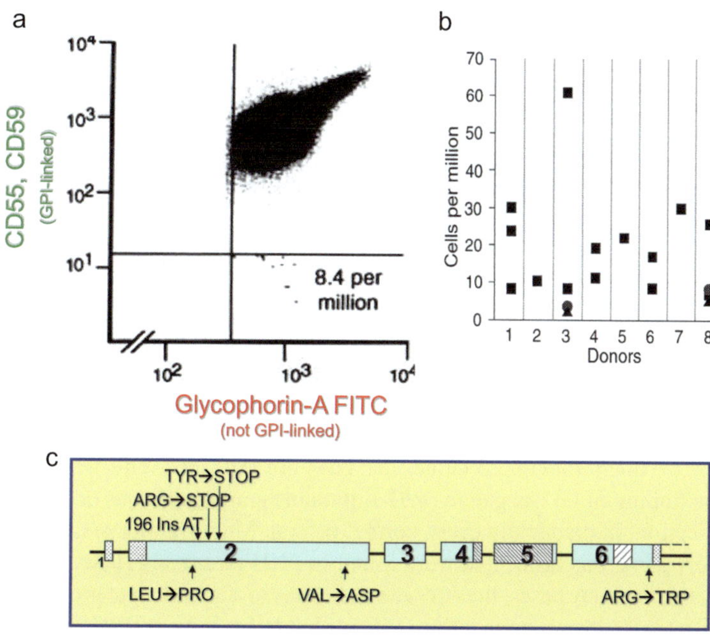

Fig. 12.4 *Blood cells with a GPI-negative (PNH-like) phenotype are found in all normal people.* (**a**) PNH red blood cells from a normal donor are positively identified by light scatter characteristics and by gating to include only events that are glycophorin A positive. PNH cells are clearly seen in the lower *right* hand quadrant at a frequency of eight per million. (**b**) Frequency of PNH granulocytes in nine normal volunteer donors. Each data point represents the results from a separate blood sample. PNH cells were identified in all 19 analyses from the 9 donors. The mean frequency of PNH cells was 22 per million. The samples from donors 1, 3, 6 and 8 were drawn over a time interval of 6–8 months. (**c**) Diagram of the *PIG-A* gene with inactivating somatic mutations observed in some of the donors of panel B (Modified from Ref. [41])

Rotoli, we formulated a model [51], at that time merely hypothetical, in which the link between AA and PNH was central. We thought that BMF was the primary event; then, if a *PIG-A* mutant stem cell appears, it is able to reconstitute haematopoiesis. Depending on circumstances, the diagnosis of AA may or may not have been made at first; then, in the same patient, once haematopoiesis is largely GPI negative, the diagnosis will be PNH [52].

In this respect, a crucial result emerged when we set up erythroid cell cultures from PNH patients. An expected result was that we obtained non-PNH (normal) erythroid bursts and PNH erythroid bursts [16], but an unexpected result was that the numbers of non-PNH bursts were markedly decreased, not only in relative terms compared to PNH bursts but especially in absolute terms compared to normal controls [53]; in spite of the fact that the patients had an active cellular bone marrow, and they did not qualify, at least at the time they were studied, for the PNH-AA syndrome. Thus, there were clearly two abnormalities: a qualitative abnormality, the PNH phenotype in the majority of the bursts, and a quantitative abnormality – a marked shortage of non-PNH bursts. This latter finding was subsequently confirmed [54] at the level of long-term culture-initiating cells (presumably closer to HSCs), a compelling indication that there is regularly an element of BMF in these patients.

In essence, one could contemplate that in a marrow in which haematopoiesis has failed, a PNH clone would expand to fill the vacant space, and a possible mechanism might be an autoimmune attack specifically directed against GPI-positive stem cells, thus sparing GPI-negative stem cells. Our notion was that of conditional Darwinian selection, i.e. a PNH clone does not have a growth advantage on its own but only in a certain bone marrow environment. The animal data summarized in the previous section are in support of this notion.

Testing this idea further was greatly facilitated once *PIG-A* was identified by Taroh Kinoshita's group as the defective gene in PNH clones [20]. If the expansion of a clone with a *PIG-A* mutant genotype and a GPI-negative phenotype depends on certain environmental conditions, we might anticipate that, in the absence of those conditions, we might find micro-clones that have not expanded. This was fully verified by the finding of GPI-negative (*PIG-A* mutant) granulocytes, as detailed in the previous section, in practically every normal person. Moreover, these micro-clones had the very same mutations that were found in PNH patients [41] (see Fig. 12.4). It is likely that in many cases, the *PIG-A* mutation is in a granulocyte progenitor cell (e.g. a CFU-GM) rather than in a true HSC [43], but if it is in an HSC, it can generate, under appropriate selection pressure, the very active haematopoiesis that we can see in PNH.

In principle, since relatively few HSCs are active in normal haematopoiesis, one *PIG-A* mutant HSC – even though it has no selective advantage – might simply by chance (genetic drift) produce a large proportion of the peripheral blood cells, and these will be GPI negative. This possibility has been explored [55]. On the other hand, in a *PIG-A* mutant clone, there may be additional mutation(s) that confer to the respective subclone(s) an intrinsic growth advantage. In two patients with PNH, a mutation of the *HMGA2* gene may have played this role [56], and *HMGA2* overexpression has been reported in additional cases [57]. However, it is unlikely that these mechanisms can account for clonal expansion in the majority of patients with PNH.

12.7 Clonal Expansion Through Immune Selection

Although many factors can cause or contribute to causing AA, there is much evidence that a major mechanism is a T cell-mediated autoimmune process [58], the molecular target of which is not known. One possibility is that, in at least a proportion of cases, the target is an epitope belonging to a GPI-linked protein (which would be expected to be MHC restricted) or GPI itself which, being a glycolipid, would be CD1d restricted [59]. Immunoscopic analysis of the length of the CDR3 region of the β chain of the T cell receptor (TCR) yielded a skewed distribution in PNH patients compared to appropriate controls, [60] consistent with the presence of discrete T cell clones. These data were confirmed on fractionated CD57+ T cells, which would include those that react to glycolipid antigens. Moreover, when the CDR3 region of these fractionated cells was sequenced, in the majority of PNH patients (but not in controls), we found identical or very similar sequences [61]. Given the estimated size (of the order of 10^{18}) of the TCR repertoire, this identity of sequences cannot be attributed to chance.

In a collaborative effort with Anastasios Karadimitris, the functional properties of T cells in PNH patients have been investigated further [62]. First, when CD8+ T cells were co-cultured with HLA negative antigen-presenting B cells (line C1R) previously transduced with a CD1d expression vector (C1R-CD1d) pulsed with trypanosomal GPI (t-GPI), significantly higher levels of reactive T cells and increased production of IFN-γ were found in PNH patients than in normal controls. This did not take place when the antigen-presenting cells did not express CD1d or when they were not competent for endogenous synthesis of GPI; however, in this case reactivity was restored by the addition of exogenous human GPI (h-GPI) produced by organic synthesis [63].

Next we have tested the reactivity of T cells from PNH patients using as APC mature dendritic cells (DCs) obtained from autologous peripheral blood monocytes from the same patients. By selecting CD14-negative cells – which are the majority in PNH patients – we took advantage of the fact that these are naturally GPI-negative APCs. In the absence of added GPI, we could not demonstrate reactive T cells; however, when the APCs were preloaded with h-GPI, we detected significant numbers of reactive T cells in 7 out of 11 PNH patients. In addition, by CD1d dimer technology, GPI-specific T cells were captured in significantly higher numbers from peripheral blood of PNH patients than from controls (see Fig. 12.5). These data provide the first direct evidence for the presence in PNH patients of GPI-reactive CD1d-restricted T cells [62].

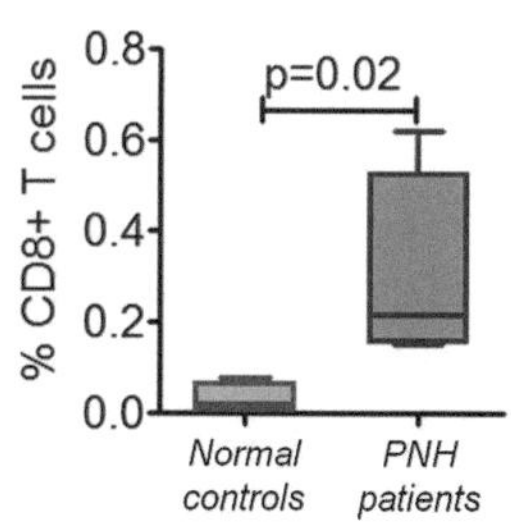

Fig. 12.5 *T cells from patients with PNH bind specifically to GPI-loaded CD1d dimers.* The data are from 6 PNH patients and 6 normal controls (Modified from Ref. [62])

12.8 Significance of Clonal Expansion in PNH *versus* Other Blood Disorders

In haematology and in oncology, the phrase clonal disease may tend to be regarded as almost synonymous with neoplastic or malignant disease, but this is not correct. Of course acute leukaemia is both clonal and highly malignant; polycythaemia vera is both clonal and neoplastic; PNH is clonal, but neither neoplastic nor malignant. From the biological point of view, in PNH we never see invasion of non-haematopoietic tissues, and erythropoiesis remains always erythropoietin dependent [16]. From the clinical point of view, PNH patients may die from thrombosis or other complications, but very rarely (estimated less than 2 % [64]) do they eventually develop AML.

Recently, the power of currently available massive parallel DNA sequencing technology has been applied to PNH [33]. The only gene that was mutated in the GPI-negative blood cells of 10 out of 10 patients was *PIG-A*; but, in addition, somatic mutations were also found in from 1 to 6 other genes. Some of these genes, notably *TET2* and *SLC20A1*, are already known to have sometimes mutations in myeloproliferative neoplasms (MPNs) or in myelodysplastic syndromes (MDS): this has led to the suggestion that PNH is just another MPN [65]. In fact, from an analysis of clonal evolution, it emerges that, whether the *PIG-A* mutation takes place early or late, it is the key to clonal expansion. At the very time when hundreds of PNH patients are having a new lease of life through anti-C5 therapy [31], it is quite wrong to amalgamate PNH with PMN (much less with acute leukaemia).

12.9 Conclusion

Just like for populations of organisms, also for populations of somatic cells the key to Darwinian selection is a particular genotype in a particular environment. The evidence that has been reviewed in this chapter (see Table 12.2) points to inactivating mutations of *PIG-A* as the genotype that enables PNH clones to expand. Darwinian selection must be favouring a certain genotype, which is perpetuated in the progeny of the original mutant (organism or somatic cell); however, what Darwinian selection sees is the phenotype, in our case the GPI-negative cells (see Fig. 12.6). This phenotype can be produced by a variety of *PIG-A* mutations [32]; in addition, even within the same patient, more than one *PIG-A* mutant clone can expand [66]: this is a good example of convergent evolution in somatic cells. The evidence from animal models reviewed in this chapter indicates that the GPI-negative phenotype does not, on its own, provide a selective advantage, and also in most humans, *PIG-A* mutant clones with a GPI-negative phenotype exist but do not expand. The environment that promotes expansion is that of aplastic anaemia, in one way, because there is room for expansion, and, in a far more specific way, because of an autoimmune attack by T cells that have specifically targeted GPI-positive HSC.

Table 12.2 Evidence for a selective autoimmune process in PNH[a]

1.	*PIG-A* mutant clones do not expand in normal people, only in PNH patients
2.	*PIG-A* mutant clones do not expand in mice
3.	Clonal expansion can take place with a variety of *PIG-A* mutations, provided they produce a GPI-negative phenotype (*convergent evolution*)
4.	Multiple clones (each one with a different *PIG-A* mutation) can coexist within the same patient (*convergent evolution*)
5.	PNH cell population has been seen to expand in patients originally diagnosed with aplastic anaemia
6.	PNH recurrence has been reported within the same patient, at an interval of more than a decade, with a new clone being involved[b]
7.	Abnormal T cell repertoire is seen in PNH patients
8.	Mouse T cells are more reactive against GPI-positive than against GPI-negative cells
9.	Clonotypically identical T cells are found in different PNH patients
10.	GPI-reactive CD1d-restricted T cells are found in PNH patients

[a]This is a summary of the evidence presented in the text, where appropriate references are also given for most of the statements listed here
[b]See Ref. [67]

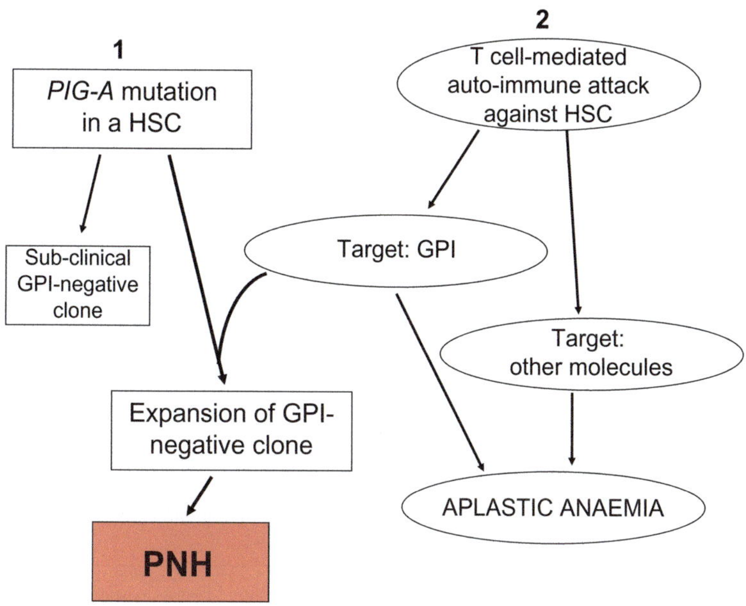

Fig. 12.6 *The Darwinian selection model of PNH pathogenesis.* The diagram shows, on the *right* hand side, the presumed pathogenesis of aplastic anaemia (AA): a T cell-mediated autoimmune attack damages HSCs. The target of the auto-reactive T cells may be the GPI molecule or another molecule expressed on HSCs. On the *left* hand side, an inactivating mutation of the *PIG-A* gene in an HSC produces a GPI-negative haematopoietic clone. In the absence of the *PIG-A* mutant clone, the autoimmune attack, even if GPI is targeted, produces AA. In the absence of the autoimmune attack, a *PIG-A* mutant clone will be of no consequence (subclinical). Only if *both* a *PIG-A* mutant clone and a GPI-targeted autoimmune attack (the two events labelled 1 and 2 in the diagram) coexist will the mutant clone expand and cause clinical PNH. In other words, Darwinian selection does not operate in favour of GPI-negative cells as such (if at all, these cells are at a disadvantage); it only operates by virtue of the presence of GPI-reactive CD1d-restricted T cells

Acknowledgement I thank all my patients with PNH and all my collaboraotors over the years in the PNH area: particularly Peter Hillmen, Monica Bessler, David Araten, Khedouja Nafa, Rosario Notaro, Luciana Gargiulo, Michela Sica.

References

1. Strübing P (1882) Paroxysmale hämoglobinurie. Dtsch Med Wocheschr 8:1–8
2. Voswinckel P (1993) Der schwarze Urin. Blackwell, Berlin
3. Marchiafava E, Nazari A (1911) Nuovo contributo all studio degli itteri cronici emolitici. Policlinico (Sez Med) 18:241
4. Ham TH, Dingle JH (1938) Studies on destruction of red blood cells. II. Chronic hemolytic mechanism with special reference to serum complement. J Clin Investig 18:657–672
5. Dacie JV, Israels MCG, Wilkinson JF (1938) Paroxysmal nocturnal haemoglobinuria of the Marchiafava type. Lancet i 231:479–482
6. Rosse WF, Dacie JV (1966) Immune lysis of normal human and paroxysmal nocturnal hemoglobinuria red blood cells. I. The sensitivity of PNH red cells to lysis by complement and specific antibody. J Clin Investig 45:736–748
7. Dacie JV (1963) Paroxysmal nocturnal haemoglobinuria. Proc R Soc Med 56:587–596
8. Lyon MF (1961) Gene action in the X chromosome in the mouse (Mus musculus L.). Nature 190:372–373
9. Beutler E, Yeh M, Fairbanks VF (1962) The normal human female as a mosaic of X-chromosome activity: studies using the gene for G6PD deficiency as a marker. Proc Natl Acad Sci U S A 48:9–16
10. Linder D, Gartler SM (1965) Glucose 6-phosphate dehydrogenase mosaicism. Utilization as a cell marker in the study of leiomyomas. Science 150:67–69
11. Luzzatto L, Allan NC (1968) Relationship between the genes for glucose 6-phosphate dehydrogenase and haemoglobin a Nigerian population. Nature 219:1041–1942
12. Oni SB, Osunkoya BO, Luzzatto L (1970) Paroxysmal nocturnal hemoglobinuria: evidence for monoclonal origin of abnormal red cells. Blood 36:145–152
13. Ghiotto G, De Sandre G (1956) Erythrocytic acetylcholinesterase. IV. Relation to some blood diseases. Acta Med Patav 16:343–362
14. Nicholson-Weller A, March JP, Rosenfeld SI, Austen KF (1983) Affected erythrocytes of patients with paroxysmal nocturnal hemoglobinuria are deficient in the complement regulatory protein, decay-accelerating factor. Proc Natl Acad Sci U S A 80:5066–5070
15. Holguin MH, Fredrick LR, Bernshaw NJ, Wilcox LA, Parker CJ (1989) Relationship between the membrane inhibitor of reactive lysis and the erythrocyte phenotypes of paroxysmal noctural hemoglobinuria. J Clin Investig 84:1387–1394
16. Rotoli B, Robledo R, Scarpato N, Luzzatto L (1984) Two populations of erythroid cell progenitors in paroxysmal nocturnal hemoglobinuria. Blood 64:847–851
17. Hirose S, Ravi L, Hazra SV, Medof ME (1991) Assembly and deacetylation of N-acetylglucosaminyl-plasmanylinositol in normal and affected paroxysmal nocturnal hemoglobinuria cells. Proc Natl Acad Sci U S A 88:3762–3766
18. Hillmen P, Bessler M, Mason PJ, Watkins WM, Luzzatto L (1993) Specific defect in N-acetylglucosamine incorporation in the biosynthesis of the glycosylphosphatidylinositol anchor in cloned cell lines from patients with paroxysmal nocturnal hemoglobinuria. Proc Natl Acad Sci U S A 90:5272–5276
19. Hillmen P, Bessler M, Bungey J, Luzzatto L (1993) Paroxysmal nocturnal hemoglobinuria: correction of abnormal phenotype by somatic cell hybridization. Somat Cell Mol Genet 19:123–129

20. Takeda J, Miyata T, Kawagoe K, Kinoshita T (1993) Deficiency of the GPI anchor caused by a somatic mutation of the PIG-A gene in paroxysmal nocturnal hemoglobinuria. Cell 73:703–711
21. Bessler M et al (1994) Paroxysmal nocturnal haemoglobinuria (PNH) is caused by somatic mutations in the PIG-A gene. EMBO J 13:110–117
22. Alfinito F et al (1996) Blood cell flow cytometry in paroxysmal nocturnal hemoglobinuria: a tool for measuring the extent of the PNH clone. Leukemia 10:1326–1330
23. Richards SJ, Hill A, Hillmen P (2007) Recent advances in the diagnosis, monitoring, and management of patients with paroxysmal nocturnal hemoglobinuria. Cytometry 72:291–298
24. Hillmen P, Hows JM, Luzzatto L (1992) Two distinct patterns of glycosylphosphatidylinositol (GPI) linked protein deficiency demonstrable in the red cells of patients with paroxysmal nocturnal haemoglobinuria. Br J Haematol 80:399–405
25. Fujioka S, Yamada T (1994) Varying populations of CD59-negative, partly positive, and normally positive blood cells in different cell lineages in peripheral blood of paroxysmal nocturnal hemoglobinuria patients. Am J Hematol 45:122–127
26. Nagakura S et al (1993) Expression of decay-accelerating factor and CD59 in lymphocyte subsets of healthy individuals and paroxysmal nocturnal hemoglobinuria patients. Am J Hematol 43:14–18
27. Vu T et al (1996) Aplastic anaemia and paroxysmal nocturnal haemoglobinuria: a study of the GPI-anchored proteins on human platelets. Br J Haematol 93:586–589
28. Rosse WF et al (1991) The erythrocytes in paroxysmal nocturnal haemoglobinuria of intermediate sensitivity to complement lysis. Br J Haematol 79:99–107
29. Hillmen P, Hows JM, Luzzatto L (1992) Two distinct patterns of glycosylphosphatidylinositol (GPI) linked protein deficiency in the red cells of patients with paroxysmal nocturnal haemoglobinuria. Br J Haematol 80:399–405
30. Rosse WF, Adams JP, Thorpe AM (1974) The population of cells in paroxysmal nocturnal haemoglobinuria of intermediate sensitivity to complement lysis: Significance and mechanism of increased immune lysis. Br J Haematol 28:181–190
31. Hillmen P et al (2006) The complement inhibitor eculizumab in paroxysmal nocturnal hemoglobinuria. N Engl J Med 355:1233–1243
32. Nafa K, Bessler M, Castro-Malaspina H, Jhanwar S, Luzzatto L (1998) The spectrum of somatic mutations in the PIG-A gene in paroxysmal nocturnal hemoglobinuria includes large deletions and small duplications. Blood Cell Mol Dis 24:370–384
33. Shen W et al (2014) Deep sequencing reveals stepwise mutation acquisition in paroxysmal nocturnal hemoglobinuria. J Clin Invest 124:4529–4538
34. Ortolan E et al (2006) CD157 plays a pivotal role in neutrophil transendothelial migration. Blood 108:4214–4222
35. Bessler M et al (2002) Glycosylphosphatidylinositol-linked proteins are required for maintenance of a normal peripheral lymphoid compartment but not for lymphocyte development. Eur J Immunol 32:2607–2616
36. Rosti V et al (1997) Murine embryonic stem cells without *pig-a* gene activity are competent for PNH-like hematopoiesis but not for clonal expansion. J Clin Investig 100:1028–1036
37. Tremml G et al (1999) Increased sensitivity to complement and a decreased red blood cell life span in mice mosaic for a nonfunctional Piga gene. Blood 94:2945–2954
38. Murakami Y, Kinoshita T, Maeda Y, Nakano T, Kosaka H, Takeda J (1999) Different roles of glycosylphosphatidylinositol in various hematopoietic cells as revealed by model mice of paroxysmal nocturnal hemoglobinuria. Blood 94:2963–2970
39. Luzzatto L (1999) Paroxysmal murine hemoglobinuria (?): A model for human PNH. Blood 94:2941–2944
40. Murakami Y et al (2002) Inefficient response of T lymphocytes to glycosylphosphatidylinositol anchor-negative cells: implications for paroxysmal nocturnal hemoglobinuria. Blood 100:4116–4122

41. Araten DJ, Nafa K, Pakdeesuwan K, Luzzatto L (1999) Clonal populations of hematopoietic cells with paroxysmal nocturnal hemoglobinuria genotype and phenotype are present in normal individuals. Proc Natl Acad Sci U S A 96:5209–5214
42. Rondelli T et al (2013) The frequency of granulocytes with spontaneous somatic mutations: a wide distribution in a normal human population. PLoS One 8:e54046
43. Hu R et al (2005) PIG-A mutations in normal hematopoiesis. Blood 105:3848–3854
44. Wang H, Chuhjo T, Yasue S, Omine M, Nakao S (2002) Clinical significance of a minor population of paroxysmal nocturnal hemoglobinuria-type cells in bone marrow failure syndrome. Blood 100:3897–3902
45. Peruzzi B, Araten DJ, Notaro R, Luzzatto L (2010) The use of PIG-A as a sentinel gene for the study of the somatic mutation rate and of mutagenic agents in vivo. Mutat Res 705:3–10
46. Miura D, Dobrovolsky VN, Kasahara Y, Katsuura Y, Heflich RH (2008) Development of an in vivo gene mutation assay using the endogenous Pig-A gene: I. Flow cytometric detection of CD59-negative peripheral red blood cells and CD48-negative spleen T-cells from the rat. Environ Mol Mutagen 49:614–621
47. Dobrovolsky VN et al (2009) Flow cytometric detection of Pig-A mutant red blood cells using an erythroid-specific antibody: Application of the method for evaluating the in vivo genotoxicity of methylphenidate in adolescent rats. Environ Mol Mutagen 51:138–145
48. Sugimori C et al (2006) Minor population of CD55-CD59- blood cells predicts response to immunosuppressive therapy and prognosis in patients with aplastic anemia. Blood 107:1308–1314
49. Okamoto M et al (2006) High frequency of several PIG-A mutations in patients with aplastic anemia and myelodysplastic syndrome. Leukemia 20:627–634
50. Lewis SM, Dacie JV (1967) The aplastic anaemia-paroxysmal nocturnal haemoglobinuria syndrome. Br J Haematol 13:236–251
51. Rotoli B, Luzzatto L (1989) Paroxysmal nocturnal haemoglobinuria. Baillières Clin Haematol 2:113–138
52. Rotoli B, Luzzatto L (1989) Paroxysmal nocturnal hemoglobinuria. Semin Hematol 26:201–207
53. Rotoli B, Robledo R, Luzzatto L (1982) Decreased number of circulating BFU-Es in paroxysmal nocturnal haemoglobinuria. Blood 60:157–159
54. Marsh JC, Elebute MO (2003) Stem cells in paroxysmal nocturnal haemoglobinuria and aplastic anaemia: increasing evidence for overlap of haemopoietic defect. Transfus Med 13:377–386
55. Dingli D, Luzzatto L, Pacheco JM (2008) Neutral evolution in paroxysmal nocturnal hemoglobinuria. Proc Natl Acad Sci U S A 105:18496–18500
56. Inoue N et al (2006) Molecular basis of clonal expansion of hematopoiesis in 2 patients with paroxysmal nocturnal hemoglobinuria (PNH). Blood 108:4232–4236
57. Murakami Y et al (2012) Deregulated expression of HMGA2 is implicated in clonal expansion of PIGA deficient cells in paroxysmal nocturnal haemoglobinuria. Br J Haematol 156:383–387
58. Young NS (2002) Acquired aplastic anemia. Ann Intern Med 136:534–546
59. Schofield L et al (1999) CD1d-restricted immunoglobulin G formation to GPI-anchored antigens mediated by NKT cells. Science 283:225–229
60. Karadimitris A et al (2000) Abnormal T-cell repertoire is consistent with immune process underlying the pathogenesis of paroxysmal nocturnal hemoglobinuria. Blood 96:2613–2620
61. Gargiulo L et al (2007) Highly homologous T-cell receptor beta sequences support a common target for auto-reactive T cells in most patients with paroxysmal nocturnal hemoglobinuria. Blood 109:5036–5042
62. Gargiulo L et al (2013) Glycosylphosphatidylinositol-specific, CD1d-restricted T cells in paroxysmal nocturnal hemoglobinuria. Blood 121:2753–2761

63. Richichi B, Luzzatto L, Notaro R, Marca G, Nativi C (2011) Synthesis of the essential core of the human glycosylphosphatidylinositol (GPI) anchor. Bioorg Chem 39:88–93
64. Socié G et al (1996) Paroxysmal nocturnal haemoglobinuria: long-term follow-up and prognostic factors. Lancet 348:573–577
65. Lee SC, Abdel-Wahab O (2014) The mutational landscape of paroxysmal nocturnal hemoglobinuria revealed: new insights into clonal dominance. J Clin Invest 124:4227–4230
66. Bessler M, Mason PJ, Hillmen P, Luzzatto L (1994) Somatic mutations and cellular selection in paroxysmal nocturnal haemoglobinuria. Lancet 343:951–953
67. Nafa K, Bessler M, Deeg HJ, Luzzatto L (1998) New somatic mutation in the PIG-A gene emerges at relapse of paroxysmal nocturnal hemoglobinuria. Blood 92:3422–3427

Chapter 13
Pathogenesis of Clonal Dominance in PNH: Selection Mechanisms in PNH

Tatsuya Kawaguchi and Hideki Nakakuma

Abstract It appears that the presence of a mutation of the *PIGA* gene alone is not sufficient for the development of paroxysmal nocturnal hemoglobinuria (PNH) and that concomitant expansion of *PIGA*-mutant clones is indispensable; however, the mechanism of such expansion is not yet fully elucidated. Because of the close association between idiopathic aplastic anemia and PNH, the prevailing hypothesis is that PNH progenitor cells can survive rather than normal progenitor cells against autoimmune attack on bone marrow cells by evading immune recognition with the aid of their membrane characteristics, leading to selective expansion of PNH clones. Various attempts have so far been made to prove this hypothesis, including examining the apoptosis resistance of PNH hematopoietic cells, involvement of conventional cytotoxic T cells or certain T-cell subsets such as CD1d-restricted T cells and natural killer receptor-expressing T cells as the immune effector cells, and involvement of natural killer cells under some stress situations. In this chapter, the results of these studies will be outlined; we will also refer to our own findings on the relationship between NKG2D-mediated immunity and the clonal selection of PNH cells.

Keywords Clonal selection • Bone marrow failure • NKG2D • ULBP

13.1 Introduction

Paroxysmal nocturnal hemoglobinuria (PNH) is an acquired hematopoietic stem cell disorder caused by a mutation(s) of the *PIGA* gene, which is characterized by the clonal expansion of PNH cells lacking glycosylphosphatidylinositol-anchored proteins (GPI-AP), leading to specific pathogenic conditions such as hemolysis

T. Kawaguchi, M.D., Ph.D. (✉)
Departments of Hematology & Infectious Diseases, Kumamoto University Graduate School of Medical Sciences, 1-1-1 Honjo, Chuoku, 860-8556 Kumamoto, Japan
e-mail: tatsu@kumamoto-u.ac.jp

H. Nakakuma
Kagoshima-Tokushukai Hospital, 3-8-1 Shimo-Arata, Kagoshima 890-0056, Japan

Y. Kanakura et al. (eds.), *Paroxysmal Nocturnal Hemoglobinuria*,
DOI 10.1007/978-4-431-56003-6_13

and thrombosis. In recent years, eculizumab, a newly introduced humanized anti-C5 antibody, has dramatically improved PNH patients in terms of not only hemolysis but also thrombosis, thereby contributing to an extremely better understanding of this disease [1]. However, the clonal dominance of PNH cells usually remains unchanged after complement inhibition by eculizumab therapy, although the percentage of PNH erythrocytes often increases. Therefore, the complement system does not seem to be directly associated with expansion of PNH clones. Even in the eculizumab era, the mechanism underlying the clonal expansion of PNH cells remains an unsolved riddle; this is an attractive and challenging topic for researchers. Because a small population of *PIGA* mutants can be detected in normal individuals [2] and a substantial expansion of the affected cells was lacking in *piga*-knockout mice [3], it is plausible that a *PIGA* mutation alone is insufficient to cause the disease and that factors other than *PIGA* mutations are required for PNH development. Currently, there are two hypotheses to explain the mechanism underlying the clonal expansion of PNH cells: one is negative selection of PNH cells under immune-mediated bone marrow injury; the other is intrinsic growth abnormality of PNH cells. These two hypotheses may not be mutually exclusive and may be cooperative to each other. This chapter reviews the potential selection mechanisms by which PNH cells can escape autoimmune attack and achieve clonal dominance.

13.2 Clinical Evidence of Immune-Mediated Bone Marrow Failure

Bone marrow failure, an essential component of clinical manifestations of PNH as well as hemolysis and thrombosis, is believed to play an important role in the pathogenesis of PNH. In fact, many patients with PNH have not only anemia but also leukocytopenia and thrombocytopenia. Since more than half a century ago when the first case report of PNH developed after idiopathic aplastic anemia (AA) was reported, many studies have demonstrated a close association between AA and PNH [4]. Based on such clinical evidence, researchers have advocated that an autoimmune mechanism is operating in the development of bone marrow failure in PNH as in AA. To support this notion, immunosuppressive agents such as cyclosporine have been found to be effective in some patients with PNH [5]. In addition, HLA-DR2, a serotype highly associated with AA, was also frequently found in PNH patients [6], and DRB1*1501 was especially shared in Japanese patients [7]. Furthermore, several attempts to clarify the characteristics of immune effector cells showed evidence of aberrant immune response in PNH: oligoclonal expansion of T cells [8], a higher degree of skewedness of the T-cell receptor V beta repertoire [9, 10], and an increased percentage of interferon-γ-producing T cells [11]. These findings suggest autoimmune-mediated insult to the bone marrow in PNH patients. Under such circumstances, how PNH cells can survive and dominate normal cells in spite of their highly vulnerable to the complement activation? To answer this question, many challenges have been done as described in the following sections.

13.3 Immune Selection Mechanisms

13.3.1 Apoptosis Resistance

The hypothesis that GPI-AP-deficient (GPI^-) cells or PNH cells are more resistant to apoptosis as compared to GPI-AP-expressing (GPI^+) normal cells is attractive, because it may better explain how PNH cells can achieve clonal dominance despite showing diminished hematopoietic activity. In the late 1990s, three research groups independently reported that granulocytes derived from PNH patients are more resistant to apoptosis induced by serum depletion, as compared to those from normal individuals [12–14]. However, two of the three studies also showed that the apoptosis resistance was not much different between patients with large PNH clones (90 % or more) and those with small PNH clones (below 10–40 %), indicating that the presence of *PIGA* mutations was not correlated with the sensitivity to apoptosis, at least in the mature blood cells in these patients [13, 14]. This conclusion is not surprising, because granulocytes despite positive or negative for GPI-AP should stem from progenitor cells surviving immune selection in the bone marrow. If this indeed is the case, the question arises as to whether the apoptosis sensitivity might differ between the normal and PNH phenotypes at the immature level of the progenitor cells before immune selection. Actually, GPI^+ $CD34^+$ cells showed higher expression levels of the Fas receptor, a greater susceptibility to apoptosis, and a greater sensitivity to killing by extrinsic Fas agonists, as compared to GPI^- $CD34^+$ cells [15, 16]. Furthermore, in vitro studies demonstrated that GPI^+ $CD34^+$ cells showed a lower proliferation potential than GPI^- $CD34^+$ cells derived from the same patient or $CD34^+$ cells from normal individuals [15, 16]. These results are consistent with the notion that GPI^- progenitor cells show clonal dominance over GPI^+ progenitor cells because of their intrinsic apoptosis resistance. This notion is supported by the results of a study comparing the gene expression profiles between GPI^+ and GPI^- $CD34^+$ cells in patients with PNH, which indicated that the former cells showed higher expression levels of the apoptosis-related genes as compared to the latter [17]. Now, the question is how does the presence or absence of GPI-AP change the sensitivity to apoptosis of the progenitor cells? One possible explanation is the difference in their responses to pro-inflammatory cytokines such as IFN-γ and TNF-α. These cytokines increase the Fas antigen expression on the bone marrow cells in vitro and suppress colony formation in normal individuals [18]. In AA, these cytokines are elevated and play a role in the pathogenesis of bone marrow failure directly or indirectly; the same is also likely to be true in patients with PNH [19].

In fact, these cytokines suppressed colony formation of the bone marrow cells from patients with PNH just as in normal individuals; however, the GPI^- progenitor cells were more resistant to the effects of the cytokines than the GPI^+ progenitor cells [20]. Such differences in their responses to the cytokines may be explained by the altered composition of the lipid rafts in GPI^- cells, which would modulate death signal transduction from external cytokines in GPI^- cells [21]. However, different sensitivities of progenitor cells to apoptosis between GPI^+ and GPI^- phenotypes could not be confirmed in the *piga*-knockout mice model. This question warrants further investigation [22].

13.3.2 Immune Escape Models

13.3.2.1 Cytotoxic T-Cell Model

In idiopathic AA, cytotoxic T lymphocytes (CTL) producing Th1 cytokines are the major effector cells responsible for immune-mediated bone marrow failure [23]. Considering the close association of AA with PNH, it can be hypothesized that GPI^- progenitor cells are less sensitive to the cytotoxic effect of CTL rather than GPI^+ progenitor cells. Several experimental models were developed to test the hypothesis (Table 13.1). First, Karadimitris et al. developed a relatively simple model to examine the role of CTL in PNH, using the Epstein-Barr virus (EBV)-transformed B-cell lines positive or negative for GPI-AP from PNH patients as the target cells and an EBV-specific cytotoxic T-cell line derived from the same patient as the effector cells. Although CTL was sufficiently activated in this model, there was no significant difference in the activation level between the GPI^+ and GPI^- target cells. Thus, they concluded that there was no GPI-AP that could modulate the CTL activation by functioning as an adhesion molecule or a costimulatory factor [24]. However, the target molecules for CTL recognition used in the study were extrinsic EBV nuclear antigen peptides, which might cause too strong immune reaction to distinguish a subtle difference in immune sensitivity between GPI^+ and GPI^- cells. On the other hand, autoantigens that could be recognized by CTL, such as kinectin- and diazepam-binding related protein-1, have been reported in patients with AA [25, 26]. Similarly, potential autoantigens have been postulated in PNH as responsible molecules for CTL to distinguish GPI^+ and GPI^- cells, though they have yet to be identified. If such autoantigens were GPI proteins, it is presumed that GPI^- cells would be spared from CTL-mediated attack because they do not process the GPI protein-derived antigen peptides [27]. To test this hypothesis, Murakami et al. examined an elaborate experimental model; they prepared a pair of GPI^- mouse thymoma cells that lacked the GPI synthesis machinery and a GPI^+ counterpart. Both cells expressed MHC class II molecules. When the synthesized GPI-linked ovalbumin was expressed in these cells, GPI^+ thymoma cells could present the antigen peptides derived from ovalbumin to the antigen-specific CTL, but GPI^- thymoma cells could not [28]. Although this model is very convincing, it has not been investigated whether such

Table 13.1 Experimental approaches by the effector-target interaction to show immune selection of PNH clone and their outcomes

Effector cells		Target cells* or molecules	Selection of GPI⁻ cells	References
Cytotoxic T cells				
Human	EBV-specific T cells	EBV-transformed B cells	No	Karadimitris, et al. [24]
	WT1-specific T cells	WT1	Yes	Ikeda, et al. [31]
	CD1d$^+$-restricted T cells	GPI	Not tested	Gargiulo, et al. [34]
	NKR$^+$ T cells	K562	Yes	Poggi, et al. [36]
	NKR$^+$ T cells	CD34$^+$ cell line, K562	Yes, but not all cases	van Bijnen, et al. [37]
Mouse	Antigen-specific CD4$^+$ T cells, alloreactive CD4$^+$ T cells	Thymoma cell line expressing GPI-anchored or transmembrane OVA	Yes	Murakami, et al. [28]
Natural killer cells		K562, ULBP1, ULBP2	Yes	Nagakura, et al. [38]
				Hanaoka, et al. [39]

*A pair of GPI-positive and GPI-negative target cells was prepared in each study
EBV Epstein-Barr virus, *WT1* Wilms' tumor 1, *NKR* natural killer cell receptors, *GPI* glycosylphosphatidylinositol, *OVA* ovalbumin

GPI proteins could serve as autoantigens in patients with PNH. Focusing on the high frequency of some MHC alleles (A*24:02, B*18:01, DRB1*04:01, DRB1*15:01) in PNH patients, Nowak et al. analyzed the current reference database on MHC molecule-eluted peptide presentation repertoires and searched for peptides that could be presented by the PNH-associated MHC alleles. Although they identified the source proteins, no GPI protein was included [29]. On the other hand, it was reported that non-GPI proteins such as Wilms' tumor 1 (WT1) protein, a human T-cell leukemia virus (HTLV) epitope, BA21, might be potential target antigens for CTL in PNH [7, 30]. In particular, Ikeda et al. observed the expression of the WT1 gene at a significantly higher frequency in the bone marrow cells of PNH patients than in those of healthy individuals. Moreover, they showed that these WT1-expressing marrow cells were susceptible to CTL in an HLA-A*24:02-restricted manner, suggesting the possible pathogenetic role of WT1 peptide-specific CD8$^+$ cells in PNH patients [31]. In their study, GPI$^-$ CD34 cells were less sensitive to cytotoxicity as compared to GPI$^+$ CD34 cells, suggesting the WT1-dependent immunologic selection of a PNH clone. However, given that the WT1 gene is abundantly expressed in both GPI$^+$ and GPI$^-$ CD34 cells, the expression level of the target antigen cannot fully explain the difference in the sensitivity of the cells to CTL-mediated cytotoxicity. In this model, the possibility that some adhesion molecules or costimulatory factors in the GPI form may affect the CTL activation is not ruled out.

13.3.2.2 CD1d-Restricted T-Cell Model

On the other hand, Luzzatto et al. pointed out the possibility that CD1d-restricted T cells recognizing lipids and glycolipids, rather than those recognizing conventional peptide antigens, may play an important role in the pathogenesis of PNH [32]. CD1d, a membrane protein with antigen-presenting ability similar to MHC molecules, is expressed on antigen-presenting cells (APCs) such as dendritic cells and B cells. It can present self-lipid antigens bound to its hydrophobic groove to CD1d-restricted T cells as well as external lipid antigens from microbes [33]. Because CD1d is also expressed on hematopoietic stem cells (HSCs), these effector cells presumably recognize and impair HSCs in a GPI-dependent manner if GPI antigens are presented by CD1d. However, in this situation, *PIGA*-mutated HSCs cannot express GPI on CD1d, as they do not have the ability to synthesize GPI, thereby escaping the GPI-dependent attack. This hypothesis is interesting and persuasive in explaining the negative selection of PNH clones in terms of GPI itself, the principal element in the pathophysiology of PNH, as a potential target antigen. Recently, Gargiulo et al. showed the presence of $CD8^+$ T lymphocytes that reacted with GPI-loaded APCs in PNH patients, using the INF-γ ELISPOT assay [34]. They also demonstrated that $CD8^+$ T lymphocytes could recognize not only extrinsic GPI but also intrinsic GPI through the invariant Vα21 T-cell receptor (TCR) and concluded that they were novel CD1d-restricted, GPI-specific T cells. Their report did not verify whether these new effector cells could distinguish between the presence and absence of GPI expression in the target cells and could exert selective cytotoxic activity on the GPI-positive cells. Advances in research on this issue are awaited.

13.3.2.3 Natural Killer Cell-Like T-Cell Model

Natural killer cell receptors (NKRs), including killer immunoglobulin-like receptors (KIRs) and C-type lectin receptors (CLRs), are expressed in some T-cell subsets as well as natural killer (NK) cells and modulate the functions of the T cells [35]. NKRs consist of both activating and inhibitory receptors. The functional directions of the cells expressing NKRs are determined according to which receptors are dominant. To define a role of such NKR^+ T cells in negative selection of PNH clones, two research groups analyzed quantitatively and qualitatively NKR^+ T cells in PNH patients [36, 37]. First, Poggi et al. compared the number of $CD3^+KIR^+$ T cells and $CD3^+CLR^+$ T cells in the peripheral blood between 13 PNH patients and healthy subjects and found no differences between the two groups of subjects. However, when KIRs or CLRs were engaged by specific antibodies in the redirected assay, T cells from PNH patients were activated much higher than those from healthy subjects, indicating an increase of the activating form of NKR^+ T cells in PNH patients [36]. Interestingly, NKR^+ T cells exerted natural killer activity, like NK cells, against GPI^+ and GPI^- K562 cells that lacked the expression of MHC class I molecules, while GPI⁻ K562 cells were less sensitive to such killer activity. Similarly, van Bijnen et al. investigated the frequency and number of T cells expressing various types of NKR in the peripheral blood of 39 PNH patients [37]. In contrast to the results by Poggi et al., they found increased number of T cells positive for CD56 and activating forms of NKR such as KIR2DS4, NKG2C, and NKG2D in PNH patients as compared with those in healthy individuals. $CD56^+$ T cells were characterized by dominance of CD8-positive, CD45RA-positive effector-memory phenotype. In addition, patient-derived $CD8^+$, $KIR2DS4^+$, and $NKG2D^+$ T-cell lines exerted cytotoxic activity against GPI-positive and GPI-negative matched pair cell lines ($CD34^+$ TF-1, KG1a, K562). Differential sensitivity of target cell pairs to each effector cell line was found depending on the degree of GPI expression, but not in all pairs.

13.3.2.4 Natural Killer Cell Model

The remaining major effector cells that have not been referred above are NK cells. To test a potential role of NK cells in the clonal selection of PNH cells, we prepared GPI-deficient *PIGA*-mutant cells (GPI^- K562) and a counterpart (GPI^+ K562) in which GPI expression was restored by the transfection of *PIGA* cDNA and determined their sensitivity to NK cells by ^{51}Cr release assay. We found that the NK sensitivity was reduced by half in GPI^- K562 cells as compared with that in GPI^+ K562 cells, showing a relative survival advantage of GPI^- cells [38]. Because the difference in NK sensitivity was determined only by the presence or absence of GPI proteins at the surface of these target cells, the responsible molecule was speculated to be a GPI protein(s) related to NK cell activation. Therefore, we focused on the most probable candidate, the human cytomegalovirus glycoprotein UL16-binding proteins (ULBPs) [39]. ULBPs are ligands of the activating NK receptor, NKG2D. To date, six isoforms of ULBP have been identified, of which ULBP1, ULBP2, ULPB3, and ULBP6 are GPI-linked proteins, while others are transmembrane proteins [40]. In our study, ULBP1–ULBP3 were detected in GPI^+ K562 cells, but not in GPI^- K562 cells. There was no difference in the gene expression of ULBP1–ULBP3 between two types of target cells, indicating that the difference in the membrane expression was only attributable to a *PIGA* mutation. The presence of antibodies to both ULBP1 and ULBP2 in this cytotoxic assay rendered GPI^+ K562 cells as less sensitive to NK cells as GPI^- K562 cells, but antibody to ULBP3 exerted no effect. In addition to the ULBP family, MHC class I-related chain A (MICA) and MHC class I-related chain B (MICB), another group of ligands for NKG2D, were expressed to the same degree in both target cells because they were type I transmembrane proteins. Antibodies to MICA/MICB decreased the NK sensitivity of both target cells, but failed to close its gap primarily found between them. Thus, we concluded that both ULBP1 and ULBP2 were key molecules that elicited differential NK sensitivity between GPI-positive and GPI-negative cells.

13.3.3 NKG2D-Mediated Immunity

13.3.3.1 NKG2D Ligands

NKG2D ligands such as ULBPs and MICA/MICB are usually undetected in most normal cells, but upregulated in the cells under various stresses such as infection, tumorigenesis, DNA damage, oxidative stress, and heat shock. Engagement of NKG2D with its ligands can activate NK cells by overriding the inhibitory signals from self-MHC class I molecules, resulting in the killing of altered cells expressing NKG2D ligands. NKG2D is expressed not only by NK cells but also by $CD8^+$ T cells, γδT cells, NKT cells, and certain $CD4^+$ T cells. In these specialized T cells, NKG2D may function as a costimulatory receptor in association with T-cell receptor (TCR)-mediated T-cell activation. Given that NKG2D ligands such as ULBPs and MICA/MICB are induced by some stress in the bone marrow cells of PNH patients, NKG2D-bearing cytotoxic lymphocytes may be strongly activated to target bone marrow cells expressing NKG2D ligands, leading to serious damage of hematopoiesis. In such a situation, PNH progenitor cells lacking ULBPs are less susceptible to cytotoxicity by NK cells or NKG2D-positive T cells as compared to normal progenitor cells, showing a survival advantage of PNH cells over normal cells (Fig. 13.1). To test this hypothesis, we analyzed expression of NKG2D ligands on blood cells of PNH patients and a pathogenetic role of NKG2D-mediated immunity as described in the following sections.

13.3.3.2 Expression of NKG2D Ligands in PNH

Membrane expressions of NKG2D ligands on blood cells were analyzed by flow cytometry in 19 PNH patients and 17 healthy subjects [41]. About a half of PNH patients carried granulocytes expressing ULBPs and/or MICA/MICB, while healthy individuals did not at all, except one who had MICA-positive granulocytes. ULBPs were also expressed in the $CD34^+$ bone marrow cells of some patients. Our results suggest that these patients had been exposed to some stress that induced the NKG2D ligands on hematopoietic cells. Importantly, in the patients positive for NKG2D ligands, normal phenotype $CD59^+$ granulocytes expressed both ULBPs and MICA/MICB, while PNH phenotype $CD59^-$ granulocytes expressed MICA/MICB alone and lacked GPI-linked ULBPs. These findings provide a pathogenetic picture similar to our hypothetic model depicted in Fig. 13.1 in terms of selection of PNH clone by NKG2D-mediated immunity.

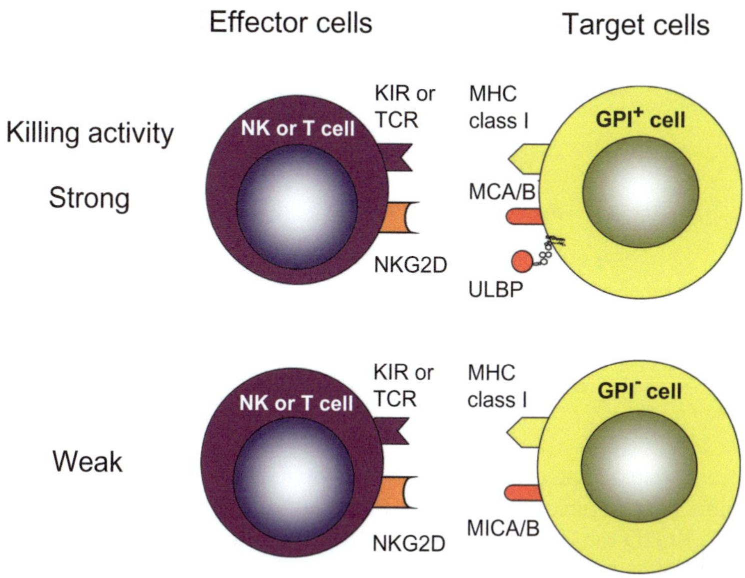

Fig. 13.1 Selection mechanism of PNH clone under NKG2D-mediated immunity. NKG2D ligands such as MICA/MICAB and ULBPs are induced by some stress on the target cells. GPI^+ cells can express both ligands, but GPI^- cells fail to express GPI-linked ULBPs. Therefore, effector cells are differentially activated by GPI^+ or GPI^- target cells through the activating NKG2D receptor after its engagement with two types or single type of ligands, respectively

13.3.3.3 Role of the NKG2D-NKG2D Ligand Interaction in PNH

We further investigated the role of NKG2D-mediated immunity in the interaction between primary target and effector cells derived from PNH patients. In fact, granulocytes expressing NKG2D ligands were killed by autologous NKG2D-bearing lymphocytes in vitro [39]. In addition, inhibitory effect of NKG2D-bearing lymphocytes on the hematopoietic colony formation by the bone marrow cells expressing NKG2D ligands was restored with the presence of anti-NKG2D antibodies. In contrast, the cytotoxic activity of NKG2D-bearing lymphocytes was not observed if the target cells either from peripheral blood or bone marrow cells were negative for NKG2D ligands. Again, these findings support our working hypothesis that NKG2D-mediated immunity is associated not only with the development of bone marrow failure but also with immune selection of PNH clones. Interestingly, NKG2D ligands were detected on granulocytes from some patients with AA or MDS, suggesting that NKG2D-mediated immunity can be shared as a potential mechanism of bone marrow failure by bone marrow failure syndromes [41]. In addition, we found some patients with AA in whom expression of NKG2D ligands was well correlated with progression of marrow failure. These cases suggest that NKG2D ligand expression may serve as a useful clinical marker for understanding

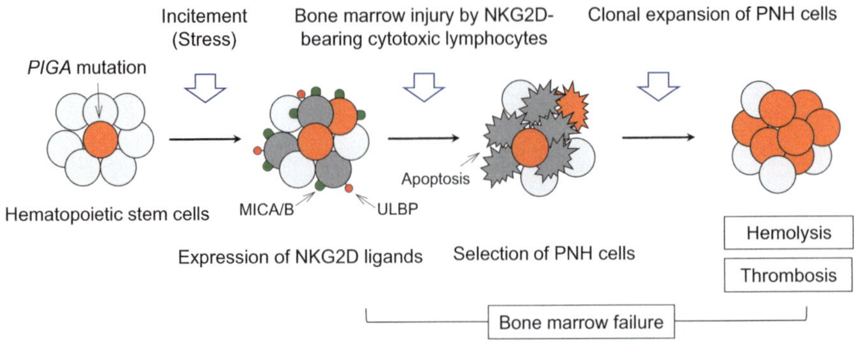

Fig. 13.2 A model of PNH pathogenesis highlighting the NKG2D-mediated immune mechanism

the disease state and predicting the disease course of immune-mediated bone marrow failure [41]. Figure 13.2 shows the PNH pathogenesis model based on the scenario of NKG2D-mediated immunity. It remains unknown why NKG2D ligands do not always express in all patients and what kind of stress induces NKG2D ligands.

13.4 Conclusion

We have outlined previous studies on the mechanisms of immune selection of PNH clones. It is presumed that the actual immune selection of PNH clones follows a very complex mechanism, because many cellular and humoral immune factors may be involved in the development of bone marrow failure in PNH. Further investigation is necessary to determine which of the models cited here most accurately reflects the PNH pathogenesis. The NKG2D-mediated immunity plays an important role not only in NK cells but also in a wide range of effector T cells expressing NKG2D, including $CD8^+$ CTL and NKR^+ T cells, as a costimulatory pathway. We believe that NKG2D-mediated immunity may be widely applicable to the explanation of the PNH clone selection, no matter which type of effector cells is a major player in PNH pathogenesis.

References

1. Hill A, Richards SJ, Hillmen P (2007) Recent developments in the understanding and management of paroxysmal nocturnal haemoglobinuria. Br J Haematol 137 (3):181–192. doi: BJH6554 [pii] 10.1111/j.1365-2141.2007.06554.x
2. Araten DJ, Nafa K, Pakdeesuwan K, Luzzatto L (1999) Clonal populations of hematopoietic cells with paroxysmal nocturnal hemoglobinuria genotype and phenotype are present in normal individuals. Proc Natl Acad Sci U S A 96(9):5209–5214

3. Rosti V, Tremml G, Soares V, Pandolfi PP, Luzzatto L, Bessler M (1997) Murine embryonic stem cells without pig-a gene activity are competent for hematopoiesis with the PNH phenotype but not for clonal expansion. J Clin Invest 100(5):1028–1036. doi:10.1172/JCI119613
4. Parker CJ (2002) Historical aspects of paroxysmal nocturnal haemoglobinuria: 'defining the disease'. Br J Haematol 117 (1):3–22. doi:3374 [pii]
5. Horikawa K, Fujisao S, Iwamoto N, Nagakura S, Kawaguchi T, Nishimura Y, Takatsuki K, Nakakuma H (1996) Cyclosporin-responsive pancytopenia and HLA class II alleles of a patient with paroxysmal nocturnal hemoglobinuria. Int J Hematol 63(2):165–166
6. Maciejewski JP, Follmann D, Nakamura R, Saunthararajah Y, Rivera CE, Simonis T, Brown KE, Barrett JA, Young NS (2001) Increased frequency of HLA-DR2 in patients with paroxysmal nocturnal hemoglobinuria and the PNH/aplastic anemia syndrome. Blood 98(13):3513–3519
7. Shichishima T, Okamoto M, Ikeda K, Kaneshige T, Sugiyama H, Terasawa T, Osumi K, Maruyama Y (2002) HLA class II haplotype and quantitation of WT1 RNA in Japanese patients with paroxysmal nocturnal hemoglobinuria. Blood 100(1):22–28
8. Risitano AM, Maciejewski JP, Muranski P, Wlodarski M, O'Keefe C, Sloand EM, Young NS (2005) Large granular lymphocyte (LGL)-like clonal expansions in paroxysmal nocturnal hemoglobinuria (PNH) patients. Leukemia 19(2):217–222
9. Karadimitris A, Manavalan JS, Thaler HT, Notaro R, Araten DJ, Nafa K, Roberts IA, Weksler ME, Luzzatto L (2000) Abnormal T-cell repertoire is consistent with immune process underlying the pathogenesis of paroxysmal nocturnal hemoglobinuria. Blood 96(7):2613–2620
10. Risitano AM, Kook H, Zeng W, Chen G, Young NS, Maciejewski JP (2002) Oligoclonal and polyclonal CD4 and CD8 lymphocytes in aplastic anemia and paroxysmal nocturnal hemoglobinuria measured by V beta CDR3 spectratyping and flow cytometry. Blood 100(1):178–183
11. Coluzzi S, Biffoni M, Pasqualetti D, Perrone MP, Vaglio S, Rahimi H, Arista MC, Laurenti L, Cerretti R, Girelli G (2004) Production of interferon-gamma by lymphocytes from paroxysmal nocturnal haemoglobinuria patients: relationship with clinical status. Br J Haematol 124(5):685–690
12. Brodsky RA, Vala MS, Barber JP, Medof ME, Jones RJ (1997) Resistance to apoptosis caused by PIG-A gene mutations in paroxysmal nocturnal hemoglobinuria. Proc Natl Acad Sci U S A 94(16):8756–8760
13. Horikawa K, Nakakuma H, Kawaguchi T, Iwamoto N, Nagakura S, Kagimoto T, Takatsuki K (1997) Apoptosis resistance of blood cells from patients with paroxysmal nocturnal hemoglobinuria, aplastic anemia, and myelodysplastic syndrome. Blood 90(7):2716–2722
14. Ware RE, Nishimura J, Moody MA, Smith C, Rosse WF, Howard TA (1998) The PIG-A mutation and absence of glycosylphosphatidylinositol-linked proteins do not confer resistance to apoptosis in paroxysmal nocturnal hemoglobinuria. Blood 92(7):2541–2550
15. Chen R, Nagarajan S, Prince GM, Maheshwari U, Terstappen LW, Kaplan DR, Gerson SL, Albert JM, Dunn DE, Lazarus HM, Medof ME (2000) Impaired growth and elevated fas receptor expression in PIGA(+) stem cells in primary paroxysmal nocturnal hemoglobinuria. J Clin Invest 106(5):689–696. doi:10.1172/JCI8328
16. Chen G, Kirby M, Zeng W, Young NS, Maciejewski JP (2002) Superior growth of glycophosphatidylinositol-anchored protein-deficient progenitor cells in vitro is due to the higher apoptotic rate of progenitors with normal phenotype in vivo. Exp Hematol 30(7):774–782. doi: S0301472X02008111 [pii]
17. Chen G, Zeng W, Maciejewski JP, Kcyvanfar K, Billings EM, Young NS (2005) Differential gene expression in hematopoietic progenitors from paroxysmal nocturnal hemoglobinuria patients reveals an apoptosis/immune response in 'normal' phenotype cells. Leukemia 19(5):862–868. doi:10.1038/sj.leu.2403678
18. Maciejewski J, Selleri C, Anderson S, Young NS (1995) Fas antigen expression on CD34+ human marrow cells is induced by interferon gamma and tumor necrosis factor alpha and potentiates cytokine-mediated hematopoietic suppression in vitro. Blood 85(11):3183–3190

19. Young NS, Maciejewski J (1997) The pathophysiology of acquired aplastic anemia. N Engl J Med 336(19):1365–1372. doi:10.1056/NEJM199705083361906
20. Barcellini W, Fermo E, Guia Imperiali F, Zaninoni A, Bianchi P, Boschetti C, Zanella A (2004) Increased resistance of PIG-A- bone marrow progenitors to tumor necrosis factor a and interferon gamma: possible implications for the in vivo dominance of paroxysmal nocturnal hemoglobinuria clones. Haematologica 89(6):651–656
21. Szpurka H, Schade AE, Jankowska AM, Maciejewski JP (2008) Altered lipid raft composition and defective cell death signal transduction in glycosylphosphatidylinositol anchor-deficient PIG-A mutant cells. Br J Haematol 142(3):413–422. doi:10.1111/j.1365-2141.2008.07203.x
22. Kulkarni S, Bessler M (2003) Effect of proinflammatory cytokines on PIGA- hematopoiesis. Exp Hematol 31(9):770–778
23. Young NS, Calado RT, Scheinberg P (2006) Current concepts in the pathophysiology and treatment of aplastic anemia. Blood 108(8):2509–2519. doi:10.1182/blood-2006-03-010777
24. Karadimitris A, Notaro R, Koehne G, Roberts IA, Luzzatto L (2000) PNH cells are as sensitive to T-cell-mediated lysis as their normal counterparts: implications for the pathogenesis of paroxysmal nocturnal haemoglobinuria. Br J Haematol 111(4):1158–1163
25. Hirano N, Butler MO, Von Bergwelt-Baildon MS, Maecker B, Schultze JL, O'Connor KC, Schur PH, Kojima S, Guinan EC, Nadler LM (2003) Autoantibodies frequently detected in patients with aplastic anemia. Blood 102(13):4567–4575. doi:10.1182/blood-2002-11-3409
26. Feng X, Chuhjo T, Sugimori C, Kotani T, Lu X, Takami A, Takamatsu H, Yamazaki H, Nakao S (2004) Diazepam-binding inhibitor-related protein 1: a candidate autoantigen in acquired aplastic anemia patients harboring a minor population of paroxysmal nocturnal hemoglobinuria-type cells. Blood 104(8):2425–2431. doi:10.1182/blood-2004-05-1839
27. Kinoshita T, Inoue N (2002) Relationship between aplastic anemia and paroxysmal nocturnal hemoglobinuria. Int J Hematol 75(2):117–122
28. Murakami Y, Kosaka H, Maeda Y, Nishimura J, Inoue N, Ohishi K, Okabe M, Takeda J, Kinoshita T (2002) Inefficient response of T lymphocytes to glycosylphosphatidylinositol anchor-negative cells: implications for paroxysmal nocturnal hemoglobinuria. Blood 100(12):4116–4122
29. Nowak J, Wozniak J, Mendek-Czajkowska E, Dlugokecka A, Mika-Witkowska R, Rogatko-Koros M, Graczyk-Pol E, Marosz-Rudnicka A, Dziopa J, Golec A, Kopec-Szlezak J, Warzocha K (2013) Potential link between MHC-self-peptide presentation and hematopoiesis; the analysis of HLA-DR expression in CD34-positive cells and self-peptide presentation repertoires of MHC molecules associated with paroxysmal nocturnal hemoglobinuria. Cell Biochem Biophys 65(3):321–333. doi:10.1007/s12013-012-9435-1
30. Nyland SB, Krissinger DJ, Clemente MJ, Irby RB, Baab KT, Jarbadan NR, Sokol L, Schaefer E, Liao J, Cuthbertson D, Epling-Burnette P, Paquette R, List AF, Maciejewski JP, Loughran TP Jr (2012) Seroreactivity to LGL leukemia-specific epitopes in aplastic anemia, myelodysplastic syndrome and paroxysmal nocturnal hemoglobinuria: results of a bone marrow failure consortium study. Leuk Res 36(5):581–587. doi:10.1016/j.leukres.2012.02.001
31. Ikeda K, Shichishima T, Yasukawa M, Nakamura-Shichishima A, Noji H, Akutsu K, Osumi K, Maruyama Y (2007) The role of Wilms' tumor gene peptide-specific cytotoxic T lymphocytes in immunologic selection of a paroxysmal nocturnal hemoglobinuria clone. Exp Hematol 35(4):618–626
32. Karadimitris A, Luzzatto L (2001) The cellular pathogenesis of paroxysmal nocturnal haemoglobinuria. Leukemia 15(8):1148–1152
33. Brennan PJ, Brigl M, Brenner MB (2013) Invariant natural killer T cells: an innate activation scheme linked to diverse effector functions. Nat Rev Immunol 13(2):101–117. doi:10.1038/nri3369
34. Gargiulo L, Papaioannou M, Sica M, Talini G, Chaidos A, Richichi B, Nikolaev AV, Nativi C, Layton M, de la Fuente J, Roberts I, Luzzatto L, Notaro R, Karadimitris A (2013) Glycosylphosphatidylinositol-specific, CD1d-restricted T cells in paroxysmal nocturnal hemoglobinuria. Blood 121(14):2753–2761. doi:10.1182/blood-2012-11-469353

35. van Bergen J, Koning F (2010) The tortoise and the hare: slowly evolving T-cell responses take hastily evolving KIR. Immunology 131(3):301–309. doi:10.1111/j.1365-2567.2010.03337.x
36. Poggi A, Negrini S, Zocchi MR, Massaro AM, Garbarino L, Lastraioli S, Gargiulo L, Luzzatto L, Notaro R (2005) Patients with paroxysmal nocturnal hemoglobinuria have a high frequency of peripheral-blood T cells expressing activating isoforms of inhibiting superfamily receptors. Blood 106(7):2399–2408
37. van Bijnen ST, Withaar M, Preijers F, van der Meer A, de Witte T, Muus P, Dolstra H (2011) T cells expressing the activating NK-cell receptors KIR2DS4, NKG2C and NKG2D are elevated in paroxysmal nocturnal hemoglobinuria and cytotoxic toward hematopoietic progenitor cell lines. Exp Hematol 39(7):751–762 e751–753. doi:S0301-472X(11)00176-7 [pii] 10.1016/j.exphem.2011.04.003
38. Nagakura S, Ishihara S, Dunn DE, Nishimura J, Kawaguchi T, Horikawa K, Hidaka M, Kagimoto T, Eto N, Mitsuya H, Kinoshita T, Young NS, Nakakuma H (2002) Decreased susceptibility of leukemic cells with PIG-A mutation to natural killer cells in vitro. Blood 100(3):1031–1037
39. Hanaoka N, Kawaguchi T, Horikawa K, Nagakura S, Mitsuya H, Nakakuma H (2006) Immunoselection by natural killer cells of PIGA mutant cells missing stress-inducible ULBP. Blood 107(3):1184–1191
40. Raulet DH, Gasser S, Gowen BG, Deng W, Jung H (2013) Regulation of ligands for the NKG2D activating receptor. Annu Rev Immunol 31:413–441. doi:10.1146/annurev-immunol-032712-095951
41. Hanaoka N, Nakakuma H, Horikawa K, Nagakura S, Tsuzuki Y, Shimanuki M, Kojima K, Yonemura Y, Kawaguchi T (2009) NKG2D-mediated immunity underlying paroxysmal nocturnal haemoglobinuria and related bone marrow failure syndromes. Br J Haematol 146(5):538–545. doi:BJH7795 [pii] 10.1111/j.1365-2141.2009.07795.x

Chapter 14
Pathogenesis of Clonal Dominance in PNH: Growth Advantage in PNH

Norimitsu Inoue and Taroh Kinoshita

Abstract Paroxysmal nocturnal hemoglobinuria (PNH) is an acquired hematopoietic disorder characterized by the clonal expansion of glycosylphosphatidylinositol (GPI)-deficient hematopoietic stem cells (HSCs). Although the deficiency in GPI caused by a somatic mutation in *phosphatidylinositol glycan-class A* (*PIGA*) can clearly account for the characteristic manifestation of intravascular hemolysis induced by complement attack in patients with PNH, additional abnormalities must be involved in the clonal expansion of GPI-deficient HSCs. Several reports have shown additional abnormalities predicted to be involved in the growth advantage of GPI-deficient HSCs in PNH. One of the best candidates is *HMGA2*, a gene encoding an architectural transcriptional regulator that is deregulated in many benign mesenchymal tumors. The aberrant expression of HMGA2 in PNH clones suggests that PNH may be viewed as a benign tumor of bone marrow cells. *WT1* transcript upregulation and *JAK2* p.V617F somatic mutation, observed in the other hematopoietic malignancies such as myeloproliferative neoplasms and myelodysplastic syndrome, have also been observed in some patients with PNH. In a recent whole-exome sequencing analysis, an average of two additional somatic mutations were observed in patients with PNH, and somatic mutations in many genes identified in other hematopoietic malignancies have been found. No gene abnormality has been found to be common to all patients with PNH. Further epigenetic and genetic analyses are necessary to clarify the general molecular mechanism involved in the expansion of PNH clones.

Keywords HMGA2 • JAK2 • TET2 • Benign tumor • Clonal expansion

---

N. Inoue (✉)
Department of Tumor Immunology, Osaka Medical Center for Cancer and Cardiovascular Diseases, 1-3-3 Nakamichi, Higahsinari-ku, 537-8511 Osaka, Japan
e-mail: inoue-no@mc.pref.osaka.jp

T. Kinoshita
Research Institute for Microbial Diseases, Osaka University, 3-1 Yamadaoka, Suita 565-0871, Osaka, Japan

WPI Immunology Frontier Research Center, Osaka University, 3-1 Yamadaoka, Suita 565-0871, Osaka, Japan

Y. Kanakura et al. (eds.), *Paroxysmal Nocturnal Hemoglobinuria*,
DOI 10.1007/978-4-431-56003-6_14

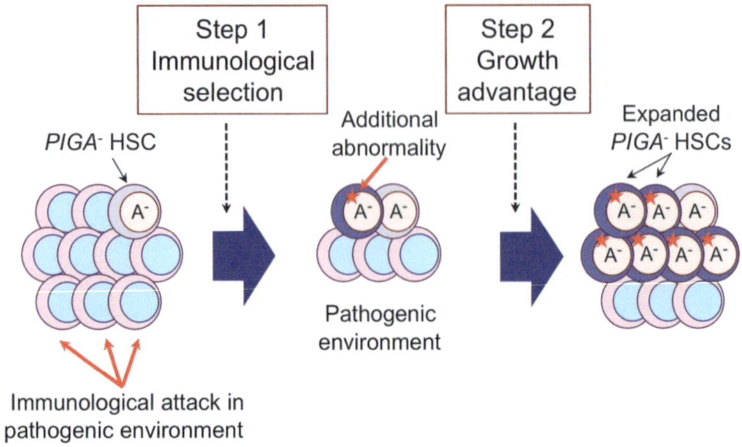

Fig. 14.1 Two-step process for clonal expansion of GPI-deficient HSCs in PNH [56]

14.1 Introduction

The clinical triad of paroxysmal nocturnal hemoglobinuria (PNH) is intravascular hemolysis, thrombophilia, and bone marrow failure. Intravascular hemolysis by complement attack is caused by a deficiency in two glycosylphosphatidylinositol (GPI)-anchored complement regulatory proteins, CD55 and CD59 [1]. Blockade of complement attack complex formation by the anti-C5 monoclonal antibody eculizumab suppresses not only intravascular hemolysis but also the peculiar thromboembolic risk in PNH. Somatic mutation of *phosphatidylinositol glycan-class A* (*PIGA*) in pluripotent hematopoietic stem cells (HSCs) impairs the synthesis of GPI in the endoplasmic reticulum, resulting in the deficiency of the cell surface expression of GPI-anchored proteins. Therefore, *PIGA* mutation fully accounts for major phenotypic manifestations such as hemolysis and thrombosis in PNH. In PNH, one or a few HSCs with a mutated *PIGA* gene clonally expand and often account for a large proportion of the granulocytes and monocytes in peripheral blood. Clonal expansion is an essential step in the pathogenesis of PNH. Many studies show evidence that both immunological selection and intrinsic growth advantage are involved in the clonal expansion of GPI-deficient HSCs (Fig. 14.1). The pathogenesis and molecular mechanisms of immunological selection in PNH are described in Chap. 13. In this chapter, we summarize the molecular mechanisms predicted to give rise to the intrinsic growth advantage of GPI-deficient HSCs.

14.2 Immunological Selection and Growth Advantage in PNH

Before the analyses of *Piga* knockout mice by several groups [2–6], since somatic mutations in the *PIGA* gene are found in HSCs in almost all patients with PNH, PNH had been considered a monogenic disorder. The deficiency in two complement regulatory GPI-anchored proteins, CD55 and CD59, caused by abnormalities in the *PIGA* gene, fully accounts for almost all of the PNH manifestations; however, the number of HSCs derived from *Piga* knockout mice remained constant and the HSCs did not clonally expand. Currently, although many researchers predict that additional abnormalities beyond *PIGA* mutation are necessary for the clonal expansion of GPI-deficient HSCs in PNH, abnormalities that fully account for clonal expansion in all PNH patients remain unknown. Two molecular mechanisms of clonal expansion have been proposed (Fig. 14.1). The first mechanism is the immunological selection of GPI-deficient HSCs in the aplastic anemia (AA) pathogenic microenvironment; an overlap between idiopathic AA and PNH has been frequently observed. It is widely accepted that the bone marrow failure in AA is caused by immunological destruction of HSCs. Indeed, immunosuppressive therapies improve prognosis in patients with severe AA. Furthermore, a small population of GPI-deficient granulocytes and/or erythrocytes (PNH-type cells, >0.003 %) was detected in many patients with AA. More than 90 % of the patients with PNH-type cells responded better to immunosuppressive therapy with antithymocyte globulin and cyclosporine than patients without PNH-type cells. Patients with an increased population of PNH-type cells in refractory anemia (RA) of myelodysplastic syndrome (MDS) have a higher probability of responding to immunosuppressive therapy than patients without this increased cell population. Thus, the appearance of GPI-deficient cells suggests the involvement of immunological mechanisms in bone marrow failure [7] and GPI-deficient cells appear resistant to immunological attack. Indeed, GPI-deficient cells can escape immunological selection in mouse and human models [8–11].

The second mechanism is the acquisition of an additional intrinsic growth advantage by GPI-deficient cells. Although a minor population of GPI-deficient granulocytes and/or erythrocytes is observed in many AA patients, the proportion of GPI-deficient cells does not change in most patients with AA who respond to immunosuppressive therapy and is maintained for more than 2 years [7]. The expanded *PIGA*-mutant clones identified in AA and MDS differ between granulocytes and monocytes and randomly change to other clones during the clinical course of the disease [12]. By contrast, the predominant GPI-deficient clones carrying the same *PIGA* mutations remain the dominant population in PNH for a long time [12, 13], and the minor clones remain minor or decline in the PNH microenvironment [13]. These results suggest that the GPI-deficient clones in PNH acquire additional characters that are different from those of the PNH-type cell population increased by immunological selection in AA and MDS.

14.3 Additional Genetic Mutations in PNH

Genetic alterations providing a growth advantage and common to all patients with PNH have not been identified yet. Several candidate genes mediate the growth advantage of GPI-deficient HSCs in PNH (Table 14.1).

14.3.1 High-Mobility Group AT-Hook 2 (HMGA2)

HMGA2 has been reported to be the most likely causative factor for the growth advantage of GPI-deficient cells in PNH. *HMGA2* was originally identified as a gene localized at the breakpoint of chromosomal rearrangements (12q13-15) in various human benign mesenchymal tumors including lipomas, uterine leiomyomas, pulmonary chondroid hamartomas, and others [14]. The breakpoints are preferentially clustered in the large intron 3 (113 kb), resulting in the upregulation of truncated or fused transcripts containing the first three exons without the 3' untranslational region (UTR) (Fig. 14.2). HMGA2 is composed of 109 amino acid residues containing amino-terminal three basic domains called AT-hooks, which bind AT-rich

Table 14.1 Genes predicted to be involved in growth advantage

Genes	Abnormalities	References
HMGA2	Chromosomal abnormalities at 12q13-15 in two patients	[15]
	Abnormal high expression in PNH granulocytes (18/24 patients, > +2SD)	[22]
	Clonal expansion of mouse HSCs expressing *HMGA2*	[21, 22, 31]
JAK2	V617F	[32, 33]
Genes around *PIGA* locus *(ASB9, ASB11)*	About 500 kb deletion of *PIGA* locus	[37]
WT1	Upregulation	[41]
Genes around *PIGT* locus *(L3MBTL1, SGK2)*	8.2 Mb deletion of *PIGT* locus	[46]
EGR1	Upregulation	[42]
RPL6		
BCL2A1	Upregulation	[44]
RAD23B		
MCL1		
RHOA		
TET2	E1250X, S1556fs and A671fs, L1514fs	[33]
MECOM	P18S, K613fs	
RIT1	Q212X, V58G	

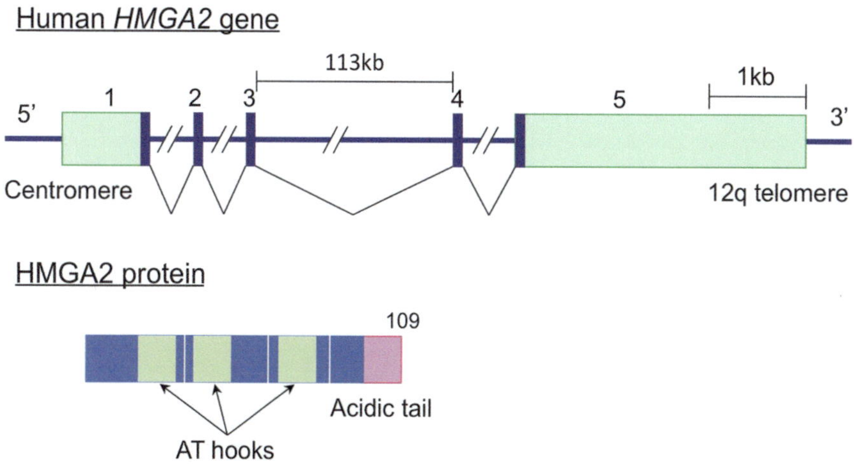

Fig. 14.2 Structure of HMGA2 gene and protein [14]

DNA in the minor groove, and an acidic carboxyl-terminal region (Fig. 14.2). HMGA2 positively or negatively regulates transcriptional activity by altering chromatin structure. HMGA2 is widely expressed in the embryo but not in most adult tissues.

14.3.1.1 Two PNH Patients with HMGA2 Abnormalities

Two PNH patients carrying abnormalities in chromosome 12 have been reported [15]. In the first case, J20, the chromosomal abnormality 46,XX,t(12;12)(q13;q15), was detected along with progress of the expansion of a PNH clone. When the karyotypes of GPI-positive and GPI-negative bone marrow-derived mononuclear cells were examined individually, the abnormal chromosome 12 karyotype was detected only in the GPI-deficient cells, while the normal karyotype was detected in all of the GPI-positive cells [16]. In this patient, a substitution mutation in the *PIGA* gene was detected, c.715G>A, resulting in an essential amino acid change (p.G239R). Therefore, two independent mutations, the abnormality in chromosome 12 and the *PIGA* mutation, coexist within one PNH clone in this patient. The chromosomal abnormality was defined as the insertion of q12 to q14.1 fragment of one chromosome 12 to q14.3 region of the other but not the translocation of chromosome 12 (Fig. 14.3) [15]. According to the Next-Gen Cytogenetic Nomenclature [17], the chromosomal abnormality of this patient, J20, is as follows:

46,XX,ins(12;12)(q14.3;q12q14.1)dn.seq[GRCh38/hg38]ins(12;12)
(12pter->12q14.3(65,964,51{0–1})::12q12q14.1(40,613,03{3–4}-59,089,35{0–1})::
12q12(40,613,1{70–69}-40,610,4{96–69})::12q14.3(65,981,3{21–48})- > 12qter;
12pter->12q12(40,610,450)::12q14.1(59,099,213)->12qter)dn

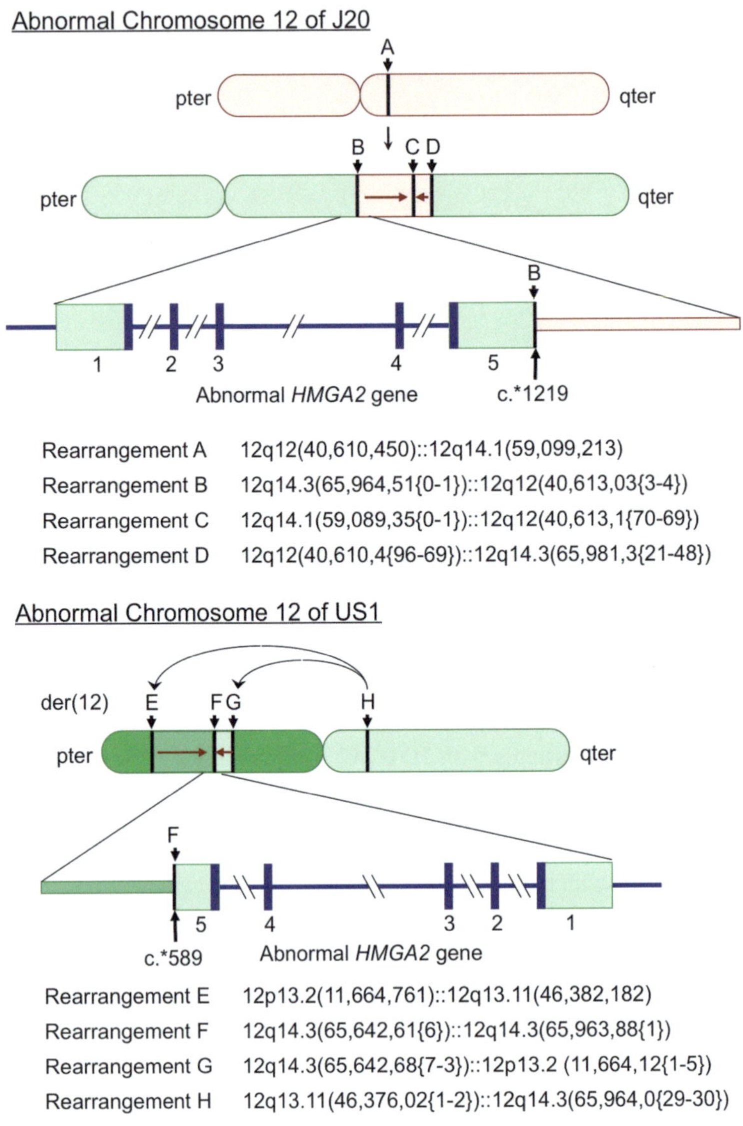

Fig. 14.3 Abnormal chromosome 12 in two patients with PNH [15]

In the second case, US1, all metaphases of bone marrow cells show the abnormal karyotype of chromosome 12, 46,XX,ins(12)(p12~13q13q12) [15]. Therefore, all of the GPI-deficient cells must have this chromosomal abnormality. The 14 bp deletion of exon 2 in the *PIGA* gene (c.693_706del) was also detected in this patient, leading to a frameshift mutation (p.Ser232fs). The chromosomal abnormality is described as follows (Fig. 14.3):

46,XX,ins(12)(p13.2q14.3q13.11)dn.seq[GRCh38/hg38]ins(12)
(12pter->12p13.2(11,664,761)::12q13.11q14.3 (46,382,182-65,642,61{6})::
12q14.3(65,963,88 {1}-65,642,68{7–3})::12p13.2(11,664,12{1–5})->
12q13.11(46,376,02{1–2})::12q14.3(65,964,0{29–30})->12qter)dn

One of the breakpoints formed by four rearrangements in the PNH patients affected the same gene, *HMGA2*. Both breakpoints in patients J20 and US1 were located within the 3' UTR of *HMGA2* (Fig. 14.3). In bone marrow cells, the *HMGA2* transcript was upregulated 2.6 times and 5.0 times in patients J20 and US1, respectively, compared to normal individuals. Furthermore, in both patients, the *HMGA2* transcripts were transcribed mainly from the truncated *HMGA2* alleles on the rearranged chromosome 12 rather than on the normal alleles. This result suggests that the *PIGA*-deficient cells in which the expression of *HMGA2* is upregulated by chromosomal abnormalities clonally expand like benign tumors. PNH and benign tumors have similar characteristics. Although the *PIGA*-mutant clones initially expand, they are maintained in a definite proportion for a long time and malignant conversion is rare, unlike in the other premalignant hematopoietic diseases (less than 3 %) [18, 19]. The clones generally do not increase beyond normal ranges and are appropriately controlled by hematopoietic factors. Furthermore, *PIGA*-mutant HSCs are maintained within the bone marrow and do not invade extramedullary tissues such as the spleen, liver, lymph node, and other nonhematopoietic tissues. Therefore, the concept of PNH as a benign tumor of bone marrow is supported in GPI-deficient HSCs with aberrant expression of *HMGA2* that acquire full clonal expansion ability.

14.3.1.2 Control of *HMGA2* Expression

In lipoma, the *HMGA2* gene is frequently fused to other genes such as the *LIM domain-containing preferred translocation partner* (*LPP*) gene on t(3;12)(q27-28;q13-15). *HMGA2* is highly expressed even in the absence of *HMGA2* gene locus rearrangement in some mesenchymal tumors. These highly expressed transcripts of *HMGA2* contain the cryptic exons localized within introns 3 and 4 without exon 5 or the 3' UTR (Fig. 14.4). The 3' UTR sequence of *HMGA2* plays an essential role in the downregulation of HMGA2 expression by inhibiting the translation and/or degrading the mRNA. The 3' UTR has seven conserved sites complementary to the *let-7* microRNA (*MIRLET7*) (Fig. 14.4) [20]. *HMGA2* transcripts lose these sites in benign mesenchymal tumors without chromosome 12 abnormalities, resulting in increased truncated HMGA2 mRNA and protein. In fact, the *HMGA2* gene in the two PNH patients with the chromosome 12 abnormality, J20 and US1, lost five and six *MIRLET7* binding sites, respectively (Fig. 14.4), and the several truncated types of HMGA2 transcripts carrying a cryptic exon were highly expressed in the PNH clones.

The pathway regulated by the Lin28b protein, the microRNA (miRNA) let-7, and its target gene *Hmga2* is critical for fetal hematopoiesis in mouse models [21].

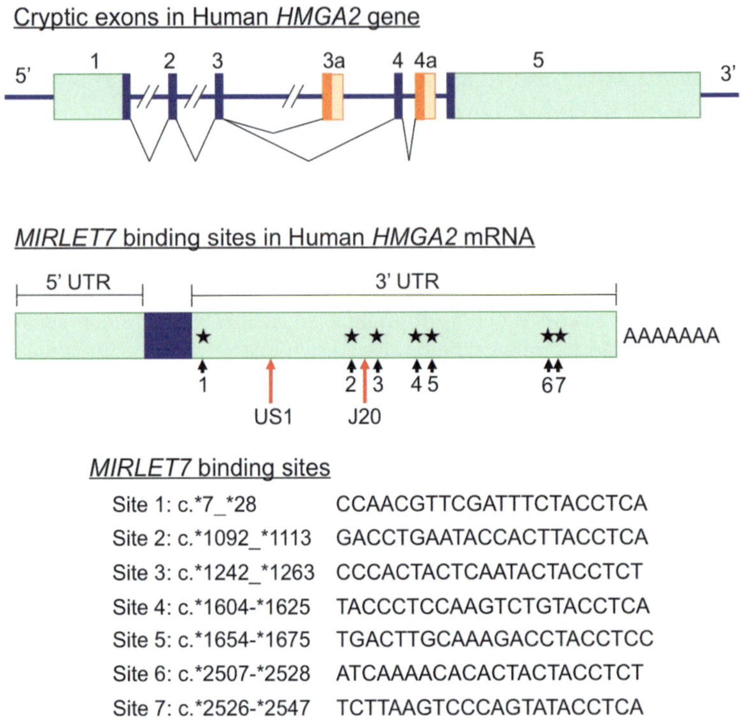

Fig. 14.4 Cryptic exons and *MIRLET7* binding sites in human *HMGA2* gene. *Orange boxes*, cryptic exons (3a and 4a). *Red arrows*, rearrangements found in PNH patients J20 and US1. *Black asterisks*, *MIRLET7* binding sites

Fetal and adult hematopoieses are regulated by distinct programs. Fetal HSCs have high self-renewal ability and predominantly generate erythroid and myeloid cells. By contrast, adult HSCs do not expand in number, but remain quiescent and generate cells of all lineages. Lin28b, *let-7* miRNA, and Hmga2 play an important role in the increased self-renewal potential of fetal HSCs. The Lin28b protein is more predominantly expressed in mouse fetal liver than in adult bone marrow and binds to the long pri-*let-7* transcripts and the approximately 70 nt stem-loop precursor miRNA (pre-*let-7* miRNA) to inhibit the posttranscriptional maturation of *let-7*. Three (*let-7b*, *c*, and *d*) among six *let-7* miRNAs (*let-7*a to f) are expressed in fetal HSCs at lower levels than in adult HSCs. The expression of four *let-7* miRNAs (*let-7a*, *b*, *d*, and *f*) was inhibited by the overexpression of Lin28b in adult bone marrow cells. Since mature *let-7* miRNA binds to the 3' UTR of *Hmga2* transcripts to inhibit the expression of Hmga2, Hmga2 is highly expressed in fetal liver via the low expression of mature *let-7* miRNA and high expression of Lin28b. This result suggests that deregulation of this pathway causes increased HSC self-renewal potential as in fetal hematopoiesis.

14.3.1.3 Overexpression of HMGA2 in PNH Patients with Normal Karyotypes

Murakami et al. reported that *HMGA2* mRNA was upregulated in whole peripheral blood cells derived from 18 of 24 patients with PNH compared to AA patients and healthy individuals [22]. Although these patients do not have any chromosomal abnormalities, truncated *HMGA2* transcripts, but not full-length transcripts, are expressed at higher levels than in normal individuals. The expression of *MIRLET7B* and *C* was significantly lower in the peripheral blood cells of PNH patients than in those of normal individuals. Although the suppression of *Let7* miRNA may upregulate other genes involved in the expansion of PNH clones, the increased level of truncated *HMGA2* transcripts in PNH patients is likely to be caused by abnormal transcriptional induction but not by the suppression of *Let7* miRNA. Recently, Lam et al. reported that the expression of *HMGA2* was transcriptionally regulated by *RUNX1* and increased in hematopoietic progenitor cells in the absence of *RUNX1* [23]. Therefore, it is necessary to identify transcription factors involved in the upregulation of *HMGA2* in patients with PNH.

The overexpression of truncated *HMGA2* and the chromosomal breakpoint within the *HMGA2* gene are also detected in patients with myeloid malignancies such as myelofibrosis with myeloid metastasis [24], MDS [25], polycythemia vera [26], and myeloproliferative neoplasm [27]. Harada-Shirado et al. also reported that the granulocytes of patients with primary myelofibrosis (PMF) show higher *HMGA2* expression than those of patients with PV or ET and those of healthy individuals [28]. Interestingly, the granulocytes of all patients with PMF mainly express full-length *HMGA2* transcripts, unlike patients with PNH, and the expression of *MIRLET7A1* and *C* was suppressed in PMF patients with high expression levels of *HMGA2*. These results suggest that the suppression of *MIRLET7* induces the upregulation of *HMGA2* in patients with PMF through different mechanisms than in patients with PNH.

14.3.1.4 Clonal Expansion of HMGA2-Expressing HSCs In Vivo

The upregulation of HMGA2 directly induces the clonal expansion of human and mouse HSCs in vivo.

In humans, Cavazzana-Calvo et al. reported that clones with lentivirus vector integration into the *HMGA2* gene locus underwent greater expansion than other clones after gene therapy against human β-thalassemia [29, 30]. The $CD34^+$ HSCs of a patient with a severe type of β^E/β^0-thalassemia were infected with a lentivirus vector carrying a functional β-globin gene driven by an erythroid-specific promoter and expanded further in vitro. The HSCs were transplanted into the patient who had received chemotherapy as a conditioning regimen before transplantation. The lentivirus vector-bearing blood cells gradually increased in number, and 13.5 % of whole bone marrow and 11.1 % of long-term culture-initiating cells (LTC-IC) contained the lentivirus vector 2 years after transplantation. Importantly, the lentivirus vector was integrated within the third intron of the *HMGA2* gene in about 50 % of the vector-bearing LTC-IC but not in lymphoid lineage cells. Furthermore, the expression of truncated *HMGA2* without exon 4 or 5 was increased specifically in erythroid cells, but not in granulocytes or monocytes by the erythroid-specific β-locus control region effect. Since the clone bearing the vector integration site within *HMGA2* increased equally in erythroid cells, granulocytes, and monocytes, truncated HMGA2 transcripts should be overexpressed in LTC-IC upon loss of *let-7* binding sites. This result would suggest that the overexpression of truncated HMGA2 increases the number of hematopoietic progenitor cells and promotes the differentiation of myeloid cells during human hematopoiesis.

Three groups reported mouse models that overexpress mouse or human *HMGA2*. Ikeda et al. established a transgenic (TG) mouse line that carries mouse *Hmga2* cDNA containing the full coding region without six of the seven *let-7* miRNA binding sites and driven by the *Pgk* promoter [31]. In this TG mouse, *Hmga2* transcript and Hmga2 protein are overexpressed in the bone marrow, spleen, and thymus compared to wild-type mice. The bone marrow of *Hmga2* TG mice was hypercellular and had a high erythroid content. Furthermore, *Hmga2* TG mice showed splenomegaly with an increase in erythroid cells in spite of a decrease in serum erythropoietin (Epo) level. When cells mixed with the bone marrow cells of wild-type and TG mice were transplanted into irradiated mice, the proportion of peripheral blood cells derived from TG mice significantly and gradually increased in all lineages. In Murakami's report, lineage-negative bone marrow cells were transduced with retrovirus vector bearing the truncated human *HMGA2* (exon 1–3) and transplanted into irradiated mice [22]. *HMGA2*-transduced cells gradually expanded in all hematopoietic lineages compared to control vector-transduced cells. Myeloid cells transduced with truncated *HMGA2* expanded to a remarkably greater extent than lymphoid cells. To assess the self-renewal activity of Hmga2- or Lin28b-expressing HSCs, Copley et al. examined the chimerism of *Hmga2*-expressing cells obtained from secondary transplanted mice [21]. *Hmga2* overexpression in adult bone marrow HSCs increased self-renewal activity.

These results suggest that HMGA2 overexpression in the HSCs of patients with PNH promotes the expansion of PNH clones like benign tumors. In the future, since HMGA2-expressing HSCs can expand with or without GPI anchor deficiency [31], it will be necessary to clarify the association between GPI deficiency and *HMGA2* overexpression.

14.3.2 JAK2^{V617F} *Mutation in PNH*

Sugimori et al. described three PNH patients with an acquired substitution mutation in the *Janus kinase 2* (*JAK2*) gene (c.1849G > T), resulting in a change from valine to phenylalanine (p.V617F) [32]. Two of these patients also have a 500 kb deletion at Xp22.2, including the *PIGA* gene (described below). Shen et al. also reported that a somatic homozygous *JAK2* mutation (p. V617F) was detected in two of three patients with a 500 kb deletion including the *PIGA* gene when 61 genes frequently affected in MDS were analyzed by targeted exome sequencing [33]. The *JAK2* mutation was also found in GPI-positive cells as well as GPI-deficient cells in the two patients Shen et al. analyzed.

JAK2 is a *Janus* family tyrosine kinase (the family comprises JAK1, 2, 3, and Tyk2) that associates with the cytoplasmic domain of cytokine receptors such as Epo, thrombopoietin, and granulocyte colony-stimulating factor (G-CSF) [34, 35]. The binding of ligands induces the cross tyrosine phosphorylation of JAK2, which phosphorylates tyrosines on the receptors, leading to the activation of signaling pathways such as signal transducer and activator of transcription (STAT), mitogen-activated protein kinase (MAPK), phosphatidylinositol-3'-kinase (PI3K), and AKT (Fig. 14.5). The activation of JAK/STAT pathways facilitates the development of lymphoid and myeloid malignancies. The somatic mutation of the pseudokinase domain (JH2) of JAK2 at codon 617 (p.V617F) is detected in more than 95 % of patients with PV and in about 50 % of those with essential thrombocythemia (ET) and PMF (Fig. 14.5). The JH2 domain has protein kinase activity and phosphorylates S523 and T570 and negatively regulates the JH1 kinase domain of JAK2 [36]. The JH2 mutation at codon 617 reduces the kinase activity, leading to increased basal kinase activity and downstream signaling.

The numbers of white blood cells (WBCs) and platelets are generally lower in patients with PNH than in normal individuals because idiopathic AA and PNH often overlap. By contrast, in the three patients with PNH carrying the *JAK2* mutation reported by Sugimori et al., the numbers of WBCs and platelets increased beyond normal ranges and almost all granulocytes, but only few red cells, were deficient in GPI anchor [32]. Most typical PNH patients harbored no *JAK2* mutation in Sugimori's analysis [32] and Shen's whole-exome sequencing [33]. In patients with the *JAK2* mutation, the disease should have characteristics of both PNH and MPN rather than present as typical PNH. These cases with PNH clones carrying the *JAK2* mutation should be classified as rare cases of PNH/MPN syndrome.

14.3.3 Microdeletion Including PIGA *Locus*

Most *PIGA* gene somatic mutations are small alterations, such as base substitutions, small deletions, or insertions of several bases. O'Keefe et al. reported three patients with PNH carrying about 500 kb deletion at Xp22.2, including the *PIGA* locus [37]. In addition to the *PIGA* locus deletion, two of the three patients also had the *JAK2* mutation described above. Shen also reported three patients with a 500 kb *PIGA* locus deletion. In addition to the *PIGA* gene deletion, these three patients had a deletion of 555 kb including *ankyrin repeat and SOCS box containing 9* (*ASB9*), *ASB11*, *c-fos-induced growth factor* (*FIGF*), and pirin (*PIR*); a deletion of 506 kb including *ASB9*, *ASB11*, *FIGF*, *PIR*, and *BMX non-receptor tyrosine kinase* (*BMX*);

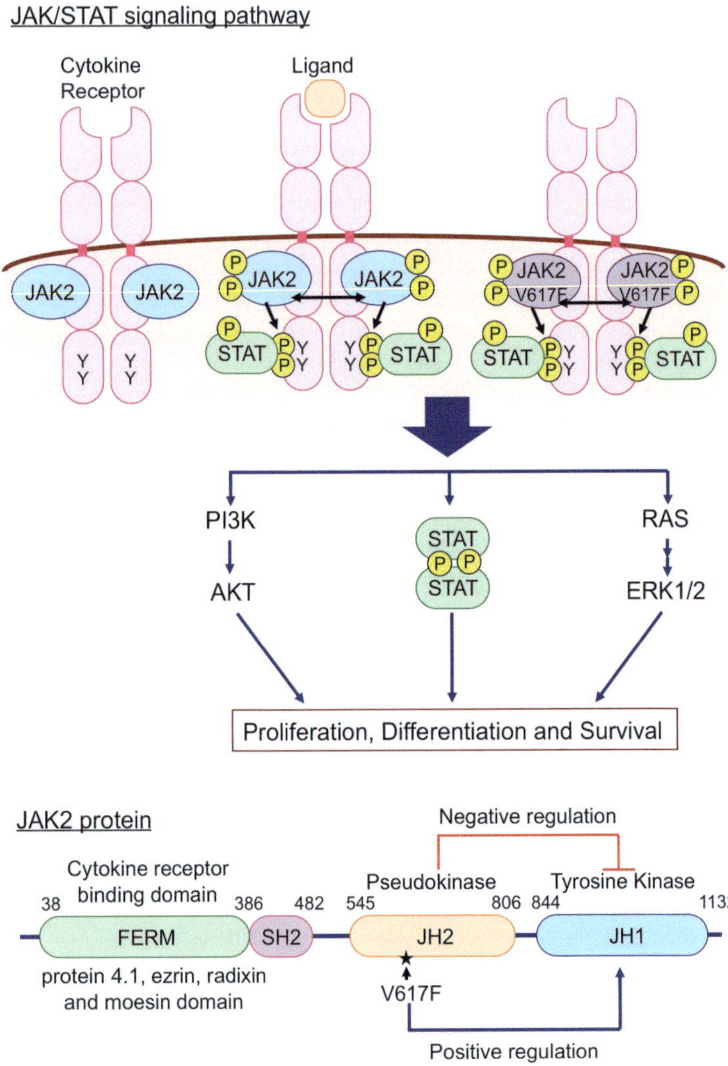

Fig. 14.5 JAK2 structure and signaling pathway [34, 35]

and a 616 kb deletion including the *PIGA* gene. Although the authors did not describe which genes are localized within the 616 kb deletion in the last patient, a common deletion in the three patients includes *ASB9* and *ASB11*, which function as a ubiquitin ligase complex. There is no report that these proteins are involved in the proliferation of HSCs. The involvement of genes such as ASB9 and ASB11 in the growth advantage of HSCs should be examined.

14.3.4 *Upregulation of* WT1

The *Wilms' tumor 1* (*WT1*) gene encodes a 55 kDa transcriptional regulator containing four zinc finger domains at the carboxyl terminus and is essential for renal development [38]. Germ line mutations in the *WT1* gene cause Wilms' tumors and renal and genitourinary abnormalities in WAGR and Denys-Drash syndrome.

The *WT1* gene is highly expressed in acute leukemia blast cells with high frequency (73–93 %) [39, 40]. Elevated expression of *WT1* is also observed in almost all types of solid tumors and in other hematopoietic malignancies such as chronic myeloid leukemia and MDS [39]. The WT1 expression level is a suitable marker of minimal residual disease in leukemia after treatment and can be used to monitor MDS disease progression. WT1 may also be a suitable immunotherapeutic target in hematopoietic malignancies and other solid tumors. When the expression of the *WT1* gene was measured in the bone marrow mononuclear cells of 21 PNH patients, 21 AA patients, and 20 healthy individuals, *WT1* levels were significantly higher in PNH patients than in AA patients (4.8 times) and healthy individuals (10.2 times) [41]. The expression of the *WT1* gene was higher in GPI anchor-deficient HSCs than in GPI anchor-positive HSCs [10]. Furthermore, $CD8^+$ T cells that recognize the WT1 peptide presented on MHC class I were detected in patients with PNH [10]. These WT1 peptide-specific CTLs may play a role in the bone marrow failure and/or immunological selection of GPI-deficient clones in PNH.

14.3.5 *Upregulation of Other Genes*

Lyakisheva et al. reported that *early growth response factor 1* (*EGR1*) and *ribosomal protein L6* [*RPL6*, called *TAX-responsive enhancer element-binding protein* (*TAXREB107*) in the paper] were specifically upregulated in granulocytes in PNH [42]. *EGR1* encodes a zinc finger protein that positively or negatively regulates transcription. The overexpression of these genes was also observed in other clonal hematopoietic diseases such as myeloproliferative syndrome, MDS, and PV; however, Joslin et al. reported that N-ethyl-nitrosourea-treated Egr1+/− and Egr1−/− mice develop T-cell lymphoma or myeloproliferative disorders [43]. *EGR1* may be a tumor suppressor gene localized in a commonly deleted region of 5q in AML and MDS. The relationship between the upregulation of these genes and the growth advantage of PNH clones has not been clarified yet. The overexpression of *BCL2-related protein A1* (*BCL2A1*), *RAD23B*, *myeloid cell leukemia 1* (*MCL1*), and *RhoA* in granulocytes in PNH was also reported [44]. *BCL2A1* and *MCL1* encode anti-apoptotic proteins that belong to the Bcl-2 family. RAD23B is involved in nucleotide excision repair. *RhoA* encodes a small GTP-binding protein that regulates cell morphogenesis and motility through actin cytoskeleton remodeling. Although the blood cells of patients with PNH are thought to be resistant to apoptosis, the upregulation of these genes has not yet been shown to be involved in such resistance.

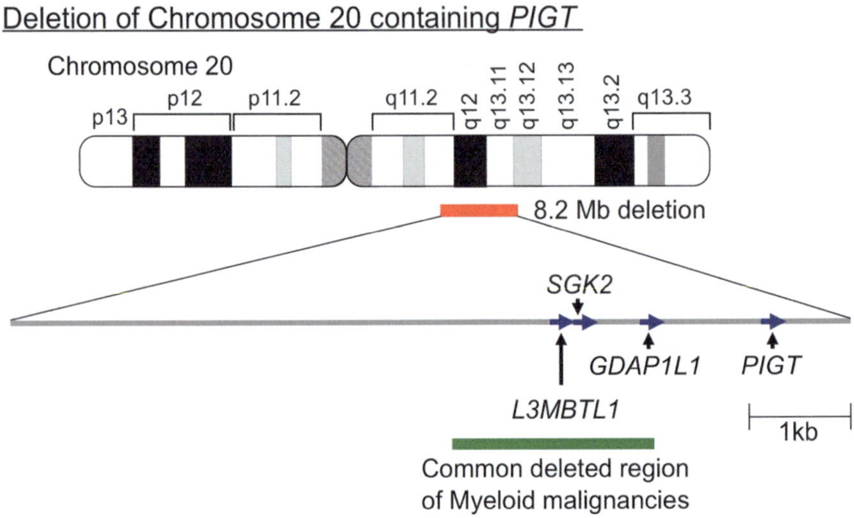

Fig. 14.6 Abnormality of PNH patient carrying *PIGT* mutation [52]

14.3.6 Microdeletion Including PIGT *Locus*

A *PIGA* gene inactivating mutation has been found in most patients with PNH [1, 45]. *PIGA* is the only gene mapped to the X chromosome among genes involved in GPI anchor biosynthesis, modification of GPI anchor, and transport of GPI-anchored proteins. Since *PIGA* is transcribed from one active X chromosome even in females, one somatic mutation in the *PIGA* gene is sufficient to cause a GPI anchor deficiency, but two somatic mutations are necessary in the other GPI anchor biosynthesis genes. Krawitz et al. described a unique patient with PNH in whom both *PIGT* alleles on chromosome 20q are mutated (Fig. 14.6) [46]. One mutation is a single nucleotide germ line substitution from A to G at the splice acceptor site of intron 10 (c.1401-2A>G), and the other is the 8.2 Mb somatic deletion including the *PIGT* gene. The PIGT protein is a subunit of the GPI transamidase complex, which is composed of five subunits (PIGK, PIGS, PIGT, PIGU, and GPAA1) and removes the carboxyl terminal GPI-attachment signal peptide from a GPI-precursor protein and transfers the protein to a mature GPI anchor [47–49]. Interestingly, this deleted region on chromosome 20q is commonly affected in chronic myeloid malignancies such as MPN and MDS [50, 51]. Three imprinted genes, *L3MBTL1*, *SGK2* (*serum-/glucocorticoid-regulated kinase 2*), and *GDAP1L1* (*ganglioside-induced differentiation-associated protein 1-like 1*), are mapped to this region [50, 51] and expressed from the paternal alleles [52]. The expression of these genes is markedly reduced in granulocytes and bone marrow of patients with chronic myeloid malignancies carrying a 20q deletion.

Only one case of PNH with both 20q deletion and *PIGT* deficiency has been reported, and there is no information about the expression of *L3MBTL1*. Therefore, it is necessary to further analyze abnormalities in PNH patients with *PIGT* deficiency. Furthermore, this patient suffered from progressive ulcerative colitis resistant to mesalazine and steroids. The possibility that this unique symptom may be associated with the 20q deletion or *PIGT* deficiency should be assessed.

14.3.7 Genetic Mutations Identified by Whole-Exome Sequencing Analysis

Recent advances in sequencing technologies and successful completion of the Human Genome Project led to the discoveries of inherited disease genes as well as somatic mutations in many cancers and premalignant diseases. To examine whether somatic mutations are acquired in PNH clones in addition to the *PIGA* mutation, Shen et al. analyzed somatic mutations in 12 patients with PNH by whole-exome sequencing (WES) and assessed alterations in 61 genes frequently affected in MDS in 36 additional patients [33]. In addition to the *PIGA* mutation, 21 non-silent mutations were detected in 10 of 12 patients analyzed by WES (an average of two additional mutations per patient). One patient had six additional mutations, but the other patients had zero to three mutations. Higher average numbers of somatic non-silent mutations per patient have been detected in other hematopoietic malignancies such as MDS (mean: 7.7) [53], PV (6.5), ET (6.5), PMF (13.0), and adult AML (17.2) [54]. Since the number of somatic mutations correlates with aggressive pathology, the lower frequencies of mutation fit with the benign phenotype of PNH. Recently, somatic mutations in AA patients were analyzed by means of WES and targeted sequencing of genes that are recurrently mutated in myeloid malignancies [55]. Somatic mutations including silent changes were detected in 25 of 52 AA patients (48 %) by WES, and the average number of somatic non-silent mutations per patient was 1.21 (the average number of total somatic mutations is 1.83). Although PNH frequently overlaps with AA, HSCs of PNH patients were more genetically affected than those of AA. Furthermore, *BCL6 corepressor* (*BCOR*) and *BCL6 corepressor-like 1* (*BCORL1*) (9.3 %), *PIGA* (7.5 %), *DNA methyltransferase 3A* (*DNMT3A*) (8.4 %), and *additional se combs-like 1* (*ASXL1*) (6.2 %) are frequently mutated in AA patients. Although clones mutated in *DNMT3A* or *ASXL1* gene, which is also frequently affected in MDS and AML patients but not in PNH, expanded, clones carrying *PIGA* somatic mutations that cause PNH and *BCOR*- and *BCORL1*-mutated clones decreased or remained stable. These results indicate that molecular mechanisms of clonal hematopoiesis should be different between PNH and AA. In Shen's study, only four genes, *Ten-Eleven Translocation methylcytosine dioxygenase 2* (*TET2*), *MDS1 and EVI1 complex locus* (*MECOM*), *Ras-like without CAAX1* (*RIT1*), and *JAK2* (described above), were affected in more than two patients with PNH. The other 28 genes were mutated in only a single patient.

The TET2 protein catalyzes the conversion of 5-methylcytosine to 5-hydroxymethylcytosine, 5-formylcytosine, and 5-carboxycytosine in the presence of 2-oxoglutarate, bivalent iron, and oxygen and is involved in the demethylation process of cytosine. TET2 is commonly affected in the initial stage of many hematopoietic malignancies.

The *MECOM* gene, which is also called EVI1, is mapped to human chromosome 3q26 and rearranged and overexpressed in AML and MDS. MECOM is a 135 kDa transcriptional regulator with zinc finger domains that inhibits myeloid differentiation and cellular apoptosis.

The RIT1 protein belongs to the RAS-related GTPase subfamily and regulates p38-MAPK-dependent signaling pathways. Germ line mutation of RIT1 causes Noonan syndrome 8, an autosomal dominant disorder characterized by short stature, distinctive facial features, developmental delay, and cardiac abnormalities. *RIT1* gene somatic mutations are frequently found in patients with MPN or mixed MDS/MPN and chronic myelomonocytic leukemia (CMML).

Shen et al. analyzed clonal composition in nine PNH patients by single-colony sequencing assay to assess the sequential incidence of somatic mutations [33]. Interestingly, they found that additional mutations were acquired before the acquisition of the *PIGA* mutation in six of nine PNH patients (initiating mutation-first patients) (Fig. 14.7b). Furthermore, somatic mutations in two additional genes were detected early on in two PNH patients. Therefore, many patients should have ancestral gene mutations other than PIGA mutations. The *PIGA* somatic mutation may be acquired in a HSC before the clone obtains clonal expansion ability (*PIGA* mutation-first patients) (Fig. 14.7a) [56]. The somatic mutations in these genes may play two possible roles in the pathogenesis of PNH. They may function as an initiating mutation as in other hematopoietic malignancies. Welch et al. reported several frequent mutations that specifically affected AML (FAB M1) with normal cytogenetics compared to APL (FAB M3 AML) carrying the fusion gene *PML-RARA* [57]. They found initiating mutations in genes mainly involved in epigenetics such as *DNMT3A*, *isocitrate dehydrogenase 1* (*IDH1*), and *TET2*. In fact, they identified a patient carrying a larger population of clones with the *TET2* somatic mutation than clones with both *TET2* and *PIGA* mutations [33]. This *TET2* somatic mutation should function as an initiating mutation providing a growth advantage to clones both with and without PIGA mutation. By contrast, these somatic mutations may be age related and irrelevant for the pathogenesis of PNH. Somatic mutations in hematopoietic stem/progenitor cells in healthy volunteers also increase with age at the rate of 0.13 ± 0.02 exonic mutations per year of life [57]. Furthermore, the somatic mutations associated with clonal expansion and malignancies such as *TET2* and *IDH2* increase with age and are detected in blood cells of 5–6 % of individuals older than 70 years of age (2 % of individuals studied) [58]; however, in 41 patients with PNH, Chotirat found neither mutations of *IDH1* at R132 or mutations of *IDH2* at R140 and R172, which have been identified in patients with low-grade glioma and AML [59].

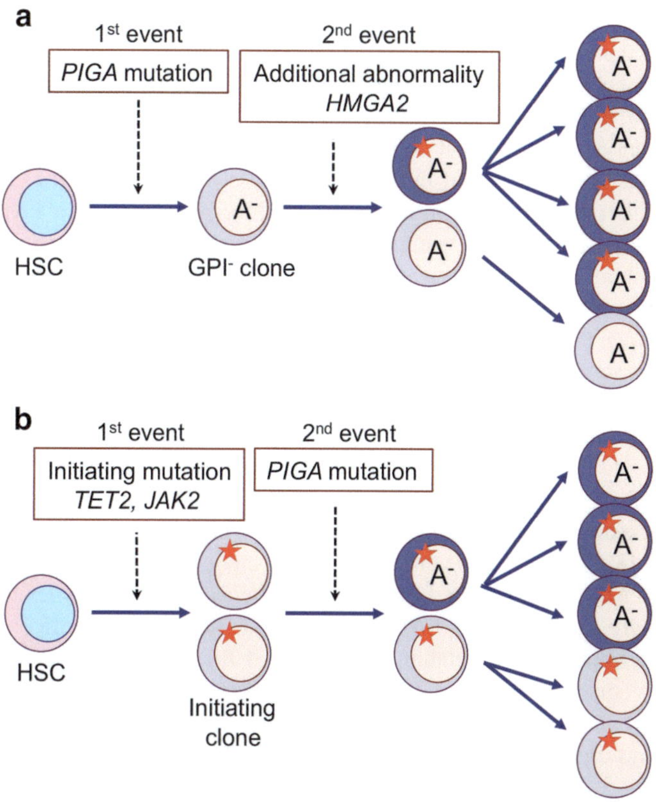

Fig. 14.7 Clonal architecture in PNH. (**a**) PIGA mutation-first patients. (**b**) Initiating mutation-first patients

14.3.8 N-RAS Mutation

Mortazavi et al. reported that a mutation of N-RAS at codon 13 (p.G13D), causing constitutive activity, was detected in a patient in whom the disease developed from AA/PNH into MDS [60]. The N-RAS mutation occurred in a multipotent HSC that can differentiate into both myeloid and lymphoid lineages, but not in a PNH clone. This result suggests that the N-RAS mutation may be involved in the development of MDS but not in the growth advantage of a PNH clone.

14.4 Considerations and Perspectives

In this chapter, several candidate genes involved in the growth advantage of PNH clones were introduced, but no abnormality accounting for the growth advantage of PNH clones in all PNH patients has been identified. Recent studies show that several genes, such as *HMGA2* and *WT1*, are upregulated in patients with PNH. To understand the molecular mechanism of this transcriptional upregulation, it is necessary to assess epigenetic alterations such as histone modifications and DNA methylation and hydroxymethylation.

WES analysis showed that somatic mutations that affect other hematopoietic malignancies are also present in the PNH clones, but it is still not clear whether these somatic mutations play important roles in the pathogenesis of PNH or function of HSCs. To identify essential genes involved in clonal expansion, young patients without age-related mutations and/or familial patients should be analyzed by WES. It is also important to analyze the differences in clonal expansion mechanisms between PNH and other myeloid malignancies such as MPN and MDS that share the same somatic mutations.

Although *PIGA* somatic mutation was thought to be the first event in PNH pathogenesis and the abnormality giving rise to clonal expansion was thought to be a second event (*PIGA* mutation-first patients) [56], WES suggests that there are patients with PNH who acquire the *PIGA* somatic mutation as a second event and who have expanded clones without GPI deficiency (initiating mutation-first patients) (Fig. 14.7) [33]. Recently, the order in which somatic mutations in two genes were acquired in MPN was analyzed by genotyping hematopoietic colonies [61]. About 10 % of patients with MPN harbor somatic mutations in both *JAK2* and *TET2*. Patients in whom *JAK2* mutations are acquired first have a greater tendency to develop PV than ET. The *JAK2* and *TET2* mutation order influences the clinical features and clonal evolution in patients with MPN. Therefore, the mutation order in *PIGA* and other genes may affect the size of the GPI-deficient cell population (Fig. 14.7).

Genetic and epigenetic analysis of GPI-deficient cells and GPI-positive cells in PNH patients will promote a better understanding of the disease and lead to therapeutic advances.

References

1. Brodsky RA (2014) Paroxysmal nocturnal hemoglobinuria. Blood 124 (18):2804–2811. doi:blood-2014-02-522128 [pii]10.1182/blood-2014-02-522128
2. Kawagoe K, Kitamura D, Okabe M, Taniuchi I, Ikawa M, Watanabe T, Kinoshita T, Takeda J (1996) Glycosylphosphatidylinositol-anchor-deficient mice: implications for clonal dominance of mutant cells in paroxysmal nocturnal hemoglobinuria. Blood 87(9):3600–3606
3. Rosti V, Tremml G, Soares V, Pandolfi PP, Luzzatto L, Bessler M (1997) Murine embryonic stem cells without pig-a gene activity are competent for hematopoiesis with the PNH phenotype but not for clonal expansion. J Clin Invest 100(5):1028–1036. doi:10.1172/JCI119613
4. Murakami Y, Kinoshita T, Maeda Y, Nakano T, Kosaka H, Takeda J (1999) Different roles of glycosylphosphatidylinositol in various hematopoietic cells as revealed by a mouse model of paroxysmal nocturnal hemoglobinuria. Blood 94(9):2963–2970
5. Tremml G, Dominguez C, Rosti V, Zhang Z, Pandolfi PP, Keller P, Bessler M (1999) Increased sensitivity to complement and a decreased red blood cell life span in mice mosaic for a nonfunctional Piga gene. Blood 94(9):2945–2954

6. Keller P, Tremml G, Rosti V, Bessler M (1999) X inactivation and somatic cell selection rescue female mice carrying a Piga-null mutation. Proc Natl Acad Sci U S A 96(13):7479–7483
7. Sugimori C, Chuhjo T, Feng X, Yamazaki H, Takami A, Teramura M, Mizoguchi H, Omine M, Nakao S (2006) Minor population of CD55-CD59- blood cells predicts response to immunosuppressive therapy and prognosis in patients with aplastic anemia. Blood 107 (4):1308–1314. doi:2005-06-2485 [pii] 10.1182/blood-2005-06-2485
8. Murakami Y, Kosaka H, Maeda Y, Nishimura J, Inoue N, Ohishi K, Okabe M, Takeda J, Kinoshita T (2002) Inefficient response of T lymphocytes to glycosylphosphatidylinositol anchor-negative cells: implications for paroxysmal nocturnal hemoglobinuria. Blood 100 (12):4116–4122. doi: 10.1182/blood-2002-06-1669 2002-06-1669 [pii]
9. Hanaoka N, Kawaguchi T, Horikawa K, Nagakura S, Mitsuya H, Nakakuma H (2006) Immunoselection by natural killer cells of PIGA mutant cells missing stress-inducible ULBP. Blood 107(3):1184–1191. doi:2005-03-1337 [pii] 10.1182/blood-2005-03-1337
10. Ikeda K, Shichishima T, Yasukawa M, Nakamura-Shichishima A, Noji H, Akutsu K, Osumi K, Maruyama Y (2007) The role of Wilms' tumor gene peptide-specific cytotoxic T lymphocytes in immunologic selection of a paroxysmal nocturnal hemoglobinuria clone. Exp Hematol 35(4):618–626. doi: S0301-472X(07)00056-2 [pii] 10.1016/j.exphem.2007.01.045
11. Gargiulo L, Papaioannou M, Sica M, Talini G, Chaidos A, Richichi B, Nikolaev AV, Nativi C, Layton M, de la Fuente J, Roberts I, Luzzatto L, Notaro R, Karadimitris A (2013) Glycosylphosphatidylinositol-specific, CD1d-restricted T cells in paroxysmal nocturnal hemoglobinuria. Blood 121(14):2753–2761. doi:blood-2012-11-469353 [pii] 10.1182/blood-2012-11-469353
12. Okamoto M, Shichishima T, Noji H, Ikeda K, Nakamura A, Akutsu K, Maruyama Y (2006) High frequency of several PIG-A mutations in patients with aplastic anemia and myelodysplastic syndrome. Leukemia 20(4):627–634. doi:2404135 [pii] 10.1038/sj.leu.2404135
13. Nishimura J, Hirota T, Kanakura Y, Machii T, Kageyama R, Doi S, Wada H, Masaoka T, Kanayama Y, Fujii H, Inoue N, Kuwayama M, Inoue N, Ohishi K, Kinoshita T (2002) Long-term support of hematopoiesis by a single stem cell clone in patients with paroxysmal nocturnal hemoglobinuria. blood 99(8):2748–2751. doi:http://dx.doi.org/10.1182/blood.V99.8.2748
14. Fusco A, Fedele M (2007) Roles of HMGA proteins in cancer. Nat Rev Cancer 7(12):899–910. doi:nrc2271 [pii]10.1038/nrc2271
15. Inoue N, Izui-Sarumaru T, Murakami Y, Endo Y, Nishimura J, Kurokawa K, Kuwayama M, Shime H, Machii T, Kanakura Y, Meyers G, Wittwer C, Chen Z, Babcock W, Frei-Lahr D, Parker CJ, Kinoshita T (2006) Molecular basis of clonal expansion of hematopoiesis in 2 patients with paroxysmal nocturnal hemoglobinuria (PNH). Blood 108(13):4232–4236. doi:blood-2006-05-025148 [pii]10.1182/blood-2006-05-025148
16. Nishimura JI, Inoue N, Azenishi Y, Hirota T, Akaogi T, Shibano M, Kawagoe K, Ueda E, Machii T, Takeda J (1996) Analysis of PIG-A gene in a patient who developed reciprocal translocation of chromosome 12 and paroxysmal nocturnal hemoglobinuria during follow-up of aplastic anemia. Am J Hematol 51(3):229–233. doi:10.1002/(SICI)1096-8652(199603)51:3<229::AID-AJH8>3.0.CO;2-Z [pii] 10.1002/(SICI)1096-8652(199603)51:3<229::AID-AJH8>3.0.CO;2-Z
17. Ordulu Z, Wong KE, Currall BB, Ivanov AR, Pereira S, Althari S, Gusella JF, Talkowski ME, Morton CC (2014) Describing sequencing results of structural chromosome rearrangements with a suggested next-generation cytogenetic nomenclature. Am J Hum Genet 94 (5):695–709. doi: S0002-9297(14)00172-4 [pii] 10.1016/j.ajhg.2014.03.020
18. Harris JW, Koscick R, Lazarus HM, Eshleman JR, Medof ME (1999) Leukemia arising out of paroxysmal nocturnal hemoglobinuria. Leuk Lymphoma 32(5–6):401–426. doi:10.3109/10428199909058399
19. Nishimura J, Kanakura Y, Ware RE, Shichishima T, Nakakuma H, Ninomiya H, Decastro CM, Hall S, Kanamaru A, Sullivan KM, Mizoguchi H, Omine M, Kinoshita T, Rosse WF (2004) Clinical course and flow cytometric analysis of paroxysmal nocturnal hemoglobinuria in the United States and Japan. Medicine (Baltimore) 83(3):193–207. doi: 00005792-200405000-00005 [pii]

20. Mayr C, Hemann MT, Bartel DP (2007) Disrupting the pairing between let-7 and Hmga2 enhances oncogenic transformation. Science 315(5818):1576–1579. doi:1137999 [pii] 10.1126/science.1137999
21. Copley MR, Babovic S, Benz C, Knapp DJ, Beer PA, Kent DG, Wohrer S, Treloar DQ, Day C, Rowe K, Mader H, Kuchenbauer F, Humphries RK, Eaves CJ (2013) The Lin28b-let-7-Hmga2 axis determines the higher self-renewal potential of fetal haematopoietic stem cells. Nat Cell Biol 15 (8):916–925. doi:ncb2783 [pii] 10.1038/ncb2783
22. Murakami Y, Inoue N, Shichishima T, Ohta R, Noji H, Maeda Y, Nishimura J, Kanakura Y, Kinoshita T (2012) Deregulated expression of HMGA2 is implicated in clonal expansion of PIGA deficient cells in paroxysmal nocturnal haemoglobinuria. Br J Haematol 156(3):383–387. doi:10.1111/j.1365-2141.2011.08914.x
23. Lam K, Muselman A, Du R, Harada Y, Scholl AG, Yan M, Matsuura S, Weng S, Harada H, Zhang DE (2014) Hmga2 is a direct target gene of RUNX1 and regulates expansion of myeloid progenitors in mice. Blood 124(14):2203–2212. doi: blood-2014-02-554543 [pii] 10.1182/blood-2014-02-554543
24. Andrieux J, Demory JL, Dupriez B, Quief S, Plantier I, Roumier C, Bauters F, Lai JL, Kerckaert JP (2004) Dysregulation and overexpression of HMGA2 in myelofibrosis with myeloid metaplasia. Genes Chromosomes Cancer 39(1):82–87. doi:10.1002/gcc.10297
25. Odero MD, Grand FH, Iqbal S, Ross F, Roman JP, Vizmanos JL, Andrieux J, Lai JL, Calasanz MJ, Cross NC (2005) Disruption and aberrant expression of HMGA2 as a consequence of diverse chromosomal translocations in myeloid malignancies. Leukemia 19(2):245–252. doi:2403605 [pii] 10.1038/sj.leu.2403605
26. Storlazzi CT, Albano F, Locunsolo C, Lonoce A, Funes S, Guastadisegni MC, Cimarosto L, Impera L, D'Addabbo P, Panagopoulos I, Specchia G, Rocchi M (2006) t(3;12)(q26;q14) in polycythemia vera is associated with upregulation of the HMGA2 gene. Leukemia 20(12):2190–2192. doi: 2404418 [pii] 10.1038/sj.leu.2404418
27. Martin SE, Sausen M, Joseph A, Kingham BF, Martin ES (2012) Identification of a HMGA2-EFCAB6 gene rearrangement following next-generation sequencing in a patient with a t(12;22)(q14.3;q13.2) and JAK2V617F-positive myeloproliferative neoplasm. Cancer Genet 205(6):295–303. doi:S2210-7762(12)00102-0 [pii] 10.1016/j.cancergen.2012.03.006
28. Harada-Shirado K, Ikeda K, Ogawa K, Ohkawara H, Kimura H, Kai T, Noji H, Morishita S, Komatsu N, Takeishi Y (2015) Dysregulation of the MIRLET7/HMGA2 axis with methylation of the CDKN2A promoter in myeloproliferative neoplasms. Br J Haematol 168(3):338–349. doi:10.1111/bjh.13129
29. Cavazzana-Calvo M, Payen E, Negre O, Wang G, Hehir K, Fusil F, Down J, Denaro M, Brady T, Westerman K, Cavallesco R, Gillet-Legrand B, Caccavelli L, Sgarra R, Maouche-Chretien L, Bernaudin F, Girot R, Dorazio R, Mulder GJ, Polack A, Bank A, Soulier J, Larghero J, Kabbara N, Dalle B, Gourmel B, Socie G, Chretien S, Cartier N, Aubourg P, Fischer A, Cornetta K, Galacteros F, Beuzard Y, Gluckman E, Bushman F, Hacein-Bey-Abina S, Leboulch P (2010) Transfusion independence and HMGA2 activation after gene therapy of human beta-thalassaemia. Nature 467(7313):318–322. doi:nature09328 [pii] 10.1038/nature09328
30. Payen E, Leboulch P (2012) Advances in stem cell transplantation and gene therapy in the beta-hemoglobinopathies. Hematol Am Soc Hematol Educ Program 2012:276–283. doi:2012/1/276 [pii] 10.1182/asheducation-2012.1.276
31. Ikeda K, Mason PJ, Bessler M (2011) 3'UTR-truncated Hmga2 cDNA causes MPN-like hematopoiesis by conferring a clonal growth advantage at the level of HSC in mice. Blood 117(22):5860–5869. doi: blood-2011-02-334425 [pii] 10.1182/blood-2011-02-334425
32. Sugimori C, Padron E, Caceres G, Shain K, Sokol L, Zhang L, Tiu R, O'Keefe CL, Afable M, Clemente M, Lee JM, Maciejewski JP, List AF, Epling-Burnette PK, Araten DJ (2012) Paroxysmal nocturnal hemoglobinuria and concurrent JAK2(V617F) mutation. Blood Cancer J 2(3):e63. doi:10.1038/bcj.2012.7

33. Shen W, Clemente MJ, Hosono N, Yoshida K, Przychodzen B, Yoshizato T, Shiraishi Y, Miyano S, Ogawa S, Maciejewski JP, Makishima H (2014) Deep sequencing reveals stepwise mutation acquisition in paroxysmal nocturnal hemoglobinuria. J Clin Invest 124(10):4529–4538. doi: 74747 [pii] 10.1172/JCI74747
34. Levine RL, Pardanani A, Tefferi A, Gilliland DG (2007) Role of JAK2 in the pathogenesis and therapy of myeloproliferative disorders. Nat Rev Cancer 7(9):673–683. doi:nrc2210 [pii] 10.1038/nrc2210
35. Vainchenker W, Constantinescu SN (2013) JAK/STAT signaling in hematological malignancies. Oncogene 32(21):2601–2613. doi: onc2012347 [pii] 10.1038/onc.2012.347
36. Ungureanu D, Wu J, Pekkala T, Niranjan Y, Young C, Jensen ON, Xu CF, Neubert TA, Skoda RC, Hubbard SR, Silvennoinen O (2011) The pseudokinase domain of JAK2 is a dual-specificity protein kinase that negatively regulates cytokine signaling. Nat Struct Mol Biol 18(9):971–976. doi: nsmb.2099 [pii] 10.1038/nsmb.2099
37. O'Keefe CL, Sugimori C, Afable M, Clemente M, Shain K, Araten DJ, List A, Epling-Burnette PK, Maciejewski JP (2011) Deletions of Xp22.2 including PIG-A locus lead to paroxysmal nocturnal hemoglobinuria. Leukemia 25(2):379–382. doi:leu2010274 [pii] 10.1038/leu.2010.274
38. Rivera MN, Haber DA (2005) Wilms' tumour: connecting tumorigenesis and organ development in the kidney. Nat Rev Cancer 5(9):699–712. doi:nrc1696 [pii] 10.1038/nrc1696
39. Sugiyama H (2010) WT1 (Wilms' tumor gene 1): biology and cancer immunotherapy. Jpn J Clin Oncol 40(5):377–387. doi: hyp194 [pii] 10.1093/jjco/hyp194
40. Owen C, Fitzgibbon J, Paschka P (2010) The clinical relevance of Wilms Tumour 1 (WT1) gene mutations in acute leukaemia. Hematol Oncol 28(1):13–19. doi:10.1002/hon.931
41. Shichishima T, Okamoto M, Ikeda K, Kaneshige T, Sugiyama H, Terasawa T, Osumi K, Maruyama Y (2002) HLA class II haplotype and quantitation of WT1 RNA in Japanese patients with paroxysmal nocturnal hemoglobinuria. Blood 100(1):22–28
42. Lyakisheva A, Felda O, Ganser A, Schmidt RE, Schubert J (2002) Paroxysmal nocturnal hemoglobinuria: Differential gene expression of EGR-1 and TAXREB107. Exp Hematol 30(1):18–25. doi:S0301472X01007639 [pii]
43. Joslin JM, Fernald AA, Tennant TR, Davis EM, Kogan SC, Anastasi J, Crispino JD, Le Beau MM (2007) Haploinsufficiency of EGR1, a candidate gene in the del(5q), leads to the development of myeloid disorders. Blood 110(2):719–726. doi:blood-2007-01-068809 [pii] 10.1182/blood-2007-01-068809
44. Heeney MM, Ormsbee SM, Moody MA, Howard TA, DeCastro CM, Ware RE (2003) Increased expression of anti-apoptosis genes in peripheral blood cells from patients with paroxysmal nocturnal hemoglobinuria. Mol Genet Metab 78(4):291–294. doi:S1096719203000477 [pii]
45. Kinoshita T, Inoue N (2002) Relationship between aplastic anemia and paroxysmal nocturnal hemoglobinuria. Int J Hematol 75(2):117–122
46. Krawitz PM, Hochsmann B, Murakami Y, Teubner B, Kruger U, Klopocki E, Neitzel H, Hoellein A, Schneider C, Parkhomchuk D, Hecht J, Robinson PN, Mundlos S, Kinoshita T, Schrezenmeier H (2013) A case of paroxysmal nocturnal hemoglobinuria caused by a germline mutation and a somatic mutation in PIGT. Blood 122(7):1312–1315. doi:blood-2013-01-481499 [pii] 10.1182/blood-2013-01-481499
47. Ohishi K, Inoue N, Maeda Y, Takeda J, Riezman H, Kinoshita T (2000) Gaa1p and gpi8p are components of a glycosylphosphatidylinositol (GPI) transamidase that mediates attachment of GPI to proteins. Mol Biol Cell 11(5):1523–1533
48. Ohishi K, Inoue N, Kinoshita T (2001) PIG-S and PIG-T, essential for GPI anchor attachment to proteins, form a complex with GAA1 and GPI8. EMBO J 20(15):4088–4098. doi:10.1093/emboj/20.15.4088

49. Hong Y, Ohishi K, Kang JY, Tanaka S, Inoue N, Nishimura J, Maeda Y, Kinoshita T (2003) Human PIG-U and yeast Cdc91p are the fifth subunit of GPI transamidase that attaches GPI-anchors to proteins. Mol Biol Cell 14(5):1780–1789. doi:10.1091/mbc.E02-12-0794 E02-12-0794 [pii]
50. Gurvich N, Perna F, Farina A, Voza F, Menendez S, Hurwitz J, Nimer SD (2010) L3MBTL1 polycomb protein, a candidate tumor suppressor in del(20q12) myeloid disorders, is essential for genome stability. Proc Natl Acad Sci U S A 107(52):22552–22557. doi: 1017092108 [pii] 10.1073/pnas.1017092108
51. Perna F, Gurvich N, Hoya-Arias R, Abdel-Wahab O, Levine RL, Asai T, Voza F, Menendez S, Wang L, Liu F, Zhao X, Nimer SD (2010) Depletion of L3MBTL1 promotes the erythroid differentiation of human hematopoietic progenitor cells: possible role in 20q- polycythemia vera. Blood 116(15):2812–2821. doi:blood-2010-02-270611 [pii] 10.1182/blood-2010-02-270611
52. Aziz A, Baxter EJ, Edwards C, Cheong CY, Ito M, Bench A, Kelley R, Silber Y, Beer PA, Chng K, Renfree MB, McEwen K, Gray D, Nangalia J, Mufti GJ, Hellstrom-Lindberg E, Kiladjian JJ, McMullin MF, Campbell PJ, Ferguson-Smith AC, Green AR (2013) Cooperativity of imprinted genes inactivated by acquired chromosome 20q deletions. J Clin Invest 123(5):2169–2182. doi: 66113 [pii] 10.1172/JCI66113
53. Nangalia J, Massie CE, Baxter EJ, Nice FL, Gundem G, Wedge DC, Avezov E, Li J, Kollmann K, Kent DG, Aziz A, Godfrey AL, Hinton J, Martincorena I, Van Loo P, Jones AV, Guglielmelli P, Tarpey P, Harding HP, Fitzpatrick JD, Goudie CT, Ortmann CA, Loughran SJ, Raine K, Jones DR, Butler AP, Teague JW, O'Meara S, McLaren S, Bianchi M, Silber Y, Dimitropoulou D, Bloxham D, Mudie L, Maddison M, Robinson B, Keohane C, Maclean C, Hill K, Orchard K, Tauro S, Du MQ, Greaves M, Bowen D, Huntly BJ, Harrison CN, Cross NC, Ron D, Vannucchi AM, Papaemmanuil E, Campbell PJ, Green AR (2013) Somatic CALR mutations in myeloproliferative neoplasms with nonmutated JAK2. N Engl J Med 369(25):2391–2405. doi:10.1056/NEJMoa1312542
54. Yoshida K, Toki T, Okuno Y, Kanezaki R, Shiraishi Y, Sato-Otsubo A, Sanada M, Park MJ, Terui K, Suzuki H, Kon A, Nagata Y, Sato Y, Wang R, Shiba N, Chiba K, Tanaka H, Hama A, Muramatsu H, Hasegawa D, Nakamura K, Kanegane H, Tsukamoto K, Adachi S, Kawakami K, Kato K, Nishimura R, Izraeli S, Hayashi Y, Miyano S, Kojima S, Ito E, Ogawa S (2013) The landscape of somatic mutations in Down syndrome-related myeloid disorders. Nat Genet 45(11):1293–1299. doi:ng.2759 [pii] 10.1038/ng.2759
55. Yoshizato T, Dumitriu B, Hosokawa K, Makishima H, Yoshida K, Townsley D, Sato-Otsubo A, Sato Y, Liu D, Suzuki H, Wu CO, Shiraishi Y, Clemente MJ, Kataoka K, Shiozawa Y, Okuno Y, Chiba K, Tanaka H, Nagata Y, Katagiri T, Kon A, Sanada M, Scheinberg P, Miyano S, Maciejewski JP, Nakao S, Young NS, Ogawa S (2015) Somatic mutations and clonal hematopoiesis in aplastic anemia. N Engl J Med 373(1):35–47. doi:10.1056/NEJMoa1414799
56. Inoue N, Murakami Y, Kinoshita T (2003) Molecular genetics of paroxysmal nocturnal hemoglobinuria. Int J Hematol 77(2):107–112
57. Welch JS, Ley TJ, Link DC, Miller CA, Larson DE, Koboldt DC, Wartman LD, Lamprecht TL, Liu F, Xia J, Kandoth C, Fulton RS, McLellan MD, Dooling DJ, Wallis JW, Chen K, Harris CC, Schmidt HK, Kalicki-Veizer JM, Lu C, Zhang Q, Lin L, O'Laughlin MD, McMichael JF, Delehaunty KD, Fulton LA, Magrini VJ, McGrath SD, Demeter RT, Vickery TL, Hundal J, Cook LL, Swift GW, Reed JP, Alldredge PA, Wylie TN, Walker JR, Watson MA, Heath SE, Shannon WD, Varghese N, Nagarajan R, Payton JE, Baty JD, Kulkarni S, Klco JM, Tomasson MH, Westervelt P, Walter MJ, Graubert TA, DiPersio JF, Ding L, Mardis ER, Wilson RK (2012) The origin and evolution of mutations in acute myeloid leukemia. Cell 150(2):264–278. doi:S0092-8674(12)00777-5 [pii] 10.1016/j.cell.2012.06.023

58. Xie M, Lu C, Wang J, McLellan MD, Johnson KJ, Wendl MC, McMichael JF, Schmidt HK, Yellapantula V, Miller CA, Ozenberger BA, Welch JS, Link DC, Walter MJ, Mardis ER, Dipersio JF, Chen F, Wilson RK, Ley TJ, Ding L (2014) Age-related mutations associated with clonal hematopoietic expansion and malignancies. Nat Med 20(12):1472–1478. doi: nm.3733 [pii] 10.1038/nm.3733
59. Chotirat S, Thongnoppakhun W, Wanachiwanawin W, Auewarakul CU (2015) Acquired somatic mutations of isocitrate dehydrogenases 1 and 2 (IDH1 and IDH2) in preleukemic disorders. Blood Cells Mol Dis 54(3):286–291. doi:S1079-9796(14)00150-8 [pii] 10.1016/j.bcmd.2014.11.017
60. Mortazavi Y, Tooze JA, Gordon-Smith EC, Rutherford TR (2000) N-RAS gene mutation in patients with aplastic anemia and aplastic anemia/ paroxysmal nocturnal hemoglobinuria during evolution to clonal disease. Blood 95(2):646–650
61. Ortmann CA, Kent DG, Nangalia J, Silber Y, Wedge DC, Grinfeld J, Baxter EJ, Massie CE, Papaemmanuil E, Menon S, Godfrey AL, Dimitropoulou D, Guglielmelli P, Bellosillo B, Besses C, Dohner K, Harrison CN, Vassiliou GS, Vannucchi A, Campbell PJ, Green AR (2015) Effect of mutation order on myeloproliferative neoplasms. N Engl J Med 372(7):601–612. doi:10.1056/NEJMoa1412098

Chapter 15
Clinical Management in PNH

Tsutomu Shichishima and Hideyoshi Noji

Abstract Paroxysmal nocturnal hemoglobinuria (PNH) is characterized by intravascular hemolysis via complement (C)-mediated hemolysis, thrombosis, and bone marrow failure. Treatment protocol of PNH is proposed from the views of degree of clinical severity; of predominant pathophysiology, described above; and of response to medication therapy. PNH patients with lower degree of clinical severity or complete remission with below 1 % of PNH-type granulocytes and erythrocytes should be observed without medication. With the progression of clinical severity and main pathophysiology and increase of above 10 % of PNH-type erythrocytes, medication therapy should be initiated because of appearance of various subjective symptoms. Although it is certain that eculizumab treatment is predominant for intravascular hemolysis, the therapy develops breakthrough hemolysis, extravascular hemolysis of C3-bound erythrocytes, and poor response to eculizumab treatment. It is controversial whether or not hemolysis in classic PNH patients should be treated with prednisolone because of its adverse effects. Then, administration of a human plasma-derived haptoglobin product may be suitable for uncontrolled hemolysis triggered by eculizumab treatment and hemolytic attack. Immunosuppressive therapy with cyclosporine A (CSA) and/or antithymocyte globulin and androgens in PNH with hypocellular bone marrow are useful as well as those for aplastic anemia and a combination of filgrastim and CSA or recombinant human erythropoietin administration results in a trilineage response of hematopoiesis or a response of anemia, respectively. As thrombotic events rarely occur even in PNH patients without receiving eculizumab and with less than 50 % of PNH granulocytes or in PNH patients receiving eculizumab, indication of warfarin should be carefully investigated.

T. Shichishima, M.D., Ph.D. (✉)
Department of Hematology and Oncology, Fukushima Medical University,
1 Hikariga-oka, Fukushima 960-1295, Japan

Fukushima Research Institute of Environment and Medicine,
16-6 Mito-uchi Houkida-aza, Fukushima 960-8560, Japan
e-mail: t-shichi@fmu.ac.jp

H. Noji, M.D., Ph.D.
Department of Hematology, Fukushima Medical University,
1 Hikariga-oka, Fukushima 960-1295, Japan

Y. Kanakura et al. (eds.), *Paroxysmal Nocturnal Hemoglobinuria*,
DOI 10.1007/978-4-431-56003-6_15

Supportive therapies, including blood transfusions, and therapies for complications, such as iron deficiency anemia and renal dysfunction, are also needed. Hematopoietic stem cell transplantation is curative therapy for PNH, but indication of it is now limited predominantly to PNH with severe bone marrow failure.

Keywords Treatment protocol of PNH • Medication therapy for PNH • Haptoglobin therapy • Supportive care for PNH • Hematopoietic stem cell transplantation

15.1 Introduction

Clinically, paroxysmal nocturnal hemoglobinuria (PNH) is characterized predominantly by intravascular hemolysis via complement (C)-mediated hemolysis, thrombosis, and bone marrow failure [1]. C-mediated hemolysis causes anemia, icterus, and grossly visible hemoglobinuria and consequently develops cholelithiasis, acute or chronic renal dysfunction, or iron deficiency anemia in PNH patients. Recently, it has been proposed that many data support the existence of a novel mechanism of human disease, hemolysis-associated smooth muscle dystonia, vasculopathy, endothelial dysfunction, and inflammation and oxidation, resulting in adverse clinical signs and symptoms by local and systemic NO (nitric oxide) deficiency through release of hemoglobin (Hb) in plasma [2]. PNH is a representative disorder with the mechanism and signs/symptoms associated with decrease of NO, like renal dysfunction, gastrointestinal dystonias and pain, pulmonary hypertension and dyspnea, thrombosis and platelet activation, and erectile dysfunction (Fig. 15.1), resulting in a diversity of clinical symptoms/signs in PNH [3], although PNH patients have not necessarily all of these symptoms/signs. In addition, extracellular Hb has been found to trigger specific pathophysiologies that are associated with adverse clinical outcomes in patients with hemolysis, such as acute and chronic vascular disease, inflammation, thrombosis, and renal impairment (Fig. 15.1), by the extracellular translocation of Hb; attenuation of NO and oxidative reactions, described above; release of free hemin; and molecular-signaling effects of hemin [4]. Thrombosis in PNH is caused by a combination of several factors, which are activation of platelets; intravascular hemolysis following depletion of NO, toxicity of free Hb, and red cell microvesicles; deficiency of urokinase-type plasminogen activator receptor; endothelial dysfunction; and thrombin production via C activation pathway [5]. It is well known that thrombosis is the most frequent cause of death in American and European patients with PNH [6, 7]. Bone marrow failure, associated with putative immunologic mechanisms [8], undertakes leukocytopenia and thrombocytopenia, resulting in infection and hemorrhage, respectively, which are the main causes of death in Japan [7, 9].

With the accumulation of clinical and pathophysiologic findings in PNH, the international PNH interest group (I-PIG) proposed that PNH is classified into three subcategories: classic PNH (subcategory A), PNH in the setting of another specified

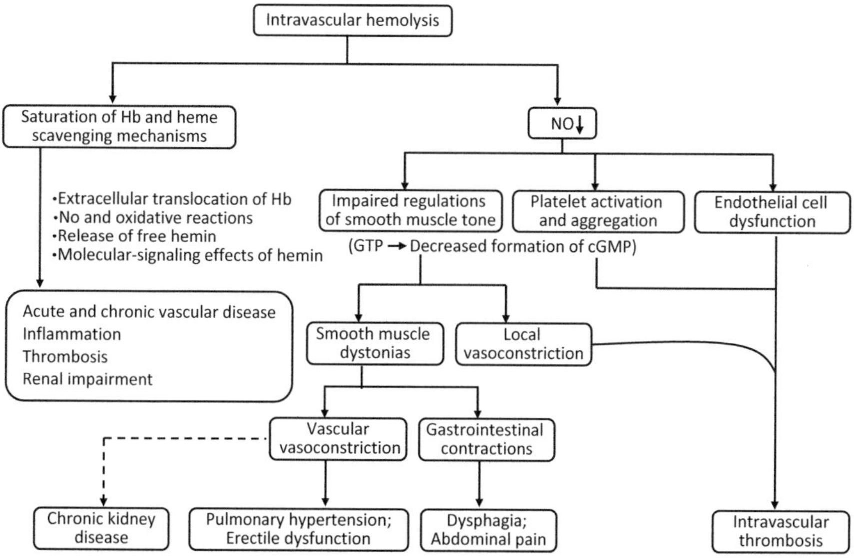

Fig. 15.1 Adverse clinical effects associated with excessive free Hb through intravascular hemolysis in PNH. Intravascular hemolysis via C-mediated hemolysis in PNH develops adverse clinical effects, including acute and chronic vascular disease, inflammation, thrombosis, renal impairment, and smooth muscle dystonias, by the following four mechanisms: (1) extravascular translocation of Hb, (2) NO and oxidative reactions, (3) release of free hemin (ferric protoporphyrin-IX group), and (4) molecular-signaling effects of hemin [2, 4]

bone marrow disorder (subcategory B), and subclinical PNH (subcategory C) [10]. In addition, eculizumab, a humanized monoclonal antibody to the fifth component of C5 that inhibits terminal C activation, has been developed with a beneficial effect on reducing C-mediated hemolysis in PNH [11]. Therefore, based on the advances of diagnostic tools and therapy for PNH, clinical management of treatment for PNH should be summed up at this time.

15.2 Treatment Protocol of PNH

It is considered to be difficult that we rigorously determine treatment algorithm of PNH, because PNH symptoms and signs are certainly derived from three chief pathophysiologies, as described above, but each PNH patient has not necessarily one main pathophysiology alone, and the proportion of PNH-type granulocytes (PNH clone size) does not necessarily determine the severity of PNH. In addition, main pathophysiology of PNH sometimes changes during the period of clinical course. However, practical hematologists need to determine the direction of treatment for PNH. Then, we tried to propose the treatment protocol of PNH by

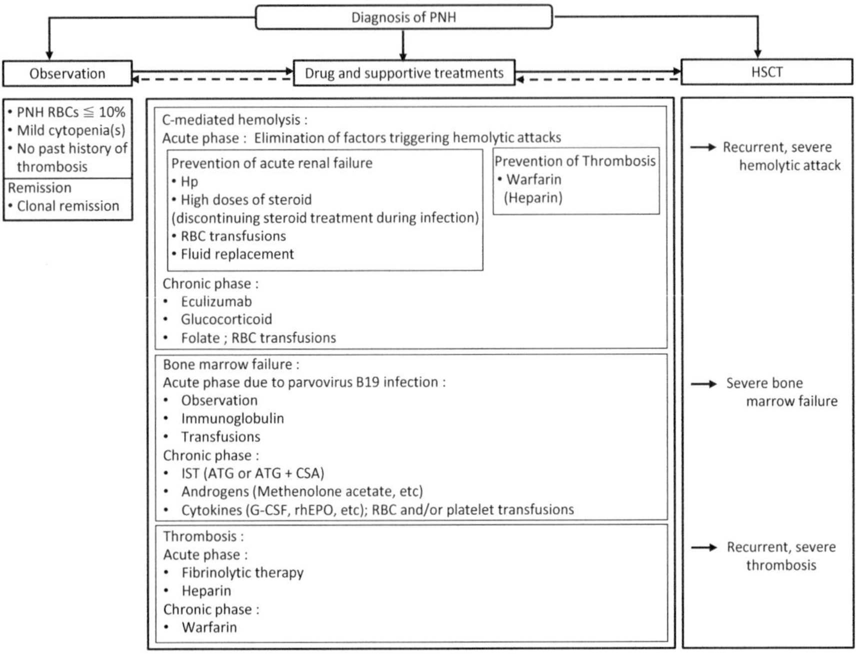

Fig. 15.2 Treatment protocol in PNH. PNH patients, who have below 10 % of GPI-AP-negative erythrocytes, mild cytopenia(s), and no past history of thrombosis at diagnosis, and PNH patients with clonal remission during their clinical courses should be observed without treatment for PNH. When PNH patients deviate from the observation group, described above, they usually need some drug or supportive care for predominant pathophysiology of PNH, including intravascular hemolysis via C-mediated hemolysis, bone marrow failure, or thrombosis. Although HSCT is curative therapy for PNH, in the eculizumab era, the indication of HSCT for may be limited mainly to patients with severe bone marrow failure

summarizing treatment options of three chief pathophysiologies, including observation, medical therapy, supportive care, and hematopoietic stem cell transplantation (HSCT), reported in the past (Fig. 15.2).

15.2.1 Observation

When diagnosing PNH, it is essential to detect PNH-type erythrocytes and granulocytes of peripheral blood by flow cytometry using antibodies to CD55 and/or CD59 of glycosylphosphatidylinositol-anchored protein (GPI-AP) or FLAER (a fluorescently labeled inactive variant of the protein aerolysin) [12, 13]. The PNH Working Group of Research Committee for the Idiopathic Hematopoietic Disorders in Japan clearly describes that over 1 % of negative and intermediate populations of GPI-AP expressions, determined by flow cytometry, in erythrocytes and granulocytes mean PNH-type ones (Table 15.1) [14], because PNH patients with over 1 % of them have

Table 15.1 Diagnostic criteria, modified in 2013, by the PNH Working Group of Research Committee for the Idiopathic Hematopoietic Disorders [14]

1.	As clinical symptoms, visible hemoglobinuria (urine with pale red to dark brown color) is observed in addition to anemia and jaundice in most settings. Venous thrombosis, hemorrhagic diathesis, and susceptibility to infection are sometimes observed. It does not occur congenitally, but occurs in wide-ranging age population centering around young and middle-aged people.
2.	The following laboratory findings are often seen:
	1) Anemia and decreased WBC and platelet counts
	2) Elevated concentrations of serum indirect bilirubin and LDH and decreased concentration of serum haptoglobin
	3) Positive reaction for Hb and hemosiderin in supernatant and sediment, respectively, of urine
	4) Reduced score of neutrophil alkaline phosphatase and low level of erythrocyte acetylcholinesterase
	5) Increased proportion of erythroblasts in bone marrow (bone marrow is hyperplastic in many cases, but is hypoplastic in some cases)
	6) Positive finding of Ham's test (acidified serum lysis test) or sugar-water test
3.	The diagnosis of PNH is suspected in the presence of clinical symptoms and laboratory findings, described above, and confirmed by the following laboratory findings:
	1) Negative finding for direct Coombs' test
	2) Detection and quantification of hematopoietic cells (especially, erythrocytes) with deficiency of GPI-APs
4.	Subcategories of PNH are determined by bone marrow aspiration, bone marrow biopsy, and its chromosomal examination, but you need not necessarily determine any subcategory in the patient:
	1) Clinical PNH (with hemolytic findings)
	(1) Classic PNH
	(2) PNH with bone marrow failure
	(3) Mixed-type PNH
	2) Bone marrow failure disorders having a thin PNH-type blood cell (the disorders in which hemolytic findings are not obvious are referred to as follows and differentiated from clinical PNH)
5.	Reference information
	1) Hemolytic findings include increases of serum LDH, indirect bilirubin, and reticulocyte count and decrease of serum haptoglobin; clinical PNH is diagnosed on the basis of >1 % of the proportion of PNH-type-III erythrocytes and over 1.5 times of the upper limit in serum LDH

some sort of hemolytic findings [15]. On the basis of the past experience, it is considered that PNH patients with below 10 % of GPI-negative erythrocytes, mild cytopenia(s), no blood cell transfusions, and no past history of thrombosis at diagnosis should be observed without treatment for PNH [16, 17].

Eight % (3/38), 15 % (12/80), and > 5 % (11/220) of PNH patients accomplished a spontaneous remission during the observation period of > 10 years, less than 20 years, and 0 and 2–39 years, respectively [6, 18, 19]. In addition, 26 % (7/29) and 13 % (4/30) of PNH patients treated with high-dose cyclophosphamide and eculizumab, respectively, achieved a clinical remission during the observation period of 1.5–11.5 years and 6–80 months, respectively [16, 17]. If PNH patients accomplish a spontaneous remission, they need not any therapy, while most PNH patients with a therapy-related remission, which almost means a clinical remission, but not a clonal remission, need to continue the drug administration.

15.2.2 Medication Therapy

When PNH patients deviate from the observation group, described above or in Fig. 15.2, they usually need some drug therapy or supportive care, indicating that it means expansion of PNH clone size or progress of bone marrow failure. In this section, we describe medical therapy for intravascular hemolysis via C-mediated hemolysis, bone marrow failure, and thrombosis in PNH.

15.2.2.1 Medical Therapy for Intravascular Hemolysis and Extravascular Hemolysis

Eculizumab Therapy

It is well known that eculizumab is very effective for hemolysis in PNH, resulting in improvement of anemia, followed by decrease of frequency of red blood cell (RBC) transfusions, and of clinical symptoms due to decrease of NO via chronic intravascular hemolysis. In the era of eculizumab, it is thought that the frequency using prednisolone for chronic hemolysis and hemolytic attacks is significantly decreased. However, eculizumab treatment has developed three important adverse effects associated with its action mechanism. First, breakthrough hemolysis, which is defined as inefficacy in blocking C-mediated hemolysis in the last days before the next drug administration [20], was observed during long-term treatment by eculizumab in 17 % (7/41) and 10.7 % (21/195) of PNH patients [20, 21]. Long-term treatment by eculizumab almost develops the increase of proportion and number of C-sensitive erythrocytes and sometimes elicits appearance of human antihuman antibodies or neutralizing antibodies to eculizumab, leading to transient or persistent breakthrough hemolysis. Although any breakthrough hemolysis did not result in the discontinuation of eculizumab, if you need, the interval of eculizumab administration should be shortened. Second, it has been reported that eculizumab elicits extravascular hemolysis of C3-bound erythrocytes following C3 opsonization associated with reduction of C5 conversion by it [20]. The mean Hb value for PNH patients with a positive Coombs' test was significantly lower that for PNH patients with a negative Coombs' test among 31 eculizumab-treated patients [22]. Although it is controversial whether glucocorticoid should be given to eculizumab-treated patients with a positive Coombs' test and progression of anemia [23, 24], the use of prednisolone might be considered for progression of anemia, which needs RBC transfusions, following a transient increase of Hb level by eculizumab treatment. Third, Nishimura et al. [25] reported that there were PNH patients with poor response to eculizumab treatment in Japan, who had single and heterozygous mutation (c.2654G > A) of C5, leading to a low affinity of eculizumab to C5. In these most patients, we are compelled to cancel eculizumab treatment and to initiate prednisolone therapy for C-mediated hemolysis. On the other hand, we have experienced two PNH patients, who had the same mutation as described above and portal and/or hepatic vein thrombosis with abdominal pain [25, 26]. Eculizumab treatment did not attenuate the value of LDH in these patients. However, abdominal pain and/or ascites have surprisingly disappeared by eculizumab treatment and then the value of D-dimer was also decreased in the PNH patients. It is considered that this effect of eculizumab treatment on thrombosis is probably associated with partially poor response due to heterozygous polymorphism of C5, suggesting that part of eculizumab may function normally even in the poor responders.

Prednisolone Therapy

Some papers have reported that prednisolone therapy, using alternate day, high-dose prednisolone or low-dose prednisolone daily, is beneficial for prevention of hemolysis in some classic PNH patients, but not in bone marrow failure PNH patients, during chronic phase [27–29]. During the acute phase of hemolysis, the dose of prednisolone is increased, leading to suppression of hemolytic attacks [27]. Although it is thought that prednisolone inhibits the activation of C, the action mode of prednisolone is not clear at all. Therefore, some hematologists take objection to the prednisolone therapy for chronic and acute hemolysis because the effect of prednisolone on hemolysis is uncertain and the adverse effects of it are great. It is controversial whether or not hemolysis in classic PNH patients should be treated with prednisolone, but this discussion may be limited to extravascular hemolysis from now because eculizumab compared with prednisolone has a more beneficial and certain effect on C-mediated hemolysis, as described above.

Haptoglobin (Hp) Therapy

Diminished plasma concentrations of Hp, hemopexin (HXP), and heme were reported in patients with various hemolytic diseases [30].Hp and CD163 receptors on macrophages coordinate Hb dimer clearance when Hb from RBCs is released during hemolysis. When heme is released into plasma, several proteins, such as HPX, high- and low-density lipoproteins, albumin, and α-microglobulin, with different affinities to heme collectively bind and clear heme from circulation [31]. All 4 mechanisms of Hb and hemin toxicity, as described in Fig. 15.1, are specifically attenuated by the natural scavenger proteins Hp and HPX [4]. However, no HPX product is available at a quality that would allow more extensive in vivo studies beyond murine models, suggesting that expanded studies with HPX treatment may not be possible in the near future for larger models of relevant clinical conditions.

A human plasma-derived Hp product was developed by the Japanese Green Cross and was approved in 1985 for the treatment of hemolysis due to extracorporeal circulation, burn injuries, and trauma with massive blood transfusions [32–34]. In addition, case reports support the successful use of Hp in patients with hemolytic anemias [35, 36], including PNH [37]. It is well known that exacerbations of hemolysis in PNH occasionally trigger severe complications, especially acute renal failure and thrombosis. In order to limit acute renal injury due to exacerbations of hemolysis, the primary clinical criteria for Hp administration are the appearance and reversal of visible hemoglobinuria. Although the total doses of Hp for acute hemolytic conditions are various according to the effect on exacerbated hemoglobinuria, the doses of Hp per day in an adult patient with PNH are usually 4000 U. One bolus of Hp 100 mL includes 2000 U of Hp. It is considered that the administration of Hp during acute hemolytic condition is also effective for thrombosis, but we have not sufficient data with this. Therefore, Hp product may be administrated, at least, for breakthrough hemolysis occasionally elicited by eculizumab treatment without changing eculizumab administration schedule or a remarkable increase of indirect bilirubin due to extravascular hemolysis triggered by eculizumab treatment, suggesting that Hp, but not prednisolone, should be commonly administered for adverse events, such as breakthrough hemolysis and extravascular hemolysis, by eculizumab treatment. In the near future, Hp should be investigated and approved as a treatment for exacerbated hemolysis or uncontrolled hemolysis due to hemolytic anemias, including PNH, not only in Japan but also in the world. The Benesis Corporation reported results of the survey that only 3 of 2483 patients, who underwent a therapy by a Hp product, had adverse events, such as fall in blood pressure (0.08 %) and vomiting (0.04 %) and that none of the patients had any virus infection.

Folate

Folate administration is recommended to compensate for the increased utilization of folate associated with the burst of erythropoiesis that is a consequence of acute or chronic hemolysis [10].

Development of New Medicines

Eculizumab treatment for intravascular hemolysis in PNH raises a varying degree of extravascular hemolysis, as described above, disturbing the increase of Hb concentration. Then, we want a better medicine that can prevent both intravascular and extravascular hemolysis in PNH. Following in vitro study with an antibody against

C3b (mAb 3E7) [38], the fusion protein TT30 that combines regulatory domain of factor H (FH) with the iC3b/C3d-binding domains of CD21 [39, 40], and a novel inhibitor that links the regulatory and surface recognition areas of FH (mini-FH) [41], has been developed. The former is currently evaluated in a phase I clinical trial enrolling PNH patients. More recently, it was demonstrated that peptide inhibitors of C3 activation effectively prevent in vitro hemolysis and C3 opsonization of PNH erythrocytes [42]. In addition, the development of several new therapeutic agents besides the drugs described above, which have different mechanisms suppressing C activation of alternative pathway and various medication methods of them, is advanced. In the future, the efficacy of these drugs, including adverse effects, should be clinically evaluated.

15.2.2.2 Treatment for Hypoplastic Bone Marrow in PNH

When considering treatment for PNH patients with hypoplastic bone marrow, immunosuppressive therapy (IST) with cyclosporine A (CSA) and/or antithymocyte globulin (ATG) and androgens, including methenolone or danazol, are useful as well as that for aplastic anemia (AA). IST using ATG is suitable for treatment of PNH patients with hypoplastic bone marrow, lower proportions of GPI-AP-negative cells, and mild hemolysis, while is not for treatment of classic PNH patients, because IST is effective only on bone marrow failure, but not the reduction of size of PNH clone [43]. In addition, IST with ATG sometimes elicits the exacerbations of hemolysis in PNH patients with higher proportions of GPI-AP-negative erythrocytes [44]. However, Alashkar et al. [45] recently reported a PNH patient with high proportion (97.4 %) of CD59-negative RBC and a hypoplastic bone marrow, who was concomitantly treated with IST and eculizumab, resulting in a partial remission hematologically without hemolytic and thrombotic events. Subsequently, in PNH patients with mild and moderate hypoplasia, it is popular to use androgens, while in those with severe and very severe hypoplasia, CSA. It is generally recommended to add methenolone to CSA treatment and then danazol to it, if they are refractory to treatment with CSA in the latter. Moreover, an efficient option for the treatment of hypoplastic PNH using a combination of filgrastim (granulocyte colony-stimulating factor, G-CSF) and CSA was proposed [46]. The treatment resulted in a trilineage response of hematopoiesis and a decrease of the proportion of GPI-negative granulocytes in all the patients treated with this regimen. The responses to recombinant human erythropoietin (rhEPO) for treatment of anemia in PNH patients with bone marrow failure have been also reported in spite of higher levels of plasma EPO [47–49]. Recently, Hill et al. [50] reported a PNH patient with bone marrow failure treated with eculizumab, followed by concurrent treatment with rhEPO. Addition of rhEPO increased Hb levels and rendered the patient transfusion independent for a long period.

15.2.2.3 Prevention of Thromboembolism by Warfarin

It is well known that the frequency of thrombotic event in Asian patients with PNH is significantly lower than that in American and European patients [6, 7, 19], although we are not able to explain this difference. It has been believed that primary prophylaxis with warfarin should be considered if the PNH clone size is larger than 50 %, the platelet count is stable at higher than 100×10^9/L, and there is no known contraindication to anticoagulation [51]. However, since it was known that eculizumab compared with warfarin has a beneficial effect on reducing thrombotic events in PNH [48], as described in 3.1.5, it is considered that prophylaxis effect on thromboembolism with warfarin in PNH is insufficient [52, 53]. Nevertheless, indication for treatment of warfarin should be reconsidered in PNH patients in the future because thrombotic events sometimes or rarely occur even in those without receiving eculizumab and with less than 50 % of PNH clone size or in those with receiving eculizumab, respectively. Also, whether warfarin can be eliminated in PNH patients receiving eculizumab is the subject of future investigation. Helley et al. [54] reported that treatment with eculizumab in 23 PNH patients was associated with significant decreases in plasma markers of coagulation activation, including prothrombin fragment 1 + 2 and D-dimers, and reactional fibrinolysis, including plasmin antiplasmin complexes, in addition to those of endothelial cell activation, suggesting useful markers when considering indication for warfarin treatment. Finally, warfarin should carefully be administered to PNH patients, who especially have thrombocytopenia, because of complication of warfarin-induced hemorrhage, including fatal hemorrhage [51].

15.2.3 Supportive Care

15.2.3.1 Blood Transfusion

When the effect of drug therapies on hemolysis or bone marrow failure in PNH, described above, is not sufficient, PNH patients need RBC and platelet transfusion for anemia and hemorrhagic diathesis, respectively. In Japan, RBC transfusions are usually performed below 7 g/dL of Hb concentrations with subjective symptoms of anemia, while platelet transfusions below $1 \times 10^4/\mu L$ with hemorrhagic diathesis. The use of saline-washed RBCs has been advocated to minimize hemolysis after transfusion to patients with PNH [27], which may be due to the infusion of activated C components present in the plasma in the stored blood. However, in 1989, Brecher and Taswell [55] indicated that the use of saline-washed RBCs is unnecessary and that patients with PNH should be transfused with group-specific blood and blood products from the experience in 23 PNH patients who had been transfused with 556 blood components, including 431 RBC products. At present, when PNH patients are transfused, physicians in most hospitals in Japan use packed RBC products supplied by the Japan Red Cross, but not saline-washed RBC products, because almost white blood cells (WBCs) and plasma of the blood donor are eliminated from the packed products. Naturally, it is allowed to use washed RBC products when PNH patients with higher proportions of PNH-type erythrocytes are transfused.

15.2.3.2 Iron Chelation Therapy for Hemosiderosis Associated with RBC Transfusions

Bird et al. [56] proposed the disorders of bone marrow failure syndromes, including myelodysplastic syndromes (MDS), primary myelofibrosis, MDS/myeloproliferative neoplasm, AA, pure red cell aplasia, and allogeneic stem cell transplant, which may develop hemosiderosis predominantly in the liver, heart, and endocrine in association with RBC transfusions. Although PNH patients develop iron deficiency anemia rather than hemosiderosis in most cases because of the increase of erythropoiesis associated with C-mediated hemolysis, there is some possibility that PNH patients with hypoplastic bone marrow, myelodysplasia or myelofibrosis may occasionally have it as a result of frequent RBC transfusions. To avoid adverse effects by hemosiderosis, iron chelation therapy should be considered and administered in these patients [57].

15.2.4 Therapy for Complications of PNH

15.2.4.1 Iron Deficiency Anemia

PNH patients often develop iron deficiency anemia due to loss of iron by hemoglobinuria and hemosiderinuria. If PNH patients have iron deficiency anemia with subjective symptoms, such as general malaise, vertigo, and palpitation, and Hb concentration of below 7 g/dL, oral administration of iron may be initiated. However, iron replenishment in most cases results in exacerbations of hemolysis probably due to the delivery to the circulation of C-sensitive erythrocytes which derive from the burst of erythropoiesis that follows iron administration [27, 29, 58]. Therefore, iron replenishment should be discontinued as soon as subjective symptoms from anemia disappear despite Hb concentration. If PNH patients with severe iron deficiency anemia wish to securely and sufficiently raise Hb concentration, they should receive RBC transfusions because they suppress the burst of erythropoiesis of C-sensitive erythrocytes.

15.2.4.2 Renal Dysfunction

Chronic kidney disease (CKD) in PNH patients is caused by some factors, such as hemosiderin deposition predominantly in the proximal tubules, diffuse vascular damage and microthrombosis indicated by autopsy findings of infarction, papillary necrosis, and interstitial scarring, and tubulointerstitial inflammation, associated with chronic exposure to free Hb and decrease of NO due to it [59, 60]. In addition, it is well known that total NO production is decreased in renal disease due to impaired endothelial and renal NO production [61]. Hillmen et al. [62] reported that prior to eculizumab treatment, 64 % of PNH patients had evidence of CKD assessed by the criteria of the National Kidney Foundation [63]. Subsequently, they demonstrated that following 36 months of treatment with eculizumab, 93.1 % of PNH patients showed either an improvement or stabilization in CKD [21]. It is generally known that patients with G3b of the CKD stage, who have below 45 mL/minute/1.73 m^2 of glomerular filtration rate, increase overall death, death by cardiovascular disorders, progress to end-stage kidney injury, and rate developing acute kidney injury [64], suggesting that eculizumab therapy for PNH patients should be initiated before they develop CKD of stage G3b. PNH patients, who have CKD with no effects of eculizumab treatment on renal injury and impairment of renal function or develop CKD of stages G3b to G5 and acute kidney injury, should be treated for various complications triggered by them with conventional and medicine therapies and hemodialysis [65]. Nishimura et al. [7] reported that CKD accounts for 8–18 % of disease-related mortality. Anemia derived from kidney disorders at the stage of G4 of the CKD stage classification is found in half of CKD patients [66].

15.2.5 HSCT

It is well known that HSCT is curative therapy for PNH [10]. In fact, if HSCT is successful, the transplanted patients have little relapse of PNH [67]. Allogeneic HSCT with myeloablative conditioning had curative, high rates (almost >20 %) of graft failure and modest overall survival (almost <60 % at 2 years). In spite of curative effect of it, the number of PNH patients, who actually underwent HSCT and were reported in the world, is much less [67–77] (Table 15.2), because long-term survival rate in patients with PNH is better than that in patients with malignant hematopoietic disorders, and there is the risk of death through HSCT, although the feasibility of non-myeloablative HSCT for PNH with a reduced intensity conditioning has been demonstrated [75–77], as shown in Table 15.2. It has been reported that 50 % survival period of PNH patients in UK, France, Japan, and USA was 10.0, 14.6, 16.0, and 23.3 years, respectively [6, 7, 9, 19]. Therefore, most PNH patients are occasionally observed and then treated with supportive procedures, like transfusion and replacement fluid, and medication. The protocol for treatment of PNH according to each pathophysiology is proposed and almost approved by specialists of PNH in Japan (Fig. 15.2). Before launching of eculizumab, prednisolone, androgens, and warfarin have played the main roles in treatment of intravascular hemolysis, bone marrow failure, and thrombosis, respectively. However, the roles of these drugs and HSCT are changing because of a beneficial effect of eculizumab on reducing C-mediated hemolysis in PNH. It has been considered that HSCT for PNH is generally applied to patients with severe bone marrow failure, severe and repeated

Table 15.2 Reports of HSCT for PNH patients

Author	Patients	Conditioning	Donor	Survival
Antin et al. [66] (1985)	4	Cy/PCZ/ATG/(n = 2) or Bu/Cy/PCZ/ATG (n = 2)	HLA-identical sibling	4/4
Kolb et al. [67] (1989)	1	Bu/Cy	HLA-identical sibling	1/1
	1	None	Syngeneic twin	1/1
Kawahara et al. [68] (1992)	6	Cy (n = 4) or Bu/Cy (n = 2)	HLA-identical sibling	6/6 *
	2	None	Syngeneic twin	2/2 *
	1	TBI/Cy	Parent	0/1
Bemba et al. [69] (1999)	16	TBI/Cy (n = 9) or Bu/Cy (n = 6) or TBI/Cy (n = 1)	HLA-identical sibling	9/16
Saso et al. [65] (IBMTR) (1999)	48	Cy (n = 3) or Bu/Cy (n = 25) or TBI/Cy (n = 20)	HLA-identical sibling	27/48
	2	TBI/Cy/Bu or CY	Syngeneic twin	2/2
	1	Bu/Cy	Parent	0/1
	6	Bu/Cy (n = 4) or TBI/Cy (n = 2)	HLA-matched unrelated	1/6
Raiola et al. [70] (2000)	7	Bu/Cy	HLA-identical sibling	7/7
Woodard et al. [71] (2001)	3	TBI/ATG/Cy/Ara-C	HLA-matched unrelated	3/3
Lee JL et al. [72] (2003)	3	Bu/Flu/ATG	HLA-identical sibling	2/3
	2	Cy/ATG	l-locus-mismatched related	2/2
Hegenbart et al. [73] (2003)	2	Flu/TBI	HLA-identical sibling	4/7
	5		HLA-matched unrelated	
Srinivasan et al. [74] (2006)	12	Cy/Fly/(ATG)	HLA-identical sibling	11/12
			Parent	
			l-antigen-mismatched sibling	
Santarone et al. [75] (2010)	26	Bu/Cy (n = 15) or Flu/Thio/Melph (n = 3)	HLA-identical unrelated	15/26
		Cy (n = 1), Cy/Thio (n = 1), Cy/Fly (n = 2), or Cy/Flu/TBI (n = 5)	HLA-matched unrelated	
			Haploidentical mother	(0/1)
			l-antigen-mismatched sibling	(0/1)
			l-antigen-mismatched unrelated	(0/1)

Abbreviations: *Cy* cyclophosphamide, *PCZ* procarbazine, *Bu* busulfan, *TBI* total body irradiation, *Ara-C* cytarabine, *Flu* fludarabine, *Thio* thiotepa, *Melph* melphalan exacerbations of hemolysis, and severe and repeated thrombosis, who have the risk of death. In the eculizumab era, the indication of HSCT for PNH may be limited predominantly to patients with severe bone marrow failure [10]. In addition, it must be evaluated whether we should add eculizumab to a conditioning regimen of HSCT and how eculizumab should be used in the regimen [78].

References

1. Shichishima T, Noji H (2002) A new aspect of the molecular pathogenesis of paroxysmal nocturnal hemoglobinuria. Hematology 7:211–227
2. Rother RP, Bell L, Hillmen P et al (2005) The clinical sequelae of intravascular hemolysis and extracellular plasma hemoglobin-A novel mechanism of human disease. JAMA 293:1653–1662
3. Hill A, Rother RP, Wang X et al (2010) Effect of eculizumab on haemolysis-associated nitric oxide depletion, dyspnea, and measures of pulmonary hypertension in patients with paroxysmal nocturnal haemoglobinuria. Br J Haematol 149:414–425
4. Schaer DJ, Buehler PW, Alayash AI et al (2013) Hemolysis and free hemoglobin revisited: exploring hemoglobin and hemin scavengers as a novel class of therapeutic proteins. Blood 121:1276–1284
5. Hill A, Kelly RJ, Hillmen P (2013) Thrombosis in paroxysmal nocturnal hemoglobinuria. Blood 121:4985–4996
6. Socié G, Mary J-Y, de Gramont A et al (1996) Paroxysmal nocturnal hemoglobinuria: long-term follow-up and prognostic factors. Lancet 348:573–577
7. Nishimura J, Kanakura Y, Ware RE et al (2004) Clinical course and flow cytometric analysis of paroxysmal nocturnal hemoglobinuria in the United States and Japan. Medicine 83:193–207
8. Young NS, Maciejewski JP (2000) Genetic and environmental effects in paroxysmal nocturnal hemoglobinuria: this little PIG-A goes Why? Why? Why? J Clin Invest 106:637–641
9. Fujioka S, Asai T (1989) Prognostic features of paroxysmal nocturnal hemoglobinuria in Japan. Acta Haematol Jpn 52:1386–1394
10. Parker C, Omine M, Richards S et al (2005) Diagnosis and management of paroxysmal nocturnal hemoglobinuria. Blood 106:3699–3709
11. Hillmen P, Hall C, Marsh JCW et al (2004) Effect of eculizumab on hemolysis and transfusion requirements in patients with paroxysmal nocturnal hemoglobinuria. N Engl J Med 350:552–559
12. Shichishima T, Terasawa T, Hashimoto C et al (1991) Heterogeneous expression of decay accelerating factor and CD59/membrane attack complex inhibition factor on paroxysmal nocturnal haemoglobinuria (PNH) erythrocytes. Br J Haematol 78:545–550
13. Brodsky RA, Mukhina GL, Li S et al (2000) Improved detection and characterization of paroxysmal nocturnal hemoglobinuria using fluorescent aerolysin. Am J Clin Pathol 114:459–466
14. The PNH Working Group in Research Committee for the Idiopathic Hematopoietic Disorders by Ministry of Health, Labor, and Welfare, Japan (2014) Guidelines for the diagnostic criteria and management of PNH. http://zoketsushogaihan.com/download.html (In Japanese)
15. Shichishima T, Ikeda K, Takahashi N et al (2010) Low concentrations of serum haptoglobin has impact on understanding complex pathophysiology in patients with acquired bone marrow failure syndromes. Int J Hematol 91:602–610
16. Pu JJ, Mukhina G, Wang H et al (2011) Natural history of paroxysmal nocturnal hemoglobinuria clones in patients presenting as aplastic anemia. Eur J Haematol 87:37–45

17. DeZern AE, Dorr D, Brodsky RA (2012) Predictors of hemoglobin response to eculizumab therapy in paroxysmal nocturnal hemoglobinuria. Eur J Haematol 90:16–24
18. Nakakuma H, Nagakura S, Kawaguchi T et al (1994) Persistence of affected T lymphocytes in long-term clinical remission in paroxysmal nocturnal hemoglobinuria. Blood 84:3925–3928
19. Hillmen P, Lewis SM, Bessler M et al (1995) Natural history of paroxysmal nocturnal hemoglobinuria. N Engl J Med 333:1253–1258
20. Risitano AM, Notaro R, Marando L et al (2009) Complement fraction 3 binding on erythrocytes as additional mechanism of disease in paroxysmal nocturnal hemoglobinuria patients treated by eculizumab. Blood 113:4094–4100
21. Hillmen P, Muus P, Roth A et al (2013) Long-term safety and efficacy of sustained eculizumab treatment in patients with paroxysmal nocturnal haemoglobinuria. Br J Haematol 162:62–73
22. Hill A, Rother RP, Amold L et al (2010) Eculizumab prevents intravascular hemolysis in patients with paroxysmal nocturnal hemoglobinuria and unmasks low-level extravascular hemolysis occurring through C3 opsonization. Haematologica 95:567–573
23. Berzuini A, Montanelli F, Prati D (2010) Hemolytic anemia after eculizumab in paroxysmal nocturnal hemoglobinuria. N Engl J Med 363:993–994
24. Risitano AM, Notaro R, Luzzatto L et al (2010) Paroxysmal nocturnal hemoglobinuria-Hemolysis before and after eculizumab. N Engl J Med 363:2270–2272
25. Nishimura J, Yamamoto M, Hayashi S et al (2014) Genetic variants in C5 and poor response to eculizumab. N Engl J Med 370:632–639
26. Yokoyama H, Itoh T, Kawajiri A et al (2013) Efficacy of eculizumab for thrombosis resistant to anticoagulant therapy alone in a case of PNH. Jpn J Clin Hematol 54:575 (Abstract)
27. Rosse WF (1982) Treatment of paroxysmal nocturnal hemoglobinuria. Blood 60:20–23
28. Issaragrisil S, Piankijagum A, Tang-naitrisorana Y (1987) Corticosteroids therapy in paroxysmal nocturnal hemoglobinuria. Am J Hematol 25:77–83
29. Shichishima T, Saitoh Y, Noji H et al (1996) In vivo effect of various therapies on complement-sensitive erythrocytes in paroxysmal nocturnal hemoglobinuria. Int J Hematol 63:291–302
30. Muller-Eberhard U, Javid J, Liem HH et al (1968) Plasma concentrations of hemopexin, haptoglobin and heme in patients with various hemolytic diseases. Blood 32:871–885
31. Schaer D, Alayash AI (2010) Clearance and control mechanisms of hemoglobin from cradle to grave. Antioxid Redox Signal 12:181–184
32. Kanamori Y, Tanabe H, Shimono T et al (1989) The effects of administration of haptoglobin for hemolysis by extracorporeal circulation. Rinsho Kyobu Gaka 9:463–467
33. Yoshioka T, Sugimoto T, Ukai T et al (1985) Haptoglobin therapy for possible prevention of renal failure following thermal injury: a clinical study. J Trauma 25:281–287
34. Gando S, Tedo I (1994) The effects of massive transfusion and haptoglobin therapy on hemolysis in trauma patients. Surg Today 24:785–790
35. Horai T, Tanaka K, Takeda M (2006) Coronary artery bypass grafting under cardiopulmonary bypass in a patient with beta-thalassemia: report of a case. Surg Today 36:538–540
36. Ohga S, Higashi E, Nomura A et al (1995) Haptoglobin therapy for acute favism: a Japanese boy with glucose-6-phosphate dehydrogenase Guadalajara. Br J Haematol 89:421–423
37. Hattori K, Hirano T, Oshimi K (2000) Protease inhibitors and haptoglobin for treatment of renal failure in paroxysmal nocturnal hemoglobinuria. Am J Hematol 63:61–62
38. Lindorter MA, Pawluczkowycz AW, Peek EM et al (2010) A novel approach to preventing the hemolysis of paroxysmal nocturnal hemoglobinuria: both complement-mediated cytolysis and C3 deposition are blocked by a monoclonal antibody specific for the alternative pathway of complement. Blood 115:2283–2291
39. Fridkis-Harell M, Storek M, Mazsaroff I et al (2011) Design and development of TT30, a novel C3d-targeted C3/C5 convertase inhibitor for treatment of human complement alternative pathway-mediated diseases. Blood 118:4705–4713
40. Risitano AM, Notaro R, Pascariello C et al (2012) The complement receptor 2/factor H fusion protein TT30 protects paroxysmal nocturnal hemoglobinuria erythrocytes from complement-mediated hemolysis and C3 fragment opsonization. Blood 119:6307–6316

41. Schmidt CQ, Bai H, Lin Z et al (2013) Rational engineering of a minimized immune inhibitor with unique triple-targeting properties. J Immunol 190:5712–5721
42. Risitano AM, Ricklin D, Huang Y et al (2014) Peptide inhibitors of C3 activation as a novel strategy of complement inhibition for the treatment of paroxysmal nocturnal hemoglobinuria. Blood 123:2094–2101
43. Panquette RL, Yoshimura R, Veiseh C et al (1997) Clinical characteristics predict response to antithymocyte globulin in paroxysmal nocturnal haemoglobinuria. Br J Haematol 96:92–97
44. Tran MH, Fadeyi E, Sheinberg P et al (2006) Apparent hemolysis following intravenous antithymocyte globulin treatment in a patient with marrow failure and a paroxysmal nocturnal hemoglobinuria clone. Transfusion 46:1244–1247
45. Alashkar F, Dührsen U, Röth A (2016) Horse anti-thymocyte globulin (hATG) and eculizumab as concomitant therapeutic approach in an aplastic PNH patient: go or no-go? Eur J Haematol 97:403–405
46. Schubert J, Scholz C, Geissler RG et al (1997) G-CSF and cyclosporine induce an increase of normal cells in hypoplastic paroxysmal nocturnal hemoglobinuria. Ann Hematol 74:225–230
47. Stebler C, Tichelli A, Dazzi H et al (1990) High-dose recombinant human erythropoietin for treatment of anemia in myelodysplastic syndromes and paroxysmal nocturnal hemoglobinuria: a pilot study. Exp Hematol 18:1204–1208
48. Balleari E, Gatti AM, Mareni C et al (1996) Recombinant human erythropoietin for long-term treatment of anemia in paroxysmal nocturnal hemoglobinuria. Haematologica 81:143–147
49. McMullin MF, Hillmen P, Elder GE et al (1996) Serum erythropoietin levels in paroxysmal nocturnal haemoglobinuria: implications. Br J Haematol 92:815–817
50. Hill A, Richards SJ, Rother RP et al (2007) Erythropoietin treatment during complement inhibitor with eculizumab in a patient with paroxysmal nocturnal hemoglobinuria. Haematologica 92:e31–e33
51. Hall C, Richards S, Hillmen P (2003) Primary prophylaxis with warfarin prevents thrombosis in paroxysmal nocturnal hemoglobinuria (PNH). Blood 102:3587–3591
52. Hillmen P, Muus P, Duhrsen U et al (2007) Effect of the complement inhibitor eculizumab on thromboembolism in patients with paroxysmal nocturnal hemoglobinuria. Blood 110:4123–4128
53. Moyo VM, Mukhina GL, Garrett ES et al (2004) Natural history of paroxysmal nocturnal haemoglobinuria using modern diagnostic assays. Br J Haematol 126:133–138
54. Helley D, de Latour RP, Porcher R et al (2010) Evaluation of hemostasis and endothelial function in patients with paroxysmal nocturnal hemoglobinuria receiving eculizumab. Haematologica 95:574–584
55. Brecher ME, Taswell HF (1989) Paroxysmal nocturnal hemoglobinuria and the transfusion of washed red cells. a myth revisited. Transfusion 29:681–685
56. Bird RJ, Kenealy M, Forsyth J et al (2012) When should iron chelation therapy be considered in patients with myelodysplasia and other bone marrow failure syndromes with iron overload? Intern Med J 42:450–455
57. Butler A, Patton WN (2012) Iron chelation therapy in myelodysplastic syndromes: we need more evidence, not more guidelines. Intern Med J 42:481–484
58. Shichishima T, Yoshida M, Yokoyama A et al (1989) Erythropoiesis of complement-sensitive cells in a PNH patient with iron deficiency anemia during iron therapy. Eur J Haematol 42:310–311
59. Clark DA, Butler SA, Braren V et al (1981) The kidneys in paroxysmal nocturnal hemoglobinuria. Blood 57:83–89
60. Nath KA, Vercellotti GM, Grande JP et al (2001) Heme-protein-induced chronic renal inflammation:suppressive effect of induced heme oxygenase-1. Kidney Int 59:106–117
61. Baylis C (2008) Nitric oxide deficiency in chronic kidney disease. Am J Physiol Renal Physiol 294:F1–F9

62. Hillmen P, Elebute M, Kelly R et al (2010) Long-term effect of the complement inhibitor eculizumab on kidney function in patients with paroxysmal nocturnal hemoglobinuria. Am J Hematol 85:553–559
63. Levin AL, Stevens PE, Bilous RW et al (2013) KDIGO 2012 clinical practice guideline for the evaluation and management of chronic kidney disease. Kidney Int Suppl 3:1–150
64. Drey N, Roderick P, Mullee M et al (2003) A population-based study of the incidence and outcomes of diagnosed chronic kidney disease. Am J Kidney Dis 42:677–684
65. Hussain S, Qureshi A, Kazi J (2013) Renal involvement in paroxysmal nocturnal hemoglobinuria. Nephron Clin Pract 123:28–35
66. Keith DS, Nichols GA, Gullion CM et al (2004) Longitudinal follow-up and outcomes among a population with chronic kidney disease in a large managed care organization. Arch Intern Med 164:659–663
67. Saso R, Marsh J, Cevreska L et al (1999) Bone marrow transplants for paroxysmal nocturnal haemoglobinuria. Br J Haematol 104:392–396
68. Antin JH, Ginsburg D, Smith BR et al (1985) Bone marrow transplantation for paroxysmal nocturnal hemoglobinuria: eradication of the PNH clone and documentation of complete lymphohematopoietic engraftment. Blood 66:1247–1250
69. Kolb HJ, Holler E, Bender-Götze C et al (1989) Myeloablative conditioning for marrow transplantation in myelodysplastic syndromes and paroxysmal nocturnal haemoglobinuria. Bone Marrow Tlansplant 4:29–34
70. Kawahara K, Witherspoon RP, Storb R (1992) Marrow transplantation for paroxysmal nocturnal hemoglobinuria. Am J Hematol 39:283–288
71. Bemba M, Guardiola P, Garderet L et al (1999) Bone marrow transplantation for paroxysmal nocturnal haemoglobinuria. Br J Haematol 105:366–368
72. Raiola AM, Lint MTV, Lamparelli T et al (2000) Bone marrow transplantation for paroxysmal nocturnal hemoglobinuria. Haematologica 85:59–62
73. Woodard P, Wang W, Pitts N et al (2001) Successful unrelated donor bone marrow transplantation for paroxysmal nocturnal hemoglobinuria. Bone Marrow Transplant 27:589–592
74. Lee J-L, Lee J-H, Lee J-H et al (2003) Allogeneic hematopoietic cell transplantation for paroxysmal nocturnal hemoglobinuria. Eur J Haematol 71:114–118
75. Hegenbart U, Niederwieser D, Forman S et al (2003) Hematopoietic cell transplantation from related and unrelated donors after minimal conditioning as a curative treatment modality for severe paroxysmal nocturnal hemoglobinuria. Biol Blood Marrow Transplant 9:689–697
76. Srinivasan R, Takahashi Y, McCoy JP et al (2006) Overcoming graft rejection in heavily transfused and allo-immunised patients with bone marrow failure syndromes using fludarabine-based haematopoietic cell transplantation. Br J Haematol 133:305–314
77. Santarone S, Bacigalupo A, Risitano AM et al (2010) Hematopoietic stem cell transplantation for paroxysmal nocturnal hemoglobinuria: long-term results of a retrospective study on behalf of the Gruppo Italiano Trapianto Midollo Osseo (GITMO). Haematologica 95:983–988
78. Taniguchi K, Okada M, Yoshihara S et al (2011) Strategy for bone marrow transplantation in eculizumab-treated paroxysmal nocturnal hemoglobinuria. Int J Hematol 94:403–407

Chapter 16
Clinical Effects of Eculizumab in PNH

Jeffrey Szer

Abstract Eculizumab is a humanized monoclonal antibody which binds with high affinity to the fifth component of complement preventing its cleavage into C5a and C5b. Given that the clinical manifestations of paroxysmal nocturnal haemoglobinuria (PNH) are based on the activity of C5b-9, (the membrane attack complex) on unprotected PNH erythrocytes, eculizumab was tested as a therapeutic in this disease in four clinical trials beginning in 2002, including a placebo-controlled double-blind study, and was found to have efficacy in reducing markers of intravascular haemolysis, improving haemoglobin levels and reducing transfusion requirements as well as improving renal impairment, decreasing the rate and risk of thromboembolic phenomena and improving many measurable quality of life parameters. Additionally, studies undertaken following the completion of the trials suggest an improvement in overall survival such that patients treated with eculizumab for up to 8 years appear to have survival very similar to an age- and sex-matched population. This well-tolerated therapy has maintained all of the clinical benefits seen in the clinical trials over long-term use.

Keywords Eculizumab • Complement • PNH

16.1 Introduction

Eculizumab is a largely humanized monoclonal antibody directed against an epitope of the fifth component of complement (C5). It binds with extreme avidity and specificity and does so irreversibly, resulting in the prevention of cleavage of the molecule to produce C5a and the active C5b-9. The initial studies with this agent as a therapeutic were directed at inflammatory diseases felt to be complement dependent such as rheumatoid arthritis and nephritis [1, 2], but given the understanding of the pathophysiology of the disease paroxysmal nocturnal haemoglobinuria (PNH),

J. Szer (✉)
Department of Clinical Haematology & BMT Service, The Royal Melbourne Hospital, 300 Grattan Street, 3050 Parkville, VIC, Australia
e-mail: jeff.szer@mh.org.au

Y. Kanakura et al. (eds.), *Paroxysmal Nocturnal Hemoglobinuria*,
DOI 10.1007/978-4-431-56003-6_16

this was felt to be an appropriate target for complement blockade. Available data suggested that most if not all of the manifestations of PNH were due to unimpeded activity of complement on red blood cells.

16.2 Clinical Trials

The clinical efficacy of eculizumab in PNH was defined by the results of four clinical trials as well as a considerable amount of posttrial experience and, more recently, output from the PNH Registry.

16.2.1 Pilot Study

A phase 2 open-label study conducted in 11 patients with clearly haemolytic (classical) PNH requiring red cell transfusion support was undertaken in Leeds, UK, from May to December 2002 [3]. The effects noticed in this population of patients were sufficiently positive to move straight to a placebo-controlled randomized study. All 11 adult patients were treated with the now-standard regimen of eculizumab, 600 mg by intravenous infusion weekly for 4 weeks followed by a 900 mg dose 1 week later and then every second week. The study period was 12 weeks (a total of eight infusions) during which time pharmacokinetic and pharmacodynamics data were collected as well as parameters of haemolysis and quality of life.

All patients completed the study during which time there were no deaths or thromboembolic episodes. All patients showed evidence of haemolysis inhibition after the first dose of eculizumab as evidenced by decreases in the serum concentration of lactate dehydrogenase.

One patient in this study showed recurrence of haemolysis before the next dose was due based on a drop in serum levels of eculizumab and rise in lactate dehydrogenase on the day the next dose was due. This was the first patient where a suboptimal response was restored by decreasing the dosing interval to 12 days.

The major conclusion of this study was to confirm the importance of complement activation as the mechanism of haemolysis in PNH.

16.2.2 TRIUMPH Study

This was a placebo-controlled, 26-week, randomized study of eculizumab in patients with haemolytic PNH conducted in many centres in nine countries around the world [4]. The patient population was 89 patients who had been treated with at least four episodes of red cell transfusion in the previous 12 months, and patients with significant marrow failure as evidence by a platelet count of less than 100×10^9/L were excluded. These criteria resulted in 89 patients being randomized of 115 patients who were formally screened for the study. Criteria for inclusion which were subsequently adopted by a number of regulatory agencies to define a suitable patient population for treatment with eculizumab included the transfusion threshold, a PNH erythrocyte clone proportion of at least 10 % and a lactate dehydrogenase concentration of at least 1.5 multiples of the upper limit of the normal range. There was an observation period of 2 weeks followed by the treatment regimen of 600 mg weekly followed 1 week later by the first of 11 doses of 900 mg of eculizumab or placebo.

The findings of the pilot study were confirmed and reinforced with additional understanding of the effect of treatment on transfusion dependence, haemoglobin levels, thrombosis and quality of life issues particularly fatigue as well as an understanding of the sustainability of effect.

16.2.3 SHEPHERD Study

The previous studies were restricted to patients with haemolytic PNH, without significant marrow failure and with a significant transfusion requirement. The SHEPHERD study [5] was a more real-world, open-label treatment trial in 97 patients with PNH defined by a clone size of more than 10 % and an elevated lactate dehydrogenase, but a platelet count as low as 30×10^9/L and a neutrophil count of at least 0.5×10^9/L were acceptable, and only a single erythrocyte transfusion was required in the previous 24 months prior to study entry. This study had a treatment duration of 52 weeks.

The major conclusions of this study was that patients with these more liberal treatment criteria (69 of the 97 would not have been eligible for TRIUMPH study) responded as well as those in previous studies similar to those with a heavy transfusion requirement and did so independent of the platelet count: patients with platelet counts of less than 65×10^9/L derived similar benefits from eculizumab treatment as those with higher counts. Thus, it was concluded that eculizumab treatment was appropriate for a broad population of patients with PNH.

16.2.4 AEGIS Study

This was a confirmatory, open-label study for 12 weeks, undertaken in Japan in which 29 patients with PNH with eligibility criteria approximately those of the SHEPHERD study were treated with the previously described regimen undertaken for registration purposes in Japan [6]. The results were consistent with those seen in the SHEPHERD study; however, it was notable that unlike the observations in previous trials, two patients in the AEGIS study showed no clinical response to eculizumab despite serum levels suggesting that complement should have been fully blocked. This was subsequently shown to be due to a complement mutation preventing the binding of eculizumab and so far only identified in the Japanese population [7].

16.2.5 Long-Term Extension Study

Patients in the pilot, TRIUMPH and SHEPHERD, studies (a total of 195 patients) were eligible to transition to the long-term extension study where treatment with eculizumab was continued in those patients on active therapy on trials or transitioned to active therapy for the placebo-treated patients in TRIUMPH [8].

16.3 Haemolysis

The importance of lactate dehydrogenase (LD) levels as a biomarker of haemolysis was demonstrated most clearly in the TRIUMPH study which mirrored each of the other trials in results but, because of the presence of a placebo-treated control group, confirmed the effectiveness of eculizumab in reducing haemolysis. Figure 16.1 clearly shows the dramatic drop in LD within 1 week of the first 600 mg dose of eculizumab. The median LD level at baseline was 2199 IU/L with a drop to

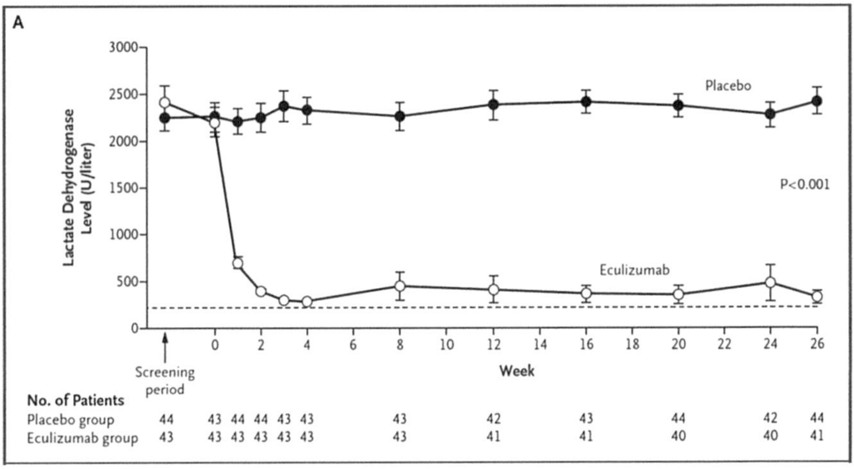

Fig. 16.1 This graph shows the degree of intravascular haemolysis according to the mean levels of lactate dehydrogenase (LD) from baseline to week 26 in the two patient groups of the TRIUMPH trial. The dashed line indicates the upper limit of the normal range for LD. In the eculizumab group, the mean level of LD was reduced to just above the upper limit of the normal range at week 26; of 41 patients in this group who completed the study, 15 had levels within the normal range. In the placebo group, all patients had levels at least five times above the upper limit of normal at week 26 (From Ref. [4])

approximately one quarter of that 1 week later and a stable median level just above the upper limit of normal at week 4 which was maintained to week 26 when the level was 327 IU/L. The South Korean group has additionally confirmed the importance of an LD level of at least 1.5 multiples of the upper limit of normal as a prognostic marker in PNH [9]. Long-term follow-up studies have demonstrated maintenance of this control of intravascular haemolysis to 5 or more years [9, 10].

While the total population of patients demonstrates stability of control, individual patients do demonstrate transient periods of heightened haemolytic activity as evidence by LD elevation. These episodes may be precipitated by other processes, most notably infection [11], surgical procedures [12] and pregnancy [13], and may require dose increases or reduction in interval of dosing during these periods. There is no reason to discontinue eculizumab during such episodes, and any such discontinuation runs the risk of precipitating massive haemolysis although few episodes of such occurrences have been documented.

An alternative measure of haemolysis is used in pharmacodynamics assays in which serum with known concentrations of eculizumab after intravenous administration is used in in vitro assays of haemolysis with a break point of 20 % haemolysis considered significant. Studies were undertaken in each of the clinical trials where a trough concentration of eculizumab of less than 35 μg/ml resulted in excessive in vitro haemolysis in a majority of cases. Of the 195 patients in the extension study, 49 patients (of 145 patients with samples available) demonstrated levels <35 μg/ml.

16.4 Transfusions and Anaemia

In each of the clinical trials, transfusion requirements were found to decrease among patients treated with eculizumab. During the 26 weeks of the randomized TRIUMPH study [4], the median number of red cell units transfused was 10 in the placebo group and 0 in the active treatment group. The mean units transfused were 11 and 3, respectively. Figure 16.2 shows that the effect on transfusion requirements continued to improve over 36 months of follow-up. The proportion of patients completely independent of transfusion requirements in the prior 6 months decreased from over 90 % at baseline to under 40 % at 6–12 months of treatment to under 20 % at 30–36 months. It was perhaps not surprising that the patients with the highest baseline transfusion requirements were less likely to achieve complete transfusion independence than those with lower requirements. Many patients in the SHEPHERD study had no transfusion requirement despite significant haemolysis as measured by LD elevation. Accordingly, while transfusion reduction is an important end point in treatment of PNH, it is not seen universally across a real-world population of PNH patients.

A significant proportion of patients with PNH is anaemic due to intravascular haemolysis and various degrees of marrow aplasia [14]. In the long-term study [9], treatment with eculizumab resulted in a steady increase in the haemoglobin

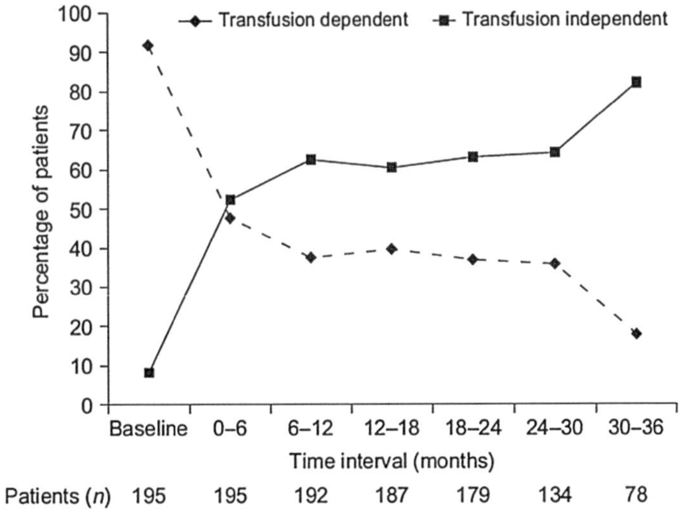

Fig. 16.2 Percentage of transfusion-independent and transfusion-dependent patients over time. Transfusion-independent patients were those who did not require a blood transfusion during the previous 6 months; transfusion-dependent patients had received at least one blood transfusion in the previous 6 months (From Ref. [8])

concentration from 93.7 g/l at baseline to 99.2 g/l after 2 weeks of treatment to 104.7 g/l by 24 months. This response was maintained after 36 months of observation. An early study showed that the addition of exogenous erythropoietic agents [15] improved haemoglobin levels and reduced transfusion rates in some patients. Such treatment has not become standard in patients with PNH but may be considered in patients with significant aplastic anaemia [16].

16.5 Thrombosis

Thrombosis is arguably the most serious complication of PNH and is the major cause of deaths of patients with this disease. Perhaps the most significant finding of the clinical trials with eculizumab was the extremely low rate of thromboembolic phenomena after treatment was initiated. There is a direct correlation between intravascular haemolysis and thrombosis in PNH, but the association is much more complicated than that as a heightened thrombosis risk is the result of interactions between the coagulation cascade, complement, PNH erythrocytes and platelets and the products of intravascular haemolysis. This has been thoroughly reviewed by Hill [17].

The use of primary prophylactic anticoagulation has been common in patients with PNH [18]. It has been variably applied to patients who are otherwise asymptomatic who have larger PNH clone populations. The clinical trials of eculizumab had in common the requirement that no change in prophylactic anticoagulation was to occur during the period of study. Thus, patients already on anticoagulants were to continue at their usual doses, while those not already receiving such therapy were prohibited from commencing it during the study period.

During the 26 weeks of the TRIUMPH study, a single thrombotic event occurred in a patient on the placebo arm of the trial. Approximately 20 % of the patients in this study had a prior history of thrombosis, and 25 % of the actively treated patients and 49 % of the placebo-treated patients were on anticoagulation during the trial. In the SHEPHERD study, two patients had thrombotic events. Both had a prior history of thrombosis, one occurred a month following early cessation of eculizumab and the other about 6 months into study period.

Detailed understanding of the effect of eculizumab on thrombotic risk came from the analysis of the extension study. Of the 195 patients, 63 had a prior history of thromboembolic events. In the period after active treatment was commenced, seven patients (five of whom had had pretreatment thrombosis and four were on anticoagulants) experienced ten episodes of thromboembolism, three in one patient. These events were observed 170–876 days after commencing eculizumab. The analysis based on time at risk of developing thrombosis both before and after commencing eculizumab showed that the institution of therapy decreased the rate of thrombosis from 11 events per 100 patient-years to 2 events per 100 patient-years.

The role of anticoagulants was also examined in this analysis. Patients were either treated with anticoagulants prior to therapy (11 patients) or both before and during therapy (84 patients), and three patients were commenced on therapeutic anticoagulants after developing a thrombosis on eculizumab therapy.

These data do not provide any evidence from which to recommend or not recommend cessation of anticoagulants after the commencement of eculizumab. It was noted that 11 patients ceased anticoagulants after commencing eculizumab, none of whom had developed a thrombosis after stopping anticoagulation. Also reported in this paper was the case of a patient who developed an ultimately fatal small bowel thrombosis 19 days after ceasing eculizumab on physician advice [19].

Eculizumab clearly reduces the risk of thromboembolic phenomena in patients with PNH. Patients who are commenced on eculizumab therapy prior to a thromboembolic event are unlikely to commence or benefit from primary thromboprophylaxis. It is less clear what should happen to patients with a prior thromboembolic event prior to commencing eculizumab therapy as well as patients stable on eculizumab who develop a potentially high thrombogenic condition such as pregnancy [13].

16.6 Quality of Life

Patients with haemolytic PNH frequently described "feeling better" soon after commencing eculizumab treatment. Objective evidence for such improvement came from the detailed quality of life assessments undertaken as primary analysis end points in the clinical trials. The major symptom experienced by these patients was fatigue, and the validated FACIT-Fatigue instrument [20] has proven to be a reliable measure of the effect of treatment. Overall quality of life was additionally assessed using the EORTC QLQ-C30 tool [21]. In the TRIUMPH study paper [4], patients treated with eculizumab had a clinically significant improvement in fatigue score of 6.4 points (4 is considered significant) by week 26, while the placebo patients deteriorated by 4.0 points. The deterioration in fatigue scores in the placebo group is attributable to frequent visits and rigorous investigations, further demonstrating the significance of the positive effect of active inhibition of complement activation on these patients. The global health scores were significantly improved in the eculizumab-treated patients as well as all five functioning scales, two of three symptom scores (fatigue and pain but not nausea and vomiting) and for three of six single-item measures (diarrhoea, anorexia and insomnia). The single-item measures that were not significantly improved were financial difficulties, constipation and diarrhoea. The same fatigue and quality of life instruments were used in the Japanese AEGIS study in which it was again demonstrated that there were significant improvements in quality of life and fatigue measures comparing pretreatment values with those after 12 weeks of treatment [6]. A Cochrane review of outcomes in patients treated for PNH suggested that future studies of quality of life issues in this patient group should be undertaken using recommendations made by the Foundation of Patient-Centered Outcomes Research [22].

Research tools built into the global PNH Registry are likely to provide robust quality of life data on these patients over an extended period of observation.

16.7 Smooth Muscle Dystonia

These symptoms in PNH are directly related to intravascular haemolysis and nitric oxide depletion by plasma-free haemoglobin and include abdominal pain, dysphagia and erectile dysfunction in males. They are observed in 25–35 % of patients. There are a number of case reports that attest to the impressive reversal of these symptoms in a majority of patients after intravascular haemolysis has been blocked by eculizumab therapy [23, 24].

16.8 Renal Function

Abnormalities of renal function affect a significant proportion of patients with PNH, and outcomes were closely monitored during the clinical trials. In the AEGIS study of 29 Japanese patients [10], 19 patients had evidence of chronic renal disease at baseline, and 12 of them had improvement in renal function, while one patient deteriorated. In addition, significantly more patients improved their stage of chronic renal failure than deteriorated, while 55 % had no change in stage. Patients with earlier stages of chronic renal disease were more likely to improve than those with higher stages, but numbers in this study were relatively small. In the extension study [8], renal function was formally assessed at a 6-month interval and was specifically addressed in a publication by Hillmen et al. [25]. Renal dysfunction or damage was observed in 65 % of the study population at baseline with 21 % of patients with later stage (stages 3–5) chronic renal disease or kidney failure. It was concluded that eculizumab treatment was safe and well tolerated in patients with renal dysfunction and resulted in statistically significant and clinically meaningful improvement (reduction) of chronic renal disease stage compared to baseline and to placebo. To confirm the AEGIS results, improvement in renal function was more commonly seen in patients with baseline chronic renal disease stages 1–2 where there was a 67.1 % improvement, although improvement was also seen in patients with stages 3–4 chronic renal disease. Improvements occurred quickly and were sustained. Forty (40) of 195 patients normalized renal function from an abnormal level after 18 months of treatment.

16.9 Pulmonary Hypertension

This less commonly considered complication of PNH has been reviewed and is known to contribute to the fatigue and dyspnoea experienced by patients with PNH, independent of anaemia [26, 27]. The mechanism of this complication, described as occurring in up to 36 % of patients with PNH and haemolysis when screened with Doppler echocardiography and levels of pro-brain natriuretic peptide (proBNP), is directly related to intravascular haemolysis and nitric oxide consumption with a contribution by definable pulmonary emboli. Seventy-three patients in the TRIUMPH study were closely evaluated for pulmonary hypertension. Almost half (47 %) of the patients had elevated levels of proBNP at baseline, and eculizumab treatment resulted in a 50 % reduction in the proportion of patients with elevated proBNP by week 26. Intriguingly, these changes began rapidly and were seen as early as to weeks after treatment commenced. These changes in proBNP were also statistically correlated with improvements in dyspnoea scores [27].

16.10 Survival

None of the clinical trials undertaken examined survival as an end point. Previous studies have shown a mortality of up to 35 % at 5 years of observation in patients with PNH [28]. During the conduct of the extension study of 195 patients, four died while on therapy with eculizumab [8]: three of these deaths were unrelated to therapy or PNH (chronic myelomonocytic leukaemia in a patient with known myelodysplastic syndrome, metastatic gastric cancer and a postsurgical cerebral event). The fourth patients died of a thrombotic complication of the small intestine after eculizumab was withdrawn by the physician as described previously.

In an ultrarare disease such as PNH, population-based studies are likely to give the best indication of impact on survival of any therapeutic intervention. From a post hoc analysis of trial data, the Cochrane analysis referred to above was unable to identify any evidence of impact of eculizumab treatment on the survival of patients with PNH [22]. A French study [29] suggested an improvement in survival of treated patients compared to historical series of patients who were untreated although untreated patients in the more recent eras had improved survival compared with those of more distant times.

Kelly conducted a case-matched controlled study of the survival of patients with PNH treated with eculizumab in the UK compared to the reported population data [30]. In this study of 79 patients followed for up to 8 years (mean 3.3 years), survival of patients with PNH treated with eculizumab was similar to the control population, very different to the natural history data previously described in this population in which survival of patients with PNH was considerably worse than the normal age- and sex-matched population [28]. The effect on survival was more obvious in patients 70 years of age or less than those more than 70 years.

16.11 Conclusion

The introduction of eculizumab into the management of patients with haemolytic PNH has resulted in demonstrated benefits in outcome with improvements in degree of anaemia, transfusion requirements, rates of thrombosis, chronic renal disease, pulmonary hypertension and symptoms of muscle dystonia. No evidence has presented to suggest that eculizumab has any benefit of underlying marrow failure or myelodysplastic syndromes which require treatment on their own merits.

The real-life clinical impact of eculizumab on patients with PNH will become clearer as data from the international PNH Registry become more complete and are appropriately analysed and published.

References

1. Tesser JKA, Fleischmann R, Mojcik C, Bombara M, Burch F (2001) Safety and efficacy of the humanized anti-C5 antibody h5G1.1 in patients with rheumatoid arthritis. Arthritis Rheum 44:S274
2. Kaplan M (2002) Eculizumab (Alexion). Curr Opin Investig Drugs 3:1017–1023
3. Hillmen P, Hall C, Marsh JC, Elebute M, Bombara MP, Petro BE, Cullen MJ, Richards SJ, Rollins SA, Mojcik CF, Rother RP (2004) Effect of eculizumab on hemolysis and transfusion requirements in patients with paroxysmal nocturnal hemoglobinuria. N Engl J Med 350:552–559
4. Hillmen P, Young NS, Schubert J, Brodsky RA, Socié G, Muus P, Röth A, Szer J, Elebute MO, Nakamura R, Browne P, Risitano AM, Hill A, Schrezenmeier H, Fu CL, Maciejewski J, Rollins SA, Mojcik CF, Rother RP, Luzzatto L (2006) The complement inhibitor eculizumab in paroxysmal nocturnal hemoglobinuria. N Engl J Med 355:1233–1243

5. Brodsky RA, Young NS, Antonioli E, Risitano AM, Schrezenmeier H, Schubert J, Gaya A, Coyle L, de Castro C, Fu CL, Maciejewski JP, Bessler M, Kroon HA, Rother RP, Hillmen P (2008) Multicenter phase 3 study of the complement inhibitor eculizumab for the treatment of patients with paroxysmal nocturnal hemoglobinuria. Blood 111:1840–1847
6. Kanakura Y, Ohyashiki K, Shichishima T, Okamoto S, Ando K, Ninomiya H, Kawaguchi T, Nakao S, Nakakuma H, Nishimura J, Kinoshita T, Bedrosian CL, Valentine ME, Khursigara G, Ozawa K, Omine M (2011) Safety and efficacy of the terminal complement inhibitor eculizumab in Japanese patients with paroxysmal nocturnal hemoglobinuria: the AEGIS clinical trial. Int J Hematol 93:36–46
7. Nishimura J, Yamamoto M, Hayashi S, Ohyashiki K, Ando K, Brodsky AL, Noji H, Kitamura K, Eto T, Takahashi T, Masuko M, Matsumoto T, Wano Y, Shichishima T, Shibayama H, Hase M, Li L, Johnson K, Lazarowski A, Tamburini P, Inazawa J, Kinoshita T, Kanakura Y (2014) Genetic variants in C5 and poor response to eculizumab. N Engl J Med 370:632–639
8. Hillmen P, Muus P, Röth A, Elebute MO, Risitano AM, Schrezenmeier H, Szer J, Browne P, Maciejewski JP, Schubert J, Urbano-Ispizua A, de Castro C, Socié G, Brodsky RA (2013) Long-term safety and efficacy of sustained eculizumab treatment in patients with paroxysmal nocturnal haemoglobinuria. Br J Haematol 162:62–73
9. Lee JW, Jang JH, Kim JS, Yoon SS, Lee JH, Kim YK, Jo DY, Chung J, Sohn SK (2013) Clinical signs and symptoms associated with increased risk for thrombosis in patients with paroxysmal nocturnal hemoglobinuria from a Korean Registry. Int J Hematol 97:749–757
10. Kanakura Y, Ohyashiki K, Shichishima T, Okamoto S, Ando KH, Kawaguchi T, Nakao S, Nakakuma H, Nishimura J, Kinoshita T, Bedrosian CL, Ozawa K, Omine M (2013) Long-term efficacy and safety of eculizumab in Japanese patients with PNH: AEGIS trial. Int J Hematol 98:406–416
11. Ueda T, Hayakawa J, Yamanishi M, Maeda M, Fukunaga Y (2013) Efficacy of eculizumab in a patient with paroxysmal nocturnal hemoglobinuria requiring transfusions 14 years after a diagnosis in childhood. J Nippon Med Sch 80:155–159
12. Kurita N, Obara N, Fukuda K, Nishikii H, Sato S, Inagawa S, Kurokawa T, Owada Y, Ninomiya H, Chiba S (2013) Perisurgical induction of eculizumab in a patient with paroxysmal nocturnal hemoglobinuria: its inhibition of surgery-triggered hemolysis and the consequence of subsequent discontinuation. Blood Coagul Fibrinolysis 24:658–662
13. Kelly RJ, Höchsmann B, Szer J, Kulasekararaj A, de Guibert S, Röth A, Weitz IC, Armstrong E, Risitano AM, Patriquin CJ, Terriou L, Muus P, Hill A, Turner MP, Schrezenmeier H, Peffault de Latour R (2015) Eculizumab in pregnant patients with paroxysmal nocturnal hemoglobinuria. N Engl J Med 373:1032–1039
14. Parker C (2009) Eculizumab for paroxysmal nocturnal haemoglobinuria. Lancet 373:759–767
15. Hill A, Richards SJ, Rother RP, Hillmen P (2007) Erythopoietin treatment during complement inhibition with eculizumab in a patient with paroxysmal nocturnal hemoglobinuria. Haematologica 92:e31–e33
16. Gurion R, Gafter-Gvili A, Paul M, Vidal L, Ben-Bassat I, Yeshurun M, Shpilberg O, Raanani P (2009) Hematopoietic growth factors in aplastic anemia patients treated with immunosuppressive therapy-systematic review and meta-analysis. Haematologica 94:712–719
17. Hill A, Kelly RJ, Hillmen P (2013) Thrombosis in paroxysmal nocturnal hemoglobinuria. Blood 121:4985–4996
18. Hall C, Richards S, Hillmen P (2003) Primary prophylaxis with warfarin prevents thrombosis in paroxysmal nocturnal haemoglobinuria. Blood 102:3587–3591
19. van Bijnen ST, van Rijn RS, Koljenovic S, Te Boekhorst P, Muus P (2012) Possible high risk of thrombotic events in patients with paroxysmal nocturnal haemoglobinuria after discontinuation of eculizumab. Br J Haematol 157:762–763
20. Cella D (1997) Manual of the functional assessment of chronic illness therapy (FACIT) measurement system. Version 4. Center on Outcomes Research and Education (CORE), Evanston Northwestern Healthcare and Northwestern University, Evanston

21. Fayers PM, Aaronson NK, Bjordal K, Groenvold M, Curran D, on behalf of the EORTC Quality of Life Study Group (2001) The EORTC QLQ-C30 scoring manual, 3rd edn. European Organisation for Research and Treatment of Cancer, Brussels
22. Martí-Carvajal AJ, Anand V, Cardona AF, Solà I (2014) Eculizumab for treating patients with paroxysmal nocturnal hemoglobinuria. Cochrane Database Syst Rev 10:CD010340
23. Hill A, Rother RP, Hillmen P (2005) Improvement in the symptoms of smooth muscle dystonia during eculizumab therapy in paroxysmal nocturnal hemoglobinuria. Haematologica 90:e111–e113
24. Grigg A, Brown M, Szer J (2010) Durable resolution of recurrent microvascular small bowel ischaemia and severe abdominal pain by eculizumab in paroxysmal nocturnal haemoglobinuria. Intern Med J 40:794–795
25. Hillmen P, Elebute M, Kelly R, Urbano-Ispizua A, Hill A, Rother RP, Khursigara G, Fu CL, Omine M, Browne P, Rosse W (2010) Long-term effect of the complement inhibitor eculizumab on kidney function in patients with paroxysmal nocturnal hemoglobinuria. Am J Hematol 85:553–559
26. Hill A, Sapsford RJ, Scally A, Kelly R, Richards SJ, Khurisgara G, Sivananthan MU, Hillmen P (2012) Under-recognised complications in patients with paroxysmal nocturnal haemoglobinuria: raised pulmonary pressure and reduced right ventricular function. Br J Haematol 158:409–414
27. Hill A, Rother RP, Wang X, Morris SM Jr, Quinn-Senger K, Kelly R, Richards SJ, Bessler M, Bell L, Hillmen P, Gladwin MT (2010) Effect of eculizumab on haemolysis-associated nitric oxide depletion, dyspnoea, and measures of pulmonary hypertension in patients with paroxysmal nocturnal haemoglobinuria. Br J Haematol 149:414–425
28. Hillmen P, Lewis SM, Bessler M, Luzzatto L, Dacie JV (1995) Natural history of paroxysmal nocturnal hemoglobinuria. N Engl J Med 333:1253–1258
29. Loschi M, Porcher R, Barraco F, Terriou L, Mohty M, de Guibert S, Mahe B, Lemal R, Dumas PY, Etienne G, Jardin F, Royer B, Bordessoule D, Rohrlich PS, Fornecker LM, Salanoubat C, Maury S, Cahn JY, Vincent L, Sene T, Rigaudeau S, Nguyen S, Lepretre AC, Mary JY, Corront B, Socie G, Peffault de Latour R (2016) Impact of eculizumab treatment on paroxysmal nocturnal hemoglobinuria: a treatment versus no-treatment study. Am J Hematol 91:366–370
30. Kelly RJ, Hill A, Arnold LM, Brooksbank GL, Richards SJ, Cullen M, Mitchell LD, Cohen DR, Gregory WM, Hillmen P (2011) Long-term treatment with eculizumab in paroxysmal nocturnal hemoglobinuria: sustained efficacy and improved survival. Blood 117:6786–6792

Chapter 17
Clinical Effects of Eculizumab in PNH: Extravascular Hemolysis After Eculizumab Treatment

Rosario Notaro and Antonio M. Risitano

Abstract The most important advance in the management of paroxysmal nocturnal hemoglobinuria (PNH) has been the introduction of eculizumab, a human monoclonal antibody against the C5 component of complement, that abrogates intravascular hemolysis by preventing the formation of the complement membrane attack complex. Complement blockade by eculizumab has proven to be clinically effective in hemolytic PNH, reducing the transfusion requirement in most of patients. However, in almost all PNH patients on eculizumab, a proportion of PNH red cells become coated with C3 and thus a potential target of phagocytosis by macrophages. This phagocytosis results in a variable degree of extravascular hemolysis that in some patients may limit the clinical benefit from eculizumab: in fact, at least one in four of transfusion-dependent PNH patients remain transfusion dependent even on eculizumab, and these patients may also have a high risk to develop iron overload. Unfortunately, there are not yet established treatments for the cases in which this extravascular hemolysis became clinically relevant: it is possible that new strategies for complement blockade could overcome this condition.

Keywords PNH • Eculizumab • Intravascular hemolysis • Extravascular hemolysis • C3 • C5

17.1 Introduction

Paroxysmal nocturnal hemoglobinuria (PNH) is characterized by the clinical triad of intravascular hemolysis, venous thrombosis, and cytopenias [1–4]. The characteristic hemolytic crisis may conceal the fact that in PNH the hemolysis is chronic and present at any time [1, 2]: in fact, Ettore Marchiafava in 1928 called the disease

R. Notaro (✉)
Core Research Laboratory, Istituto Toscano Tumori, Viale Pieraccini 6, 50139 Florence, Italy
e-mail: rosario.notaro@ittumori.it

A.M. Risitano, M.D., Ph.D.
Hematology, Department of Clinical Medicine and Surgery, Federico II University of Naples, Via Pansini 5, 80131 Naples, Italy

Y. Kanakura et al. (eds.), *Paroxysmal Nocturnal Hemoglobinuria*,
DOI 10.1007/978-4-431-56003-6_17

PNH with perpetual hemosiderinuria [5]. PNH intravascular hemolysis and, likely, the high risk of thrombosis are secondary to the inability of blood cells with the PNH phenotype to cope with activated complement. Thus, it was conceivable that the inhibition of complement could prevent hemolysis (and, likely, thrombosis). However, this idea became a reality only at the beginning of this century with the clinical development of a humanized anti-C5 monoclonal antibody, eculizumab [6]. The treatment with eculizumab has proved to be safe and highly effective in controlling the intravascular hemolysis [7–9]. Thus, this treatment with a single agent has radically changed the standard of care for PNH [10]. However, any therapy, even when effective, may have limitations and in some case these limitations may provide new insights into the pathophysiology of the disease, and the therapy with eculizumab is not an exception.

17.2 The Impaired Response to Eculizumab

It is really impressive that eculizumab is able to stop or, at least, to markedly reduce intravascular hemolysis in almost all treated patient. Despite the excellent control of the intravascular hemolysis, testified by the almost normal LDH levels, the hematological response to eculizumab is variable. Indeed, some patients remain transfusion dependent, even though their transfusion requirement may decrease [11, 12]. In the registrative clinical trial, after 6 months of follow-up, and in a subsequent trial, after 12 months of follow-up, the transfusion independence was obtained in 51 % of patients [7, 8]: the long-term analysis of these trials found that transfusion independence was reached in 65 % of the 134 patients who reached 30 months of follow-up and in 82.1 % of the 78 patients who reached 36 months of follow-up [13]. In other series, that may include also a fraction of patients enrolled in the above trials, the transfusion independence was obtained in a variable proportion of transfused patients: from 13 % of 30 patients [12] up to 84 % of 51 patients (update of Risitano et al. 2009) [14].

Transfusion independence was the main criterion of response in the initial registrative trials. More recently, different reports have tried to associate clinical response to eculizumab with the actual hematological benefit that PNH patients experience after long-term treatment with eculizumab. Indeed, persistent need of RBC transfusions identifies the minority of patients who have a limited benefit from eculizumab; however, it does not track the fraction of patients who, even if do not require regular transfusions, continue to suffer from chronic anemia. Unfortunately, the issue of hematological benefit during eculizumab treatment has not been systematically addressed in large clinical trials, and the attempts to categorize hematological response remain somehow elusive. We have proposed a classification of hematological response, where transfusion independence associated with stable normal-like Hb values (an arbitrary cutoff of 11 gr/dL was utilized) is defined as optimal hematological response [11]. All the remaining suboptimal responders are further grouped in three response categories: (i) major hematological response is characterized

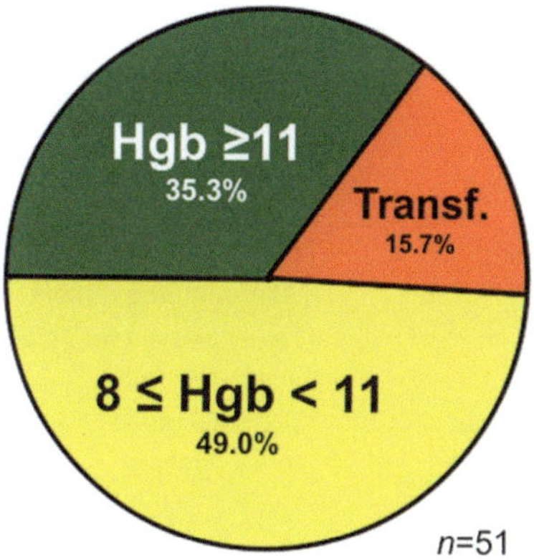

Fig. 17.1 Heterogeneity of hematological benefit during eculizumab treatment. Patients differ in their pattern of response to eculizumab. In this series, over 80 % of patients are transfusion independent on eculizumab. This is a higher proportion than in the registration trial, and it may reflect selection in that trial for patients who had a high transfusion requirement. About one-half of patients on eculizumab still have significant anemia, and unfortunately about 15 % still require blood transfusion (Transf.), more or less frequently (Updated from data reported by Risitano et al. [11] and Luzzatto et al. [14])

by transfusion independence with stable moderate anemia (Hb >8 g/dL); (ii) partial hematological response is defined by >50 % reduction of transfusion needs; and (iii) minor hematological response is defined as <50 % reduction of transfusion needs. Notably, all these response categories imply an adequate control of intravascular hemolysis, defined as marked reduction in LDH levels (patients with no reduction in LDH levels are defined as nonresponders, but likely they are limited to the few subjects carrying mutations in the C5 gene [15]. According to these categories, in our original cohort described in 2009, 15 patients (37 %) achieved an optimal response, 18 (44 %) a major response, 5 (12 %) a partial response, and 3 a minor response (attributed to progression to aplastic anemia, Fig. 17.1).

Since some degree of bone marrow failure (BMF) is present in any PNH patient, BMF may influences the clinical presentation of PNH. It is obvious that complement blockade is ineffective in PNH/AA patients in which there is a high degree of BMF and little or none hemolysis. However, there are patients in which the impaired production of red cells cooperates with hemolysis in causing the anemia: it is very likely that in these patients, complement inhibition by eculizumab reduces but not prevents the need for transfusions.

17.3 Causes of Reduced Hematological Response

The therapy with eculizumab results in the strong control of intravascular hemolysis and the consequent marked reduction of LDH levels in almost all PNH patients treated with eculizumab. The only significant exception is the patients with a rare

Table 17.1 Cause of reduced hematological response

Impaired red cell production	Bone marrow failure
	Iron and vitamin deficiency
	Inadequate Epo production (Hill, Haematologica 2007)
Persistent intravascular hemolysis	Lack of C5 inhibition because of C5 variants
	Aberrant drug turnover ("breakthrough")
	Acute and/or chronic increased complement activation.
De novo extravascular hemolysis	PNH red blood cells opsonization due to C3 binding

inherited polymorphism of C5 [15] (see below and Chap. 18 of this book) [16]. The regular administration of eculizumab at 14 days intervals maintains the complement blockade and effectively controls the intravascular hemolysis; nevertheless, hematological response is extremely heterogeneous among patients, and several factors may contribute to reduced hematological benefit. Roughly, three major causes may hamper hematological response in PNH during eculizumab treatment: (i) impaired red cell production, (ii) persistent intravascular hemolysis, and (iii) de novo extravascular hemolysis (Table 17.1).

17.3.1 Impaired Red Cell Production

As a hemolytic condition, in PNH the increased red cell turnover triggers compensatory erythropoiesis, which may eventually require vitamin and especially iron supplementation (in the absence of complement blockade, iron deficiency is common in PNH due to the "perpetual hemosiderinuria" described by Marchiafava) [5]. In addition, since some degree of bone marrow failure (BMF) is present in any PNH patient, it may also contribute to anemia of PNH patients, up to assume the form of the aplastic anemia (AA)/PNH syndrome [3, 4]. Indeed, the degree of BMF has to be considered in the context of eculizumab treatment, since it is obvious that complement blockade is ineffective (and thus not indicated) in PNH/AA patients in which there is a high degree of BMF and little or none hemolysis. However, there are patients in which the impaired production of red cells cooperates with hemolysis in causing the anemia: it is very likely that in these patients, complement inhibition by eculizumab reduces but not abolishes the need for transfusions. In these patients, adequate vitamin and/or iron supplementation may improve hematological benefit when the impaired red cell production is mostly due to deficiencies; the use of recombinant erythropoietin has also been proven effective in some patients [17]. However, in the case of a concomitant immune-mediated BMF, additional etiological treatments have to be considered (e.g., immunosuppression or even bone marrow transplantation, according to the severity of AA).

17.3.2 Persistent Intravascular Hemolysis

Even if eculizumab results in sustained control of intravascular hemolysis, in a small proportion of patients, complement blockade fades quicker, and it fails in controlling intravascular hemolysis before a new dose of eculizumab: this results in hemolytic crisis and, frequently, in transfusion requirement. It is likely that in these patients, there is a faster drug turnover of eculizumab that causes its insufficient concentration (pharmacokinetic breakthrough hemolysis) [18]: in fact, in these patients the reduction of the intervals between ECU infusions or the increase of ECU dosage usually is able to overcome the hemolysis and the subsequent transfusion requirement. However, to date, formal demonstration of increased drug turnover in these patients is lacking, even because the mechanism of clearance of eculizumab has not been described. Indeed, given that the majority of eculizumab should be circulating as complex with its target C5, it is conceivable that its turnover should parallel that of circulating immune complexes (which might be somehow modulated by genetic factors).

In addition to this pharmacokinetic breakthrough, some PNH patients on eculizumab may experience episodes of intravascular hemolysis associated with infection or inflammation, when the activation of complement (possibly via its distinct activation pathways) [12, 14, 19] generates high levels of C5 convertase activity that can overcome the eculizumab blockade of C5 (pharmacodynamic breakthrough hemolysis) [20]. Although, this may produce a drop of hemoglobin, it should not be classified as a reduced response: in fact, usually it does not require blood transfusion, and it does not benefit from increasing eculizumab. In any event, in PNH patients on eculizumab, the most frequent reason of a reduced response to eculizumab and for persistent blood transfusion requirement is chronic hemolysis with elevated reticulocyte count.

17.3.3 De Novo Extravascular Hemolysis

Irrespective of the control of intravascular hemolysis and of impaired red blood cell production, another mechanism has emerged as the main reason for suboptimal hematological response in PNH patients on eculizumab. In almost all PNH patients on eculizumab, a significant fraction of GPI-negative red blood cells (RBC) is opsonized by complement component 3 (C3) with the previously negative Coombs test becoming positive; and the red cells so opsonized may undergo extravascular hemolysis through C3-specific receptors expressed on splenic and hepatic macrophages [11]. C3 decoration on PNH red blood cells is mechanistically linked to the interception of complement cascade at the level of C5; indeed, even if PNH erythrocytes are spared from hemolysis because of the blockade of the terminal effector complement (which in some way compensate the lack of CD59), they remain unable to

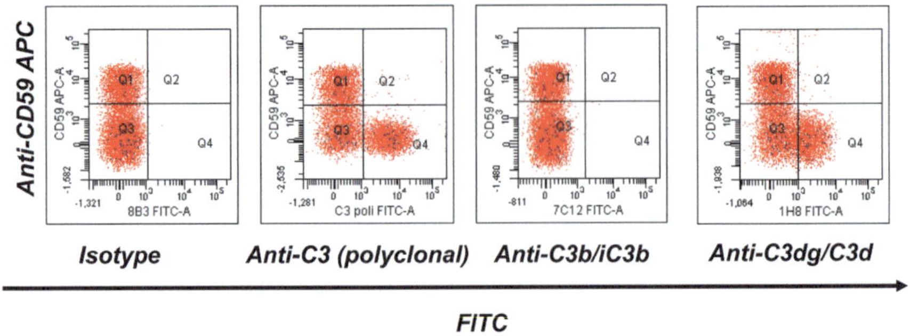

Fig. 17.2 C3 deposition in PNH during eculizumab treatment. Example of C3 deposition detected by flow cytometry in a PNH patient on eculizumab. A: isotypic control (FITC) vs. CD59 (APC, clone 59-APC, Valter Occhiena). B: C3 (FITC; Ab4214, Abcam) vs. CD59 (APC, clone 59-APC, Valter Occhiena). C: C3b/iC3b (FITC, clone 7C12) vs. CD59 (APC, clone 59-APC, Valter Occhiena). D: C3dg/C3d (FITC, clone 1H8) vs. CD59 (APC, clone 59-APC, Valter Occhiena)

control early complement activation on their surface . As a consequence, PNH erythrocytes continue to suffer from surface C3 activation and progressively accumulate C3 fragments on their surface, as easily detectable by flow cytometry (Fig. 17.2) (or even by direct antiglobulin test) [19, 21]. Basically all PNH patients on eculizumab exhibit some degree of C3 accumulation on their erythrocytes; and the majority of them eventually suffer from some extent of C3-mediated extravascular hemolysis, as testified also by a persistent reticulocytosis. However, C3-mediated extravascular hemolysis becomes clinically relevant only in 25–50 % of them, eventually resulting in suboptimal hematological response. In fact, 25–35 % of patients still need transfusions [11, 12, 14, 22, 23]; and the size of the fraction of RBC with bound C3 seems to correlate with transfusion requirement (Fig. 17.3) [11, 21]. The reason why C3 opsonization and even more the clearance of C3-opsonized erythrocytes are different among PNH patients is currently under investigation, as discussed below. However, it has to be remarked that, irrespective of its clinical relevance, this phenomenon represents a major switch in the pathophysiology of the disease; indeed, a condition typically characterized by intravascular hemolysis during eculizumab treatment may change into another one where extravascular hemolysis becomes dominant. This change in the pathogenic mechanism may also have additional clinical consequences; for instance, the typical iron deficiency consequence of perpetual hemosiderinuria is no longer detectable due to the prevention of intravascular hemolysis. Rather, it has been reported that during eculizumab treatment, iron overload may develop, especially in case of persistent transfusion need [19, 24, 25]; notably, preliminary data suggest that some degree of iron overload may become evident even in the absence of transfusions, possibly

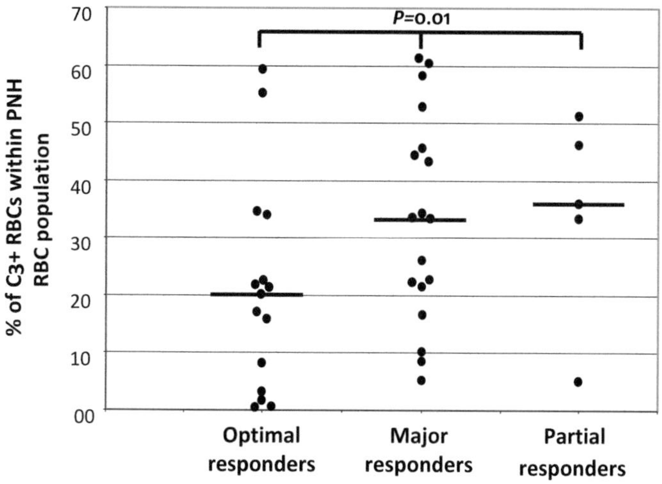

Fig. 17.3 C3 deposition and hematological response to eculizumab. Percentage of C3+ RBCs within the PNH RBC population in eculizumab-treated PNH patients achieving optimal (n = 15), major (n = 18), or partial (n = 5) hematologic response. Each dot represents a single case; bars represent median values. Kruskal-Wallis *U* test; P = 0.01 (From Risitano et al. [11])

due to extravascular hemolysis and continuous increased iron intake triggered by persistent anemia (similarly to thalassemias and myelodysplastic syndromes) (Fig. 17.4).

17.4 Genetic Determinants of Response to Eculizumab

The heterogeneity of response to eculizumab has raised the possibility that genetically determined differences may account for inter-patient variability. The most obvious evidence for this comes from the observation that patients carrying a rare inherited genetic variant of C5, c.2654G → A, harbor an intrinsic resistance to eculizumab [15]. This *C5* variant prevents the binding of eculizumab that, eventually, does not control intravascular hemolysis; this rare genetic variant has been found only in people of Far East Asian origin with an allelic frequency of 0.017 in Japanese population and of 0.004 in Han Chinese population [15]. Furthermore, it is possible to hypothesize, but not yet demonstrated, that genetic variants of *C5* could account for possible leakage in the control of intravascular hemolysis: however, *C5* genetic variants should not explain differences in C3 opsonization or in the degree of extravascular hemolysis.

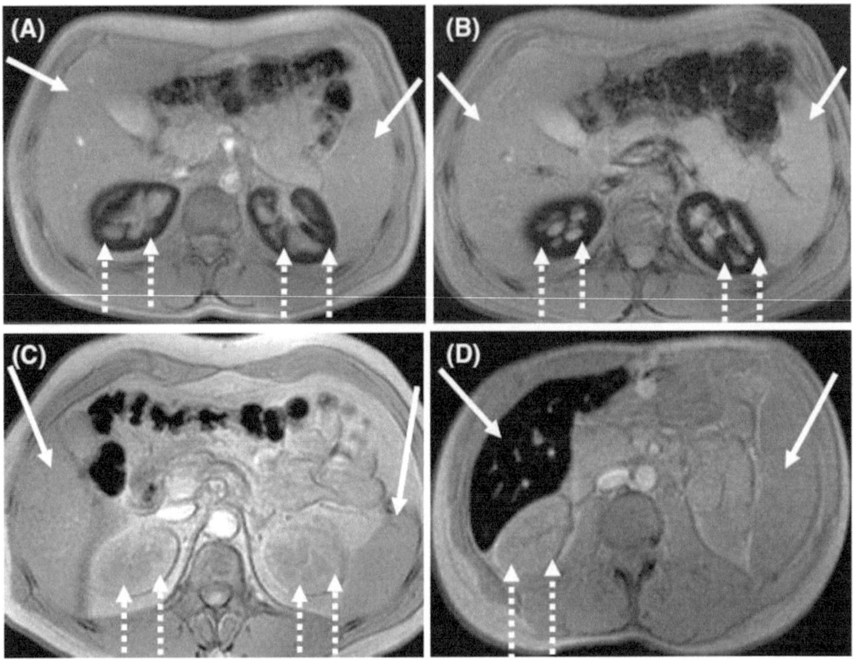

Fig. 17.4 Iron compartmentalization by magnetic resonance imaging (MRI) in PNH patients. After informed consent, T2* MRI was performed as described in Risitano et al. [24]. (**a**) Example of an untreated PNH patient (UPN NA111): MR image demonstrates a high renal CIC (*dashed white arrows*) and normal hepatosplenic CIC (*white arrows*). (**b**) Example of a PNH patient on eculizumab experiencing breakthrough (UPN NA102): MR image demonstrates a high renal CIC (*dashed white arrows*) and normal hepatosplenic CIC (*white arrows*), similarly to untreated patients. (**c**) Example of a PNH patient on eculizumab with complete blockade of intravascular hemolysis (UPN NA006): MR image demonstrates normal CIC in the kidneys (*dashed white arrows*), liver, and spleen (*white arrows*). (**d**) Example of a PNH patient on eculizumab with iron overload (UPN RM003): MR image demonstrates a normal renal CIC (*dashed white arrows*) and high hepatic CIC (*white arrow*) (From Risitano et al. [24])

The variability of mechanisms controlling C3 binding and/or removal of C3+ PNH red cells are likely to account for the variability of the proportion of C3+ PNH red cells and of the degree of extravascular hemolysis among PNH patients. It possible hypothesizes that most of this variability results from genetic diversity in genes coding for protein of the complement system and of its regulators.

Recently, we found that the *Hind* III polymorphism of the complement receptor 1 (*CR1*) gene is associated with the need of blood of transfusion of patients on eculizumab [26]. Two codominant alleles of *Hind* III polymorphism are known: the H (common) allele and the L (rare) allele that are associated, respectively, with high and with low expression of CR1 on red cells. Patients on eculizumab who still need blood transfusion were 18 % among H/H homozygotes (high CR1 levels), 33 % among H/L heterozygotes (intermediate CR1 levels), and 68 % among L/L homozygotes (low CR1 levels) (P = 0.016). Thus, higher the density of CR1 molecules on

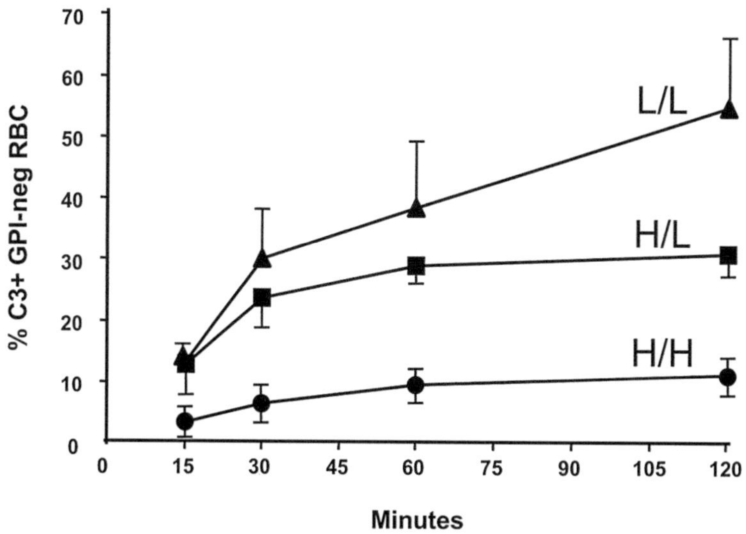

Fig. 17.5 Kinetics of in vitro C3 binding according to *CR1* genotype. *Hind* III *CR1* genotype dictates the rate of C3 binding to PNH red cells in vitro. When eculizumab-containing sera are added to red blood cells, the rate of novel C3 binding to PNH red blood cells is significantly different depending on the *CR1* genotype: H/H ($n = 6$) *vs.* H/L ($n = 3$), $P = 0.0425$; H/L ($n = 3$) *vs.* L/L ($n = 2$), $P = 0.0173$; for the comparison H/H ($n = 6$) *vs.* L/L ($n = 2$), $P < 0.0001$. Standard deviation is reported for each experimental point. H/H: homozygotes for the high expression allele of *CR1 Hind* III polymorphism. L/L: homozygotes for the low expression allele of *CR1 Hind* III polymorphism. H/L: heterozygotes for *CR1 Hind* III polymorphism (From Rondelli et al. [26])

red blood cells better is the response to eculizumab likely through the modulation of the C3 binding on red blood cells. In fact, CR1 *Hind* III genotype correlates, in vivo, with the abundance of PNH red cells that have bound C3 and, in vitro, with the kinetics of C3 binding (Fig. 17.5).

These results are consistent with the notion that the *CR1* genotype may affect the regulation of C3 activation (and thus C3 opsonization) at the level of red blood cell surface, eventually leading to differences in C3-mediated extravascular hemolysis and hematological response to eculizumab treatment. This emerges as a novel example of pharmacogenetics, which on the other hand seems do not fully explain the extreme heterogeneity of hematological response to eculizumab. Mutations, that may reach polymorphic frequency, are known in several other complement and complement-related genes, and all together they may potentially shape the individual genetic background affecting the response to eculizumab treatment in each PNH patient. Genetic variations in complement factor H (and complement factor H-related proteins), complement factor I, membrane cofactor protein, and complement component 3 (C3) have been associated to other complement-mediated disease, such as atypical hemolytic-uremic syndrome and age-related macular degeneration.

Limited data related to these genes are available in PNH patients. We have found no correlation between the C3 genotype and the need for blood transfusion, even if another group has reported that different C3 genotypes may account for different likelihood of transfusion independence during eculizumab treatment [27]. Data about the other genes commonly involved in complement-mediated diseases are lacking.

17.5 Management of Extravascular Hemolysis

Since the C3-mediated extravascular hemolysis is present in almost all PNH patients on eculizumab, a relevant clinical problem is how to manage that fraction of patients in whom it creates persistent transfusion dependence (or of persistent symptomatic anemia). It has been suggested to treat this condition by using the corticosteroid. However, it is really questionable whether corticosteroids might be effective: in fact, apart from a clinical report with short follow-up [28], our and others' experience in more than 15 patients, suggests that it is not effective [29]. In addition, the serious long-term side effects of corticosteroid should prevent their use in patients with such a chronic disease. The usage of other forms of immunosuppression and of intravenous immunoglobulin has been proposed, but there are no data (as well as limited rationale).

Splenectomy and selective splenic artery embolization have been anecdotally reported effective in three patients. In two patients on eculizumab with persistent requirement of blood transfusions, the selective splenic artery embolization splenectomy was performed mainly because of pancytopenia and splenomegaly; the pancytopenia improved in both patients, and the transfusion requirement was reduced in one and abolished in the other [30]. In one case a video-laparoscopic splenectomy has been performed in a patient with normal white cells and platelet counts because of the persistent blood transfusion requirement on eculizumab and a documented spleen and liver captation of 51Cr-labeled RBC: the procedure was uneventful, and the patients remain free of transfusion after more than 7 years (Fig. 17.6) [31]. For long-term complications (increased risk of infection and thrombosis), one would never recommend it as a standard measure.

However, it could be indicated in patients in which the splenomegaly and/or the splenic captation of RBC is well documented; in these case the selective splenic artery embolization should be chosen over surgical splenectomy because of the reduced risk of complication and the maintenance of some splenic tissue that could reduce the risk of infections.

Speculative approaches for the future might include (a) targeting the complement cascade upstream of C5, (b) interfering with the interactions between C3-opsonized red cells and macrophages, and (c) targeting the interaction between C3 and the red cells themselves. Of course it is unlikely that we can safely get rid of

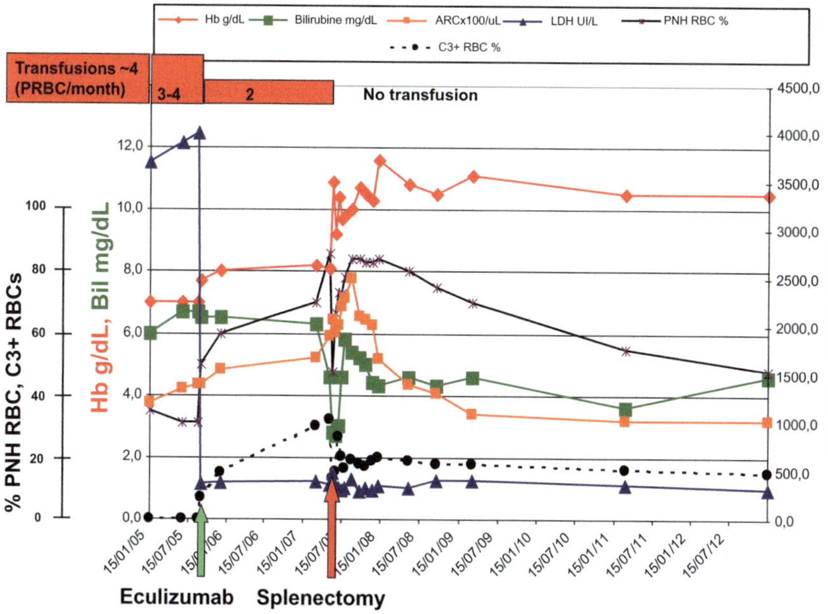

Fig. 17.6 Effect of splenectomy on C3-mediated extravascular hemolysis. Laboratory parameters in relation to anticomplement treatment and splenectomy. Eculizumab (Soliris, Alexion Pharmaceuticals) was started in September 2005 (*red arrow*), according to the standard schedule (600 mg weekly × 4 weeks, then 900 mg fortnightly). Splenectomy was performed in May 2006 (*black arrow*), by video laparoscopy, supported by vaccinations and antibiotics. No infections or other clinical complications have been recorded to date. The red squares depict the transfusional requirement (as number of packed red cell units per month); the need for transfusion (17 units in the previous 12 months) remained stable during the TRIUMPH study (placebo arm) and was significantly reduced after introduction of eculizumab, which resolved intravascular hemolysis with LDH normalization (*blue line*). However, transfusion independence with hemoglobin stabilization (*red line*) was achieved only after splenectomy, and Hb levels remained stable over time even at 9 years from splenectomy, with subsequent reduction of erythropoietic response (reticulocyte count, *orange line*). Bilirubinemia (*green line*) was persistently elevated (almost entirely unconjugated) with some fluctuations, in part due to associated Gilbert syndrome (genetically confirmed by the presence of homozygous (TA)7 polymorphism of the UGT1A1 gene) (update of Risitano et al. [31])

complement altogether, and it remains to be seen whether such modes of complement blockade will be as safe as blocking just C5. This topic is extensively covered in the Chap. 18 of this book [32].

Acknowledgments PNH studies has been in part funded by the Associazione Italiana Emoglobinuria Parossistica Notturna (RN) and the Aplastic Anemia & MDS International Foundation (RN and AMR).

We thank all the colleagues within and outside our national PNH network for sharing their experience and their thoughts.

Finally we are particularly grateful to all of our patients and their families.

References

1. Risitano AM (2012) Paroxysmal nocturnal hemoglobinuria. In: Silverberg DS (ed) Anemia. InTech, Rijeka, Croatia. pp 331–374
2. Luzzatto L, Notaro R (2003) Paroxysmal nocturnal hemoglobinuria. In: Handin RI, Lux SE, Stossel TP (eds) Blood, principles and practice of hematology, 2nd edn. Lippincot Williams & Wilkins, Philadelphia, pp 319–334
3. Parker C, Omine M, Richards S et al (2005) International PNH interest group. Diagnosis and management of paroxysmal nocturnal hemoglobinuria. Blood 106(12):3699–3709
4. de Latour RP, Mary JY, Salanoubat C, Terriou L, Etienne G, Mohty M, Roth S, de Guibert S, Maury S, Cahn JY, Socié G, French Society of Hematology, French Association of Young Hematologists (2008) Paroxysmal nocturnal hemoglobinuria: natural history of disease subcategories. Blood 112(8):3099–3106
5. Marchiafava E (1928) Anemia emolitica cronica con emosiderinuria perpetua. Il Policlinico. Sezione medica 35:105–117
6. Rother RP, Rollins SA, Mojcik CF et al (2007) Discovery and development of the complement inhibitor eculizumab for the treatment of paroxysmal nocturnal hemoglobinuria. Nat Biotechnol 25:1256–1264
7. Hillmen P, Hall C, Marsh JC, Elebute M, Bombara MP, Petro BE, Cullen MJ, Richards SJ, Rollins SA, Mojcik CF, Rother RP (2004) Effect of eculizumab on hemolysis and transfusion requirements in patients with paroxysmal nocturnal hemoglobinuria. N Engl J Med 350:552–559
8. Hillmen P, Young NS, Schubert J et al (2006) The complement inhibitor eculizumab in paroxysmal nocturnal hemoglobinuria. N Engl J Med 355:1233–1243
9. Brodsky RA, Young NS, Antonioli E et al (2008) Multicenter phase III study of the complement inhibitor eculizumab for the treatment of patients with paroxysmal nocturnal hemoglobinuria. Blood 114:1840–1847
10. Hillmen P, Muus P, Duhrsen U et al (2007) Effect of the complement inhibitor eculizumab on thromboembolism in patients with paroxysmal nocturnal hemoglobinuria. Blood 110:4123–4128
11. Risitano AM, Notaro R, Marando L et al (2009) Complement fraction 3 binding on erythrocytes as additional mechanism of disease in paroxysmal nocturnal hemoglobinuria patients treated by eculizumab. Blood 113:4094–4100
12. DeZern AE, Dorr D, Brodsky RA (2013) Predictors of hemoglobin response to eculizumab therapy in paroxysmal nocturnal hemoglobinuria. Eur J Haematol 90(1):16–24
13. Hillmen P, Muus P, Röth A, Elebute MO, Risitano AM, Schrezenmeier H, Szer J, Browne P, Maciejewski JP, Schubert J, Urbano-Ispizua A, de Castro C, Socié G, Brodsky RA (2013) Long-term safety and efficacy of sustained eculizumab treatment in patients with paroxysmal nocturnal haemoglobinuria. Br J Haematol 162(1):62–73
14. Luzzatto L, Gianfaldoni G, Notaro R (2011) Management of paroxysmal nocturnal haemoglobinuria: a personal view. Br J Haematol 153(6):709–720
15. Nishimura J, Yamamoto M, Hayashi S et al (2014) Genetic variants in C5 and poor response to eculizumab. N Engl J Med 370(7):632–639
16. Nishimura J, Yamamoto M, Kanakura Y (2015) Clinical effects of eculizumab in PNH; Poor-responders to eculizumab. In: Yuzuru Kanakura Y, Kinoshita T, Nishimura J (ed) PNH; from bench to bedside (in press)
17. Hill A, Richards SJ, Rother RP et al (2007) Erythropoietin treatment during complement inhibition with eculizumab in a patient with paroxysmal nocturnal hemoglobinuria. Haematologica 92:ECR14
18. Hill A, Hillmen P, Richards SJ, Elebute D, Marsh JC, Chan J, Mojcik CF, Rother RP (2005) Sustained response and long-term safety of eculizumab in paroxysmal nocturnal hemoglobinuria. Blood 106(7):2559–2565

19. Röth A, Hock C, Konik A, Christoph S, Dührsen U (2011) Chronic treatment of paroxysmal nocturnal hemoglobinuria patients with eculizumab: safety, efficacy, and unexpected laboratory phenomena. Int J Hematol 93(6):704–714
20. Risitano AM, Ricklin D, Huang Y et al (2014) Peptide inhibitors of C3 activation as a novel strategy of complement inhibition for the treatment of paroxysmal nocturnal hemoglobinuria. Blood 123(13):2094–2101
21. Hill A, Rother RP, Arnold L et al (2010) Eculizumab prevents intravascular hemolysis in patients with paroxysmal nocturnal hemoglobinuria and unmasks low-level extravascular hemolysis occurring through C3 opsonization. Haematologica 95(4):567–573
22. Luzzatto L, Risitano AM, Notaro R (2010) Paroxysmal nocturnal hemoglobinuria and eculizumab. Haematologica 95:523–526
23. Kelly RJ, Hill A, Arnold LM et al (2011) Long-term treatment with eculizumab in paroxysmal nocturnal hemoglobinuria: sustained efficacy and improved survival. Blood 117:6786–6792
24. Risitano AM, Imbriaco M, Marando L, Seneca E, Soscia E, Malcovati L, Iori AP, Pane F, Notaro R, Matarazzo M (2012) From perpetual haemosiderinuria to possible iron overload: iron redistribution in paroxysmal nocturnal haemoglobinuria patients on eculizumab by magnetic resonance imaging. Br J Haematol 158(3):415–418
25. Höchsmann B, Leichtle R, von Zabern I, Kaiser S, Flegel WA, Schrezenmeier H (2012) Paroxysmal nocturnal haemoglobinuria treatment with eculizumab is associated with a positive direct antiglobulin test. Vox Sang 102(2):159–166
26. Rondelli T, Risitano AM, Peffault de Latour R et al (2014) Polymorphism of the complement receptor 1 gene correlates with the hematologic response to eculizumab in patients with paroxysmal nocturnal hemoglobinuria. Haematologica 99(2):262–266
27. Kaudlay P, Hua H, He G, Newton DJ, Varghese AM, Munir T, Hill A, Kelly RJ, Richards SJ, Hillmen P (2013) Red cell complement loading in PNH patients on eculizumab is associated with a C3 polymorphism which influences C3 function, predicts for increased extravascular hemolysis and provides a rationale for C3 inhibition. Blood 122(21):2466
28. Berzuini A, Montanelli F, Prati D (2010) Hemolytic anemia after eculizumab in paroxysmal nocturnal hemoglobinuria. N Engl J Med 363:993–994
29. Risitano AM, Notaro R, Luzzatto L et al (2010) Paroxysmal nocturnal hemoglobinuria: hemolysis before and after eculizumab. N Engl J Med 363:2270–2272
30. Araten DJ, Iori AP, Brown K, Torelli GF, Barberi W, Natalino F, De Propris MS, Girmenia C, Salvatori FM, Zelig O, Foà R, Luzzatto L (2014) Selective splenic artery embolization for the treatment of thrombocytopenia and hypersplenism in paroxysmal nocturnal hemoglobinuria. J Hematol Oncol 7:27
31. Risitano AM, Marando L, Seneca E, Rotoli B (2008) Hemoglobin normalization after splenectomy in a paroxysmal nocturnal hemoglobinuria patient treated by eculizumab. Blood 112(2):449–451
32. Risitano AM (2015) Future strategies of complement inhibition in paroxysmal nocturnal hemoglobinuria. In: Yuzuru Kanakura Y, Kinoshita T, Nishimura J (ed) PNH; from bench to bedside (in press)

Chapter 18
Clinical Effects of Eculizumab in PNH: Poor Responders to Eculizumab

Jun-ichi Nishimura, Taroh Kinoshita, and Yuzuru Kanakura

Abstract Eculizumab is a humanized monoclonal antibody that targets the terminal complement protein C5 and inhibits terminal complement-mediated hemolysis associated with paroxysmal nocturnal hemoglobinuria (PNH). Seventeen Japanese patients and one native Argentinian patient were identified as having a poor response to eculizumab. C5 gene analyses of patients with PNH who had a good or poor response to eculizumab were compared, and recombinant C5 (rC5) proteins were assessed. A single missense C5 heterozygous mutation, c.2654G > A, which predicts p.Arg885His, was commonly identified in the Japanese poor responders but not in the good responders. Among the approximately 500 Japanese patients treated with eculizumab, 17 (3.4 %) were identified as poor responders; a similar prevalence of the polymorphism was also observed in healthy volunteers (3.5 %). This polymorphism had spread to at least one other East Asian country. Comparative studies of wild-type rC5 with mutant rC5 (rC5 m) showed eculizumab did not block the hemolytic activity supported by rC5 m; rather, it was completely blocked by N19/8, an anti-C5 monoclonal antibody that binds to a different site on C5 than eculizumab. Furthermore, rC5 m was also found to be incapable of binding to eculizumab. A separate poor responder (from Argentina) also had a mutation in this region, c.2653C > T, which predicts p.Arg885Cys, further supporting the importance of this site in C5 and the potential for ethnic diversity with respect to this phenomenon. These data are consistent with the hypothesis that the functional capacity of the rC5 m, together with its inability to bind to and undergo blockade by eculizumab, explains the poor response in patients carrying this mutation. The research article entitled "Genetic Variants in C5 and Poor Response to Eculizumab"

J.-i. Nishimura (✉) • Y. Kanakura
Department of Hematology and Oncology, Osaka University Graduate School of Medicine, 2-2 Yamadaoka, Suita 565-0871, Osaka, Japan
e-mail: junnishi@bldon.med.osaka-u.ac.jp

T. Kinoshita
Research Institute for Microbial Diseases, Osaka University, 3-1 Yamadaoka, Suita 565-0871, Osaka, Japan

WPI Immunology Frontier Research Center, Osaka University, 3-1 Yamadaoka, Suita 565-0871, Osaka, Japan

Y. Kanakura et al. (eds.), *Paroxysmal Nocturnal Hemoglobinuria*,
DOI 10.1007/978-4-431-56003-6_18

was originally published in the "New England Journal of Medicine" (Original Article, Nishimura J, et al., Genetic Variants in C5 and Poor Response to Eculizumab, 370, 632–639, Copyright © (2014) Massachusetts Medical Society. Reprinted with permission.), and it is reviewed herein with some updated data.

Keywords Eculizumab • Complement-mediated hemolysis • Paroxysmal nocturnal hemoglobinuria • Polymorphism

18.1 Introduction

Paroxysmal nocturnal hemoglobinuria (PNH) arises as a consequence of clonal expansion of hematopoietic stem cells that have acquired a somatic mutation in the *phosphatidylinositol glycan class A (PIGA)* gene [1–3]. The resulting hematopoietic cells are deficient in the glycosylphosphatidylinositol (GPI)-anchored regulatory proteins CD55 and CD59, which account for the intravascular hemolysis that is the primary clinical manifestation of PNH [4–6]. PNH frequently arises in association with bone marrow failure disorders, particularly aplastic anemia. Thrombosis is a major cause of morbidity and mortality, particularly in Caucasian patients with PNH [7–9].

Eculizumab is a humanized monoclonal antibody that specifically binds to the terminal complement protein C5, inhibiting its cleavage into C5a and C5b by C5 convertases. It thereby prevents the release of the inflammatory mediator C5a and the formation of the cytolytic pore C5b-9 [10, 11]. C5 blockade preserves the critical immunoprotective and immunoregulatory functions of upstream components that culminate in C3b-mediated opsonization and immune clearance. As such, eculizumab is highly effective in reducing intravascular hemolysis in PNH. It decreases or eliminates blood transfusion requirements and improves quality of life and reduces the risk of thrombosis in patients with classic PNH and in those who develop PNH secondary to aplastic anemia [12–16]. Since the approval of eculizumab by authorities outside of Japan, more than 99 % of patients administered the drug have responded to treatment, as measured by a decrease in hemolysis. However, in the Japanese AEGIS PNH-eculizumab study, 2 of the 29 treated patients (6.9 %) were identified as poor responders [17, 18]. Poor response is defined as a condition in which levels of lactate dehydrogenase (LDH) remain markedly high during treatment with eculizumab, regardless of improvements in other laboratory tests or clinical symptoms. Recently, approximately 500 Japanese patients were treated with eculizumab, 17 of which were identified as poor responders (3.4 %), all of whom share the same single polymorphism. In an original article, our group sought to elucidate the molecular basis for the poor response in this small subset of Japanese patients with PNH by applying a bedside-to-bench approach. In doing so, a C5 mutation was identified in these poor responders that prevents binding and blockade by eculizumab, thereby retaining its functional capacity to cause hemolysis. Herein, the original research article entitled "Genetic Variants in C5 and Poor Response to Eculizumab" is reviewed with some updated data [19]. All blood samples were collected by venipuncture after obtaining informed consent according to the Declaration of Helsinki. Approval was obtained for these studies from the Institutional Review Board at the institutes taking care of the poor responders as well as Osaka University.

18.2 Japanese Poor Responders from the AEGIS Clinical Study

During the 12-week eculizumab treatment period in the AEGIS study, two patients exhibited markedly elevated levels of LDH that did not decrease, suggesting that eculizumab did not protect their erythrocytes from uncontrolled complement activation (Fig. 18.1a). This was confirmed in a subsequent pharmacokinetic/pharmacodynamic analysis. Despite the fact that peak and trough levels of eculizumab during this study remained well above the minimum level (>35 μg/ml) required to completely inhibit complement-mediated hemolysis in PNH patients (Fig. 18.1b), the rates of hemolysis in the two poor responders were unaffected under conditions in which hemolysis in responders was completely suppressed (Fig. 18.1c).

These observations were corroborated through further studies on the effect of exogenous eculizumab on the hemolytic activity of patient serum sampled before administration of the drug. Although in vitro hemolytic activity in sera collected from a healthy volunteer and an eculizumab responder were completely inhibited by eculizumab at serum concentrations of 6.25 μg/ml and 12.5 μg/ml, respectively, levels as high as 2000 μg/ml eculizumab did not inhibit in vitro hemolysis in the sera of the two poor responders (Fig. 18.2a). In contrast, results with N19/8 (an anti-C5 monoclonal antibody that binds to a different site on C5 than eculizumab) showed that suppression of complement-mediated hemolysis was similar in the healthy volunteer, an eculizumab responder, and the two poor responders (Fig. 18.2b).

18.3 Nature and Prevalence of the C5 Mutation Identified in AEGIS Poor Responders

All 41 exons of the *C5* gene were amplified with primer sets specifically designed for each exon, using genomic DNA prepared from mononuclear cells of poor responders. All resultant polymerase chain reaction (PCR) products were then directly sequenced. A single missense C5 heterozygous mutation was identified in both poor responders at exon 21, c.2654G > A, which predicts p.Arg885His. This mutation was not seen in the seven eculizumab responders (Fig. 18.3a). In addition,

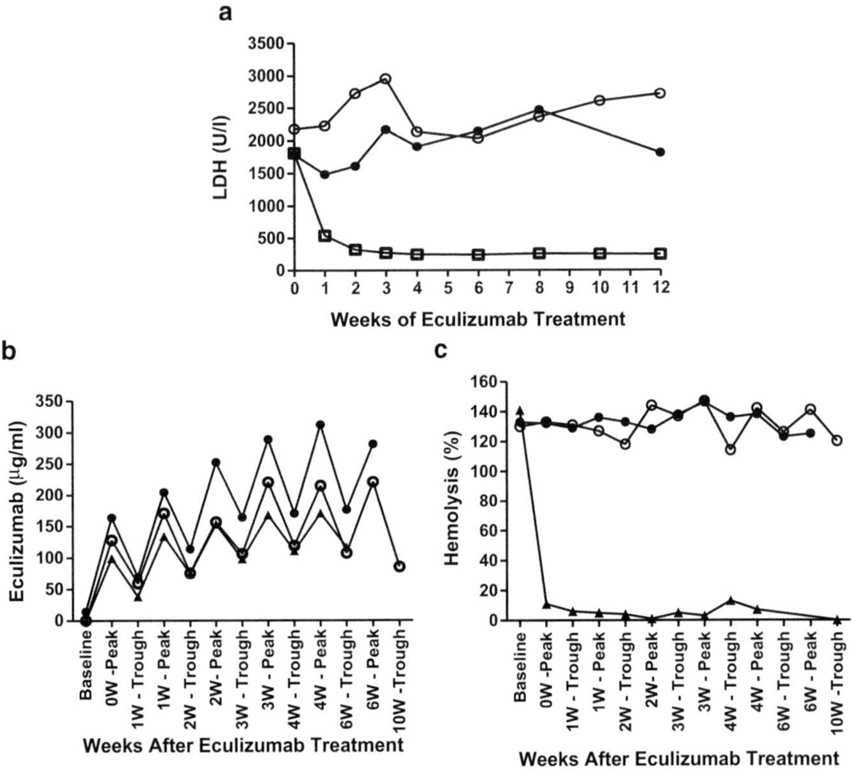

Fig. 18.1 Pharmacokinetic and pharmacodynamic analyses of two poor responders from the AEGIS study (Original Article, Nishimura J, et al., Genetic Variants in C5 and Poor Response to Eculizumab, 370, 632–639, Copyright © (2014) Massachusetts Medical Society. Reprinted with permission). *Panel A* shows LDH levels in the two poor responders, UPN1 (●) and UPN2 (○), which were not reduced during the 12-week treatment period, as well as in all 29 patients with PNH enrolled in the AEGIS study (□), in whom LDH was normalized. *Panel B* shows levels of eculizumab in the two poor responders, which were consistently >50 μg/ml throughout the treatment period; a typical responder (▲) is also shown. *Panel C* shows in vitro hemolytic activity in serum samples from the two poor responders, which, like LDH, was unaffected by treatment with eculizumab, whereas the typical responder had completely suppressed hemolytic activity throughout the treatment period

it was confirmed that the 15 other poor responders identified in Japan following the launch of eculizumab had the same C5 gene mutation. As noted above, the 17 poor responders who share this mutation have been identified from a total of approximately 500 Japanese patients administered eculizumab (3.4 %).

Next, the prevalence of this mutation was analyzed in the healthy Japanese population using a gel-based assay in conjunction with DNA samples. It was determined that 10 of 288 healthy volunteers in Japan had the same heterozygous mutation (3.5 %), which is consistent with the prevalence observed in the Japanese PNH patient population (Table 18.1). To determine the distribution of this polymorphism

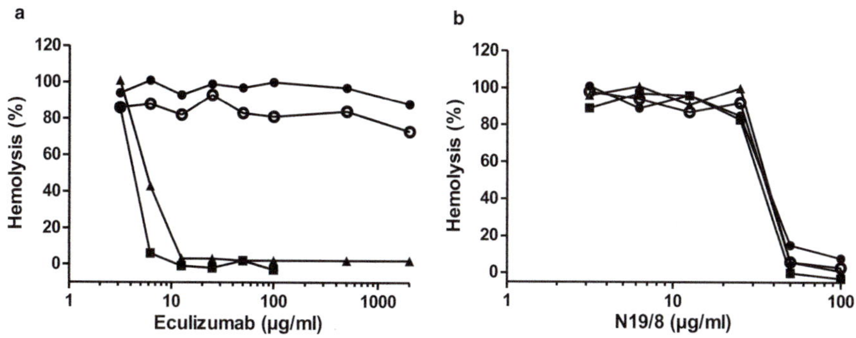

Fig. 18.2 The effect of exogenous eculizumab and a different anti-C5 antibody (N19/8) on the hemolytic activity of patient sera before drug administration (Original Article, Nishimura J, et al., Genetic Variants in C5 and Poor Response to Eculizumab, 370, 632–639, Copyright © (2014) Massachusetts Medical Society. Reprinted with permission). *Panel A* shows the effect of exogenously added eculizumab on in vitro hemolysis; exogenous eculizumab up to a final concentration of 2000 μg/ml did not inhibit in vitro hemolysis in the predrug sera of the two poor responders, UPN1 (●) and UPN2 (○), whereas a response was seen in serum from a responder (▲) and a healthy volunteer (■). *Panel B* shows the effect of an anti-C5 antibody to a different epitope (N19/8), which suppressed complement-mediated hemolysis in sera from the healthy subject, the responder, and the two poor responders shown in panel A

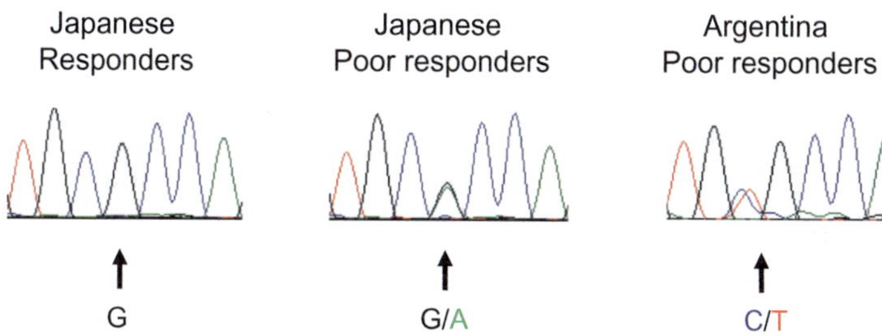

Fig. 18.3 Genetic polymorphism of C5 found in Japanese and Argentinian poor responders (Original Article, Nishimura J, et al., Genetic Variants in C5 and Poor Response to Eculizumab, 370, 632–639, Copyright © (2014) Massachusetts Medical Society. Reprinted with permission). The panel shows the sequence of the C5 polymorphism found in Japanese and Argentinian poor responders in comparison with the more frequently observed sequence in responders. A heterozygous missense mutation in the exon 21, c.2654G > A, predicting p.Arg885His, was identified in all Japanese poor responders but not in responders. A very similar mutation, c.2653C > T, which predicts p.Arg885Cys, was identified in an Argentinian poor responder

in other ethnic populations, several DNA panels were screened. The c.2654G > A polymorphism was identified in 1 out of 120 Han Chinese volunteers, but was not present in samples from 100 British people or in samples from 90 people of Mexican ancestry (Table 18.1).

Table 18.1 Ethnic distribution of the C5 polymorphisms

Origin	Analyzed numbers	Japanese c.2654G > A	Argentinian c.2653C > T
Japanese	288	10 (3.5 %)	–
British from England and Scotland	100	0 (0 %)	0 (0 %)
Han Chinese	120	1 (0.8 %)	0 (0 %)
Native Mexican American	90	0 (0 %)	0 (0 %)

18.4 Functional Properties of Mutant C5 Identified in Japanese Poor Responders

To close the genotype-phenotype loop, electrophoretically pure recombinant C5 (rC5) and mutant C5 (rC5 m) containing c.2654G > A were generated and functionally compared in various in vitro experiments. As a preliminary experiment, it was confirmed that native human (n)C5, rC5, and rC5 m restored classical pathway lysis at equivalent levels when added to C5-depleted serum (data not shown). Eculizumab did not block classical pathway lysis reconstituted with rC5 m but did block rC5 and nC5-dependent lysis (Fig. 18.4a). By contrast, as observed with patient sera, N19/8 inhibited lysis reconstituted with nC5, rC5, and rC5 m (Fig. 18.4b). Finally, although eculizumab bound rC5 in nanomolar concentrations using surface plasmon resonance, including clear association and dissociation phases, there was no detectable binding with rC5 m in the same assay up to the highest concentration (1 μM) of eculizumab tested (Fig. 18.4c).

18.5 Nature and Prevalence of a C5 Mutation Identified in a Native Argentinian Poor Responder

A poor responder whose level of LDH remained markedly high during treatment with eculizumab was referred to us from Argentina. Although the known C5 polymorphism, c.2654G > A, was not identified in this patient, a new mutation, c.2653C > T, which predicts p.Arg885Cys, was found in the nucleotide next to the known polymorphism (Fig. 18.3). To analyze the prevalence and distribution of this new polymorphism, the same DNA panels described above were also screened. This mutation was not identified in the 120 Han Chinese, the 100 British, or the 90 people of Mexican ancestry, suggesting that the prevalence of this polymorphism might be too low to be detected with this small sample size (Table 18.1).

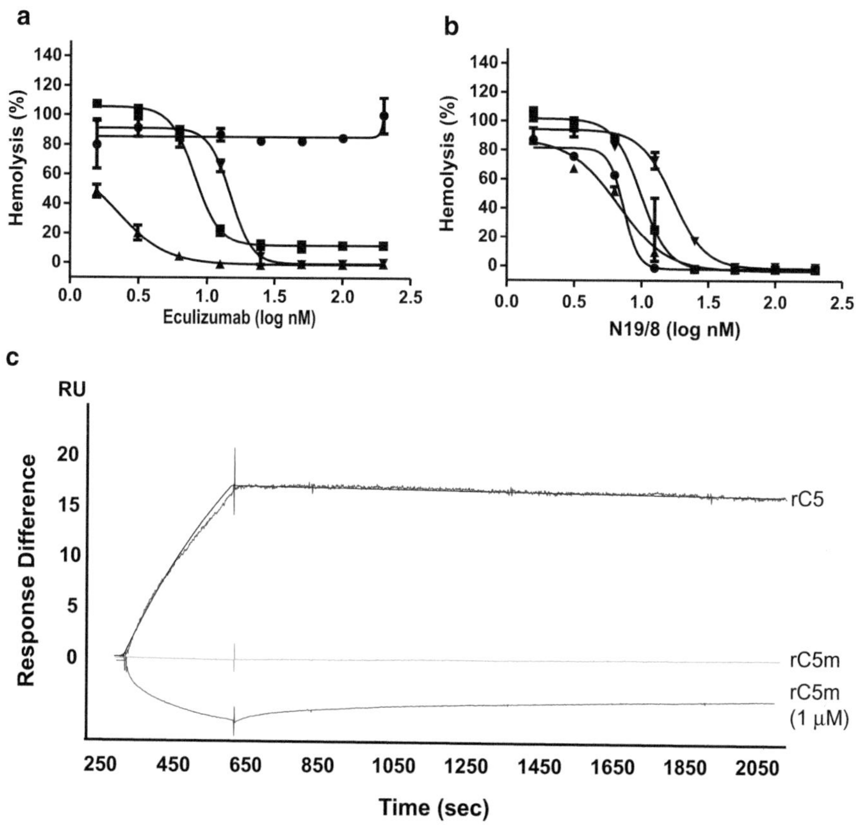

Fig. 18.4 The effect of the Japanese C5 polymorphism on the functional properties of C5 (Original Article, Nishimura J, et al., Genetic Variants in C5 and Poor Response to Eculizumab, 370, 632–639, Copyright © (2014) Massachusetts Medical Society. Reprinted with permission). *Panels A* and *B* show the effect of exogenous eculizumab and N19/8, respectively, on in vitro hemolytic activity reconstituted with either normal human serum (▼) or C5-depleted serum containing either native human C5 (nC5, ▲), recombinant C5 (rC5, ■), or recombinant mutant C5 (rC5 m, ●). Eculizumab did not block lysis reconstituted with rC5 m but did block rC5- and nC5-dependent lysis. In contrast, N19/8 inhibited lysis reconstituted with nC5, rC5, and rC5 m. *Panel C* shows the binding by surface plasmon resonance (Biacore 3000) of eculizumab to rC5 with or without the mutation. Eculizumab bound rC5 but did not bind rC5 m at concentrations of less than 5 nM. Increasing the concentration of eculizumab up to 1 μM failed to elicit detectable binding to rC5 m

18.6 Conclusions

Two patients with PNH enrolled in the Japanese AEGIS study did not exhibit the characteristic response to eculizumab treatment. Sera from these poor responders exhibited hemolytic activity even in the presence of high concentrations of exogenously added eculizumab. However, the hemolytic activity was completely blocked

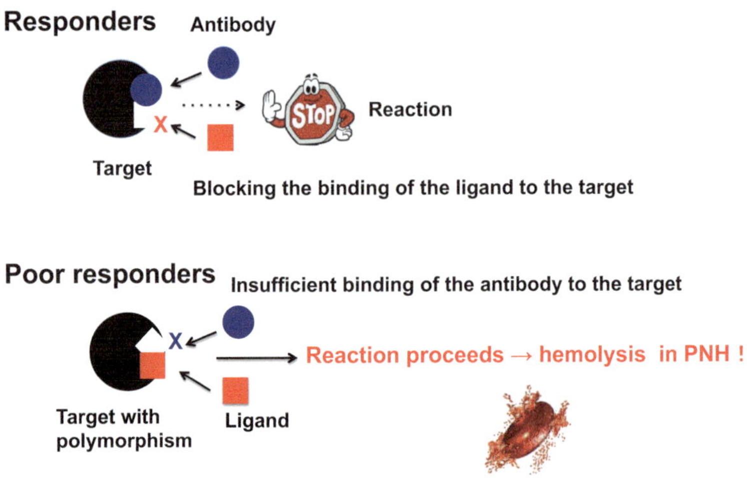

Fig. 18.5 The mechanism of poor response to antibody therapeutics by genetic polymorphisms of the target molecule

by an anti-C5 monoclonal antibody (N19/8), which binds to a different site than eculizumab. A single missense C5 heterozygous mutation, c.2654G > A, was identified in all of the 17 Japanese poor responders and in none of the responders. This polymorphism exhibited a very similar prevalence in patients with PNH (3.4 %) and the healthy population (3.5 %) and has been identified in one other Asian country. It was then showed that the hemolytic activity supported by this structural variant in vitro was not blocked by eculizumab, but was fully blocked by N19/8, and that the variant was incapable of binding eculizumab. Collectively, these data support the hypothesis that the functional capacity of the mutant C5, together with its inability to bind to eculizumab, accounts for the poor response in patients carrying this mutation.

A new polymorphism, c.2653C > T, which predicts p.Arg885Cys, was independently identified in a native Argentinian, thus indicating the importance of this site in C5 recognition by eculizumab and the potential for ethnic diversity with respect to this phenomenon. The Arg885His/Cys mutations are proximal to the C5 MG7 domain, which is near the known epitope for the binding of eculizumab [20] and is within the contact region between C5 convertase and bound C5 substrate, as inferred by Laursen et al. [21]. Evidently, considering the high specificity of monoclonal antibody binding, although these mutations disrupt the eculizumab epitope, they maintain the capacity of rC5 m to undergo cleavage by C5 convertase. Therefore, it was concluded that poor response to eculizumab in a subset of Japanese patients could be explained by the inability of a subset of lysis-competent C5 in these patients to bind and undergo blockade by eculizumab. Polymorphisms in the target proteins of antibody-based treatments that are used for other diseases might also be a point of consideration for poor responder cases (Fig. 18.5) [22–24].

Acknowledgment Supported by Alexion Pharmaceuticals, JSPS KAKENHI Grant Number JP 26461447, and a grant from SENSHIN Medical Research Foundation.

References

1. Miyata T, Takeda J, Iida Y et al (1993) The cloning of PIG-A, a component in the early step of GPI-anchor biosynthesis. Science 259:1318–1320
2. Takeda J, Miyata T, Kawagoe K et al (1993) Deficiency of the GPI anchor caused by a somatic mutation of the PIG-A gene in paroxysmal nocturnal hemoglobinuria. Cell 73:703–711
3. Miyata T, Yamada N, Iida Y et al (1994) Abnormalities of PIG-A transcripts in granulocytes from patients with paroxysmal nocturnal hemoglobinuria. N Engl J Med 330:249–255
4. Parker C, Omine M, Richards S et al (2005) Diagnosis and management of paroxysmal nocturnal hemoglobinuria. Blood 106:3699–3709
5. Brodsky RA (2009) How I treat paroxysmal nocturnal hemoglobinuria. Blood 113:6522–6527
6. Luzzatto L, Gianfaldoni G, Notaro R (2011) Management of paroxysmal nocturnal haemoglobinuria: a personal view. Br J Haematol 153:709–720
7. Hillmen P, Lewis SM, Bessler M et al (1995) Natural history of paroxysmal nocturnal hemoglobinuria. N Engl J Med 333:1253–1258
8. Socié G, Mary JY, de Gramont A et al (1996) Paroxysmal nocturnal haemoglobinuria: long-term follow-up and prognostic factors. French Society of Haematology. Lancet 348:573–577
9. Nishimura J, Kanakura Y, Ware RE et al (2004) Clinical course and flow cytometric analysis of paroxysmal nocturnal hemoglobinuria in the United States and Japan. Medicine 83:193–207
10. Rother RP, Rollins SA, Mojcik CF et al (2007) Discovery and development of the complement inhibitor eculizumab for the treatment of paroxysmal nocturnal hemoglobinuria. Nat Biotechnol 25:1256–1264
11. Parker C (2009) Eculizumab for paroxysmal nocturnal haemoglobinuria. Lancet 373:759–767
12. Hillmen P, Hall C, Marsh JC et al (2004) Effect of eculizumab on hemolysis and transfusion requirements in patients with paroxysmal nocturnal hemoglobinuria. N Engl J Med 350:552–559
13. Hill A, Hillmen P, Richards SJ et al (2005) Sustained response and long-term safety of eculizumab in paroxysmal nocturnal hemoglobinuria. Blood 106:2559–2565
14. Hillmen P, Young NS, Schubert J et al (2006) The complement inhibitor eculizumab in paroxysmal nocturnal hemoglobinuria. N Engl J Med 355:1233–1243
15. Hillmen P, Muus P, Dührsen U et al (2007) Effect of the complement inhibitor eculizumab on thromboembolism in patients with paroxysmal nocturnal hemoglobinuria. Blood 110:4123–4128
16. Brodsky RA, Young NS, Antonioli E et al (2008) Multicenter phase 3 study of the complement inhibitor eculizumab for the treatment of patients with paroxysmal nocturnal hemoglobinuria. Blood 111:1840–1847
17. Kanakura Y, Ohyashiki K, Shichishima T et al (2011) Safety and efficacy of the terminal complement inhibitor eculizumab in Japanese patients with paroxysmal nocturnal hemoglobinuria: the AEGIS Clinical Trial. Int J Hematol 93:36–46
18. Kanakura Y, Ohyashiki K, Shichishima T et al (2013) Long-term efficacy and safety of eculizumab in Japanese patients with PNH: AEGIS trial. Int J Hematol 98:406–416
19. Nishimura J, Yamamoto M, Hayashi S et al (2014) Genetic variants in C5 and poor response to eculizumab. N Engl J Med 370:632–639

20. Zuber J, Fakhouri F, Roumenina LT et al (2012) Use of eculizumab for atypical haemolytic uraemic syndrome and C3 glomerulopathies. Nat Rev Nephrol 8:643–657
21. Laursen NS, Andersen KR, Braren I et al (2011) Substrate recognition by complement convertases revealed in the C5–cobra venom factor complex. EMBO J 30:606–616
22. Wu J, Edberg JC, Redecha PB et al (1997) A novel polymorphism of FcgammaRIIIa (CD16) alters receptor function and predisposes to autoimmune disease. J Clin Invest 100:1059–1070
23. Cartron G, Dacheux L, Salles G et al (2002) Therapeutic activity of humanized anti-CD20 monoclonal antibody and polymorphism in IgG Fc receptor FcgammaRIIIa gene. Blood 99:754–758
24. Treon SP, Hansen M, Branagan AR et al (2005) Polymorphisms in FcgammaRIIIA (CD16) receptor expression are associated with clinical response to rituximab in Waldenstrom's macroglobulinemia. J Clin Oncol 23:474–481

Chapter 19
Hematopoietic Stem Cell Transplantation in PNH

Gérard Socié and Régis Peffault de Latour

Abstract The only curative treatment for PNH is hematopoietic stem cell transplantation (HSCT). However, the risk of treatment-related mortality after HSCT is relatively high, with graft-versus-host disease (GvHD) accounting for most of the transplant-related deaths. In recent years, the introduction of eculizumab, a humanized monoclonal antibody directed against the terminal complement protein C5, has had a major impact on the management of PNH. Eculizumab is highly effective in reducing intravascular hemolysis and seems to reduce the risk of thrombosis markedly. The decision to perform an HSCT in PNH has usually been deferred until disease progression to recurrent, life-threatening thromboembolism, refractory or transfusion-dependent hemolytic anemia, or development of severe aplastic anemia. Indications for HSCT should weight the natural history of the disease, the prognostic risk factors, as well as specific complications related to transplantation. Here we reviewed both single-center studies and registry studies to identify the best candidates eligible for an HSCT in patients with PNH in the complement inhibitors era.

Keywords Hematopoietic stem cell transplantation • Paroxysmal nocturnal hemoglobinuria • Thrombosis • Aplastic anemia • Hemolytic anemia

---

G. Socié, M.D., Ph.D. (✉)
Hematology-Transplantation, Hospital Saint-Louis, Assistance Publique – Hôpitaux de Paris, 1 Avenue Claude Vellefaux, 75475 Paris CEDEX 10 Paris, France

University Paris VII, Denis Diderot, Paris, France

Inserm UMR 1160, Paris, France
e-mail: gerard.socie@sls.aphp.fr

R.P. de Latour, M.D., Ph.D.
Hematology-Transplantation, Hospital Saint-Louis, Assistance Publique – Hôpitaux de Paris, 1 Avenue Claude Vellefaux, 75475 Paris CEDEX 10 Paris, France

University Paris VII, Denis Diderot, Paris, France

Y. Kanakura et al. (eds.), *Paroxysmal Nocturnal Hemoglobinuria*,
DOI 10.1007/978-4-431-56003-6_19

19.1 Introduction

Although allogeneic hematopoietic stem cell transplantation (HSCT) is the only curative treatment for paroxysmal nocturnal hemoglobinuria (PNH), its place, timing, and modalities are still highly controversial. It has been over 40 years since the first report by the Seattle group of a patient transplanted from his twin brother [1]. In the era of eculizumab, identifying patients with PNH who may benefit from allogeneic stem cell transplantation is challenging. A systematic search for reports of HSCT for PNH through the National Library of Medicine (PubMed) disclosed as of August 1, 2014, 279 articles matching the criteria "paroxysmal nocturnal hemoglobinuria" and "transplantation." Of these 279 articles, meaningful information on patients' data was available from 33 articles that have been used for the purpose of this chapter [2–33]. Since PNH is a rare disease, a number of patients in each series are limited with only three single-center studies involving more than 15 patients [4, 16, 33]. Registry data from the International Bone Marrow Transplant Registry (IBMTR) [20], from the Italian group for research in HSCT (Gruppo Italiano Trapianto Midollo Osseo or GITMO) [28], and from the European Group for Blood and Marrow Transplantation (EBMT) [31] are also summarized. Finally, current issues in 2014 on HSCT for PNH are discussed.

19.2 Transplantation for PNH: Single-Center Experience

Data on 108 patients could be traced from the literature with special attention to duplicate patient reporting [2–33].

From these 108 patients, 8 have been transplanted from a twin donor [1, 5, 7, 11, 14, 16, 17]. In these syngeneic transplants, four patients have been transplanted without conditioning, and four either rejected their graft or relapsed posttransplant. It is of note that the first patient transplanted [1] with a twin in the 1970s had very late relapse and that relapse of PNH was associated with the emergence of a new mutation in the PIG-A gene [34]. Other authors have used conditioning regimen before HSCT from twin donors ($n=3$) of whom only one showed evidence of relapse. Thus, from this limited data set, it appears that before syngeneic transplantation, conditioning regimen seems to be mandatory.

Among the 100 patients who underwent an allogeneic transplant, 69 have been transplanted from an HLA-identical sibling, 17 from an unrelated donor, 9 from unrelated cord blood, and 5 from a haploidentical family member.

Fifty-two patients received a myeloablative conditioning that was irradiation based in 20 (38 %), busulfan based in 18 (34 %), and used cyclophosphamide/ATG as in aplastic anemia in 7 patients (13 %) (other various conditionings were delivered in 7 patients). The follow-up of these patients transplanted after a myeloablative conditioning ranges from a few months to over 15 years. Most recently, the use of non-myeloablative conditioning (NMA) [13, 22, 24] has been advocated in this disease ($n=34$ patients) using either fludarabine and 2 Gy total body irradiation [13] ($n=7$) or fludarabine cyclophosphamide ($n=27$) [24, 33]. Although the preliminary results of these non-myeloablative regimens are really interesting, the follow-up of these patients is still short, and graft-versus-host disease (GvHD) remains a problem.

Both after myeloablative and NMA conditioning, the indication for transplantation seemed to be mainly aplastic anemia in 60 % of the case and mainly hemolysis/thrombosis in 40 % of the case. Severe acute GvHD of grade II or more was reported in 37 % of the case and was, as expected, the major cause of death. From all these studies, 75 % of the patients have been reported to be alive at last follow-up (months to years). Only one study provided a Kaplan-Meier estimates of 58 +/−13 % overall survival at 5 years [4], a figure far less optimistic than the one depicted from the 75 % crude incidence from all other reports. It is highly likely that this is related with publication bias, with centers who did not report small numbers of patients with bad outcome.

19.3 Transplantation for PNH: Registry Studies

The outcome of 57 consecutive allogeneic bone marrow transplants for PNH, median age 28 (range 10–47) years, reported to the IBMTR between 1978 and 1995 by 31 centers was analyzed in 1999 [20]. Source of hematopoietic cells consisted of matched related donor ($n=48$), syngeneic ($n=2$), or alternative donors (6 matched unrelated donor and 1 haploidentical donor). The majority of patients received a myeloablative conditioning regimen (busulfan plus cyclophosphamide, 53 %, and total body irradiation plus cyclophosphamide, 21 %). Sixteen were grafted for an aplastic anemia/PNH syndrome. The incidence of acute GvHD of grade II or more was 34 %, and that of chronic GvHD of 33 %. The 2-year probability of survival in 48 recipients of HLA-identical sibling transplants was 56 % (95 % confidence interval 49–63 %), and the median follow-up was 44 months. Two recipients of identical twin transplants remained alive 8 and 12 years after treatment. Only 1 of 7 alternative donor allograft recipients was alive at the 5-year follow-up. The most common causes of treatment failure were graft failure ($n=7$) and infections ($n=3$). This study suggested that TRM may be more pronounced in recipients of alternative donor allografts. Nonetheless, the study was limited by its retrospective nature and the relative small sample size.

More recently, Santarone et al. on behalf of the Gruppo Italiano Trapianto Midollo Osseo (GITMO), report on a retrospective study of 26 patients (median age, 32 years) who received an HSCT for PNH (4 AA/PNH) in Italy between 1988 and 2006 [28]. HLA-matched sibling donors were used for 22 patients; one patient received stem cells from a matched unrelated donor, and three received stem cells from mismatched donors (two related and one unrelated). A myeloablative conditioning regimen (busulfan+cyclophosphamide) was used for 15 patients. The remaining 11 patients received a variety of different reduced intensity conditioning regimens, most being cyclophosphamide or fludarabine based. Graft-versus-host disease prophylaxis was highly variable but largely cyclosporine based. Acute graft-versus-host disease greater than stage 2 occurred in 3 of the 26 patients; chronic graft-versus-host disease occurred in 10 of 20 evaluable patients with 4 (16 %) experiencing extensive chronic graft-versus-host disease. The 10-year probability of survival was 57 % for all patients, with a median follow-up of 131 months. There was one primary graft failure in a patient receiving a myeloablative conditioning regimen and one secondary graft failure in a patient who received a reduced intensity conditioning bone marrow transplantation; both patients eventually died from complications of a second transplant. The transplant-related mortality at 1 year was 26 % in patients receiving a myeloablative conditioning regimen and 63 % in the group that received a reduced intensity conditioning regimen.

The largest study published so far was the report of the European group for Blood and Marrow Transplantation (EBMT) experience in 2012 [31]. The characteristics and overall survival of 211 patients transplanted for PNH in 83 EBMT centers from 1978 to 2007 were analyzed. The three main indications for SCT were aplastic anemia ($n=100$, 48 %), severe recurrent hemolytic crisis ($n=64$, 30 %), and thrombosis ($n=47$, 22 %). Engraftment failed in 14 (7 %) of the 202 transplanted patients for whom there was documentation on this aspect. Eighty-five patients developed acute GvHD leading to a CIF of grade II–IV acute GvHD of 40 % (95% CI 34–47 %). Fifty-seven patients developed chronic GvHD (extensive, $n=24$) leading to a CIF of 29 % (95% CI 23–36 %) at 5 years. After a median (±standard error) follow-up time of 61 ± 6 months, 64 patients had died, and the 5-year OS probability was 68 % ± 3 % (Fig 19.1a). Infections and GvHD were the main causes of death. None of the variables investigated for an association with transplant outcome was a statistically significant predictor of survival, except for the indication for HSCT with outcome being worse if the indication for HSCT was thromboembolism ($p=0.03$). The 5-year OS probability was 54 ± 7 % in the case of TE, 69 ± 5 % in the case of AA without TE, and 86 ± 6 % in the case of recurrent hemolytic anemia without TE or AA (Fig. 19.1b). Of note, donor type (unrelated versus sibling) led to similar results. Risk factors for survival were also analyzed in patients who were transplanted for TE ($n=47$) or for AA without TE ($n=100$). In multivariate analysis, no factor related to survival was identified in patients transplanted for TE. A long delay (>1 year between the diagnosis of AA and transplantation) ($P=0.007$) and transplantation performed before or in 2002 ($p=0.05$) were associated with poor survival in patients transplanted for AA.

In this large study, a comparison with a cohort of 402 non-transplanted patients with PNH diagnosed between 1950 and 2005 in 92 French centers was conducted. The occurrence of complications (i.e., thromboembolism and aplastic anemia) using either an individual or a stratum-matching procedure was compared between both cohorts. Twenty-four pairs of transplanted and non-transplanted patients with thromboembolism were identified for the matched comparison, with worse overall survival for the transplanted patients (hazard ratio = 10.0; 95 % confidence interval, 1.3–78.1; $P=0.007$). This was confirmed by the global matching procedure ($P=0.03$). As regards aplastic anemia without thromboembolism, 30 pairs were

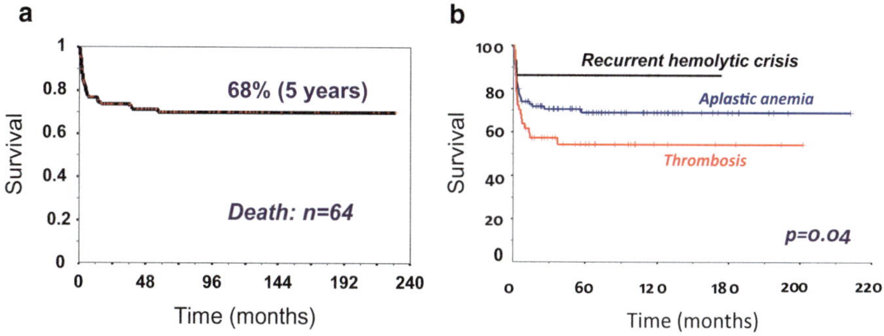

Fig. 19.1 Overall survival (panel **a**) and risk factors associated with overall survival (panel **b**) in 211 patients transplanted for PNH (EBMT study). Panel **a**: all patients are presented. Median follow-up is 61 months. Panel **b**: overall survival according to indications for transplantation is presented. Sixty-four patients were transplanted because of recurrent hemolytic crisis, 100 for aplastic anemia and 47 for thrombosis

identified for the matched comparison. It was not observed that transplanted patients had a significantly worse overall survival (hazard ratio = 4.0; 95 % confidence interval, 0.9–18.9; $P = 0.06$). A global matching procedure was not feasible.

The conclusions of this large study were as follows: (1) HSCT could no longer be considered as a standard of care of PNH patients with thromboembolism when eculizumab is available. (2) regarding the good results of HSCT in the case of recurrent hemolytic crises, HSCT can be a valuable option for patients living in countries which cannot afford eculizumab regardless of the type of donor, and (3) AA-PNH patients still seem to be appropriate candidates for SCT if they have severe disease.

19.4 Current Issues in Transplantation for PNH

The main issue for transplantation in PNH is the highly polymorphic presentation of the disease and its often unpredictable course. Data from the French Society of Hematology on 460 patients represent today the largest data set on PNH analyzed, so far [35]. The analysis of the French cohort showed that the median survival time of patients with PNH is 22 years, thus making the hazardous decision on HSCT hard to take. However, this study also pointed out some risk factors associated with a worse outcome. Although some of the risk factors are of little help for transplant decision (diagnosis before 1996, hazard ratio 2.6; age older than 40 years, HR 2.2), other factors may help physicians in their decision such as blood count at time of PNH diagnosis (hemoglobin level less than or equal to 100 g/L (10 g/dL) with an HR of 3.0 and neutropenia with an HR of 1.7) as well as severe complications occurring during follow-up such as progression to bicytopenia or pancytopenia

(HR, 3.5), development of thrombosis (HR, 15.4), and myelodysplastic syndrome or acute myeloid leukemia (HR, 15.2).

This large retrospective study has also allowed analyzing, for the first time, the disease subcategories at diagnosis and their complications during follow-up. Although clinical presentation and prognosis factors are different between classic PNH and AA-PNH syndrome, outcomes do not appear to be clearly different and are affected mainly by post-diagnosis complications, notably thrombosis, which is the main prognosis factor in all disease subcategories. Myelodysplastic syndrome and acute myeloid leukemia are classic but rare complications of PNH. Overall, speaking about indication for HSCT in PNH depends on which disease subcategories (i.e., classic PNH or AA-PNH) and/or complications (i.e., thrombosis or secondary MDS/AML) the patients are presented at time of HSCT.

19.4.1 HSCT and AA-PNH Syndrome

The introduction of flow cytometry (FC) in the 1990s as a diagnostic tool allows the detection of small clones that would otherwise not be identified. Of note, not only have diagnostic tools changed since the 1990s but also clinical presentations (R. Peffault de Latour, unpublished data, March 2007). The use of FC has thus made it possible to more frequently diagnose patients with PNH, compared with the classic Ham test, especially for patients with AA-PNH in the recent period.

In patients with overt AA-PNH syndrome (i.e., aplastic anemia with a "small" PNH clone) and no hemolysis, the reference treatment is the same than patients with AA and no PNH. Bone marrow transplantation (BMT) from a HLA-identical related donor is thus the treatment of choice for young patients with a severe disease. Cyclophosphamide (CY) with antithymocyte globulin (ATG) as conditioning regimen and the association of cyclosporine plus methotrexate as graft-versus-host disease prophylaxis represent an effective treatment, with rate of engraftment of 95 % and overall survival near 90 % [36]. All these aspects, marrow source, conditioning with CY+ATG, and GVHD prophylaxis by cyclosporine+methotrexate represent the gold standard in transplantation for acquired aplastic anemia in patients transplanted from an HLA-identical sibling donors. All deviations from this standard lead to poorer outcomes. Given these excellent results, survival is thus no more the sole concern in this situation, and prevention/early detection of late complications after BMT is currently the main objective of allogeneic BMT in this setting. For patients who lack an HLA-identical sibling donor, immunosuppressive therapy (IST) remains the treatment of choice which has been just reviewed [37]. However, 30–40 % of the patients will eventually relapse or be refractory to IST and will thus be considered for transplantation using an alternative donor. A molecularly HLA-matched unrelated donor is in this situation the best alternative possibility (Fig. 19.2). The use of other alternative sources of stem cells including cord blood or haploidentical familial donor has been recently reviewed [38].

19.4.2 HSCT and Recurrent Hemolytic Crisis and/or Thrombosis

In recent years, the introduction of eculizumab, a humanized monoclonal antibody directed against the terminal complement protein C5, has had a major impact on the management of PNH. Eculizumab is highly effective in reducing intravascular hemolysis and seems to reduce the risk of thrombosis markedly and eventually improved overall survival [39–42]. However, roughly 50 % of patients will require transfusions under eculizumab [40]. It increases the risk of meningococcal sepsis, and the very long-term survival with eculizumab is not yet well known. Moreover, eculizumab is expensive (around € 300,000 per year for each patient), does not eradicate the PNH clone, and must be given lifelong. As previously described, HSCT offers a chance for cure, but rates for mortality and morbidity are high.

The excellent overall survival [42] and the benefit in terms of quality of life [40] in patients with PNH and recurrent hemolytic crisis favor the use of eculizumab in this situation (Fig. 19.2). However, in the large retrospective study of the EBMT, 64 patients were transplanted because of recurrent hemolytic crisis with an excellent 5-year overall survival of 86 ± 6 %. However, those latter patients may be exposed in the future to a 30 % risk of chronic GvHD at 5 years post-HSCT. HSCT can thus be a valuable option for patients living in countries, which cannot afford eculizumab regardless of the type of donor.

Regarding thrombosis complication, the results of the matching comparison in the EBMT before eculizumab era suggested that HSCT can no longer be considered a standard of care for PNH patients with thromboembolism due to an unacceptable high rate of toxicity. The place of a reduced intensity-conditioning regimen in PNH, especially for patients with moderate organ dysfunction who may not tolerate a myeloablative regimen, is still unknown. Published studies on the subject are scarce to draw any meaningful conclusion. Moreover, In the EBMT study, 42 patients received a fludarabine-based reduced intensity conditioning regimen and showed no difference in terms of treatment-related mortality or OS [31]. However, the retrospective setting of this study as well as the heterogeneity of the conditioning regimens precluded further analyses. Overall, HSCT should be considered in this situation only for patients with thromboembolism while on eculizumab (Fig. 19.2).

19.4.3 HSCT and Myelodysplastic Syndrome or Acute Myeloid Leukemia I Patients with PNH

Myelodysplastic syndrome and acute myeloid leukemia are classic but rare complications of PNH, with a more than 100-fold increased risk compared with age-matched controls. The association with poor prognosis of this complication in PNH has been extensively reported [35, 43, 44]. However, only two series have analyzed the outcomes of those patients more precisely, mainly in the context of AA [45, 46].

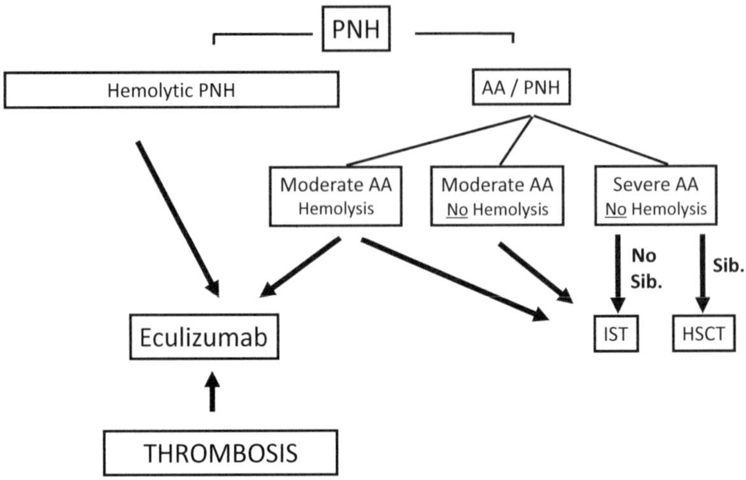

Fig. 19.2 PNH treatment algorithm in 2014. *AA* aplastic anemia, *IST* immunosuppressive treatment, *HSCT* hematopoietic stem cell transplantation

Overall, data indicate that allogeneic HSCT leads to prolonged survival in close to one-half of the patients transforming to MDS or AML from SAA, with better outcome for patients untreated at time of HSCT and patients in remission compared with patients with refractory disease.

19.5 Conclusions and Perspectives

In conclusion, given the results of the comparison between transplantation and best supportive care before eculizumab was available for patients with PNH and TE complications [31], HSCT can no longer be considered as a standard of care of PNH patients with TE when eculizumab is available. The same conclusion can be made regarding hemolytic PNH without TE. However, regarding the good results of HSCT in the case of recurrent hemolytic crises, HSCT can be a valuable option for patients living in countries, which cannot afford eculizumab, regardless of the type of donor. AA-PNH patients are candidates for HSCT if they have a severe disease and a matched family donor available. In the absence of an HLA-identical sibling donor, the current standard, first-line treatment for AA-PNH syndrome is IST combining horse antithymocyte globulins and cyclosporine. If refractory to IST, a matched unrelated donor can be proposed whatever the PNH status is.

Some questions are still open. Should we give eculizumab to a young patient (less than 18 years old) with recurrent hemolytic crisis without thrombosis and an available matched family donor? Eculizumab does not eradicate the PNH clone and must be given lifelong. Moreover, mortality and morbidity are classically low for young patients transplanted from siblings. In case of recurrent thrombosis under eculizumab and anticoagulation, it is difficult not to proceed to HSCT since thrombosis remains in PNH the most important risk factor associated with survival.

Although the preliminary results of non-myeloablative regimens are really interesting, the follow-up of these patients is still short, and graft-versus-host disease (GvHD) remains a problem. More work is on the way, and progress should be done quickly in this field. Finally, experimental transplantation is also emerging in PNH patients with few publications on both haplo and cord blood HSCT reported. For the moment, patients with PNH transplanted in this setting should be included only in experimented centers within well-designed prospective trials.

Disclosure of Conflicts of Interest GS and RPL are consultants for Alexion Pharmaceuticals.

References

1. Storb R, Evans RS, Thomas ED et al (1973) Paroxysmal nocturnal haemoglobinuria and refractory marrow failure treated by marrow transplantation. Br J Haematol 24:743–750
2. Antin JH, Ginsburg D, Smith BR, Nathan DG, Orkin SH, Rappeport JM (1985) Bone marrow transplantation for paroxysmal nocturnal hemoglobinuria: eradication of the PNH clone and documentation of complete lymphohematopoietic engraftment. Blood 66:1247–1250
3. Appelbaum FR, Fefer A, Cheever MA et al (1980) Treatment of aplastic anemia by bone marrow transplantation in identical twins. Blood 55:1033–1039
4. Bemba M, Guardiola P, Garderet L et al (1999) Bone marrow transplantation for paroxysmal nocturnal haemoglobinuria. Br J Haematol 105:366–368
5. Cho SG, Lim J, Kim Y et al (2001) Conditioning with high-dose cyclophosphamide may not be sufficient to provide a long-term remission of paroxysmal nocturnal hemoglobinuria following syngeneic peripheral blood stem cell transplantation. Bone Marrow Transplant 28:987–988
6. de Souza MH, Abdelhay E, Silva ML et al (1992) Late marrow allograft rejection following alpha-interferon therapy for hepatitis in a patient with paroxysmal nocturnal hemoglobinuria. Bone Marrow Transplant 9:495–497
7. Doukas MA, Fleming D, Jennings D (1998) Identical twin marrow transplantation for venous thrombosis in paroxysmal nocturnal hemoglobinuria; long-term complete remission as assessed by flow cytometry. Bone Marrow Transplant 22:717–721
8. Endo M, Beatty PG, Vreeke TM, Wittwer CT, Singh SP, Parker CJ (1996) Syngeneic bone marrow transplantation without conditioning in a patient with paroxysmal nocturnal hemoglobinuria: in vivo evidence that the mutant stem cells have a survival advantage. Blood 88:742–750
9. Fefer A, Freeman H, Storb R et al (1976) Paroxysmal nocturanal hemoglobinuria and marrow failure treated by infusion of marrow from an identical twin. Ann Intern Med 84:692–695
10. Flotho C, Strahm B, Kontny U et al (2002) Stem cell transplantation for paroxysmal nocturnal haemoglobinuria in childhood. Br J Haematol 118:124–127
11. Graham ML, Rosse WF, Halperin EC, Miller CR, Ware RE (1996) Resolution of Budd-Chiari syndrome following bone marrow transplantation for paroxysmal nocturnal haemoglobinuria. Br J Haematol 92:707–710
12. Grosskreutz C, Ross V, Scigliano E, Fruchtman S, Isola L (2003) Low-dose total body irradiation, fludarabine, and antithymocyte globulin conditioning for nonmyeloablative allogeneic transplantation. Biol Blood Marrow Transplant 9:453–459

13. Hegenbart U, Niederwieser D, Forman S et al (2003) Hematopoietic cell transplantation from related and unrelated donors after minimal conditioning as a curative treatment modality for severe paroxysmal nocturnal hemoglobinuria. Biol Blood Marrow Transplant 9:689–697
14. Hershko C, Gale RP, Ho WG, Cline MJ (1979) Cure of aplastic anaemia in paroxysmal nocturnal haemoglobinuria by marrow transfusion from identical twin: Failure of peripheral-leucocyte transfusion to correct marrow aplasia. Lancet 1:945–947
15. Jehn U, Sauer H, Kolb HJ et al (1983) Bone marrow transplantation in adults in acute leukemia, aplastic anemia and paroxysmal nocturnal hemoglobinuria. Results of the Medical Clinic IIi of LMU (Ludwig-Maximilians University) Munich. Klin Wochenschr 61:321–328
16. Kawahara K, Witherspoon RP, Storb R (1992) Marrow transplantation for paroxysmal nocturnal hemoglobinuria. Am J Hematol 39:283–288
17. Kolb HJ, Holler E, Bender-Gotze C et al (1989) Myeloablative conditioning for marrow transplantation in myelodysplastic syndromes and paroxysmal nocturnal haemoglobinuria. Bone Marrow Transplant 4:29–34
18. Lee JL, Lee JH, Lee JH et al (2003) Allogeneic hematopoietic cell transplantation for paroxysmal nocturnal hemoglobinuria. Eur J Haematol 71:114–118
19. Raiola AM, Van Lint MT, Lamparelli T et al (2000) Bone marrow transplantation for paroxysmal nocturnal hemoglobinuria. Haematologica 85:59–62
20. Saso R, Marsh J, Cevreska L et al (1999) Bone marrow transplants for paroxysmal nocturnal haemoglobinuria. Br J Haematol 104:392–396
21. Shaw PH, Haut PR, Olszewski M, Kletzel M (1999) Hematopoietic stem-cell transplantation using unrelated cord-blood versus matched sibling marrow in pediatric bone marrow failure syndrome: one center's experience. Pediatr Transplant 3:315–321
22. Suenaga K, Kanda Y, Niiya H et al (2001) Successful application of nonmyeloablative transplantation for paroxysmal nocturnal hemoglobinuria. Exp Hematol 29:639–642
23. Szer J, Deeg HJ, Witherspoon RP et al (1984) Long-term survival after marrow transplantation for paroxysmal nocturnal hemoglobinuria with aplastic anemia. Ann Intern Med 101:193–195
24. Takahashi Y, McCoy JP Jr, Carvallo C et al (2004) In vitro and in vivo evidence of PNH cell sensitivity to immune attack after nonmyeloablative allogeneic hematopoietic cell transplantation. Blood 103:1383–1390
25. Woodard P, Wang W, Pitts N et al (2001) Successful unrelated donor bone marrow transplantation for paroxysmal nocturnal hemoglobinuria. Bone Marrow Transplant 27:589–592
26. Markiewicz M, Wojciechowska M, Wylezol I et al (2005) First two successful unrelated donor bone marrow transplantations for paroxysmal nocturnal hemoglobinuria in Poland. Ann Transplant 10:26–30
27. Brodsky RA, Luznik L, Bolanos-Meade J, Leffell MS, Jones RJ, Fuchs EJ (2008) Reduced intensity HLA-haploidentical BMT with post transplantation cyclophosphamide in nonmalignant hematologic diseases. Bone Marrow Transplant 42:523–527
28. Santarone S, Bacigalupo A, Risitano AM et al (2010) Hematopoietic stem cell transplantation for paroxysmal nocturnal hemoglobinuria: long-term results of a retrospective study on behalf of the Gruppo Italiano Trapianto Midollo Osseo (GITMO). Haematologica 95:983–988
29. Peffault de Latour R, Purtill D, Ruggeri A, et al (2011) Influence of nucleated cell dose on overall survival of unrelated cord blood transplantation for patients with severe acquired aplastic anemia: a study by eurocord and the aplastic anemia working party of the European group for blood and marrow transplantation. Biol Blood Marrow Transplant 17:78–85
30. Taniguchi K, Okada M, Yoshihara S et al (2011) Strategy for bone marrow transplantation in eculizumab-treated paroxysmal nocturnal hemoglobinuria. Int J Hematol 94:403–407
31. Peffault de Latour R, Schrezenmeier H, Bacigalupo A, et al (2012) Allogeneic stem cell transplantation in paroxysmal nocturnal hemoglobinuria. Haematologica 97:1666–1673
32. Munoz-Linares C, Ojeda E, Fores R et al (2014) Paroxysmal nocturnal hemoglobinuria: a single Spanish center's experience over the last 40 yr. Eur J Haematol 93:309–319

33. Pantin J, Tian X, Geller N et al (2014) Long-term outcome of fludarabine-based reduced-intensity allogeneic hematopoietic cell transplantation for debilitating paroxysmal nocturnal hemoglobinuria. Biol Blood Marrow Transplant 20:1435–1439
34. Nafa K, Bessler M, Deeg HJ, Luzzatto L (1998) New somatic mutation in the PIG-A gene emerges at relapse of paroxysmal nocturnal hemoglobinuria. Blood 92:3422–3427
35. Peffault de Latour R, Mary JY, Salanoubat C, et al (2008) Paroxysmal nocturnal hemoglobinuria: natural history of disease subcategories. Blood 112:3099–3106
36. Socie G (2013) Allogeneic BM transplantation for the treatment of aplastic anemia: current results and expanding donor possibilities. Hematology Am Soc Hematol Educ Program 1:82–86
37. Young NS (2013) Current concepts in the pathophysiology and treatment of aplastic anemia. Hematology Am Soc Hematol Educ Program 1:76–81
38. Marsh JC, Kulasekararaj AG (2013) Management of the refractory aplastic anemia patient: what are the options? Blood 122:3561–3567
39. Hillmen P, Hall C, Marsh JC et al (2004) Effect of eculizumab on hemolysis and transfusion requirements in patients with paroxysmal nocturnal hemoglobinuria. N Engl J Med 350:552–559
40. Hillmen P, Young NS, Schubert J et al (2006) The complement inhibitor eculizumab in paroxysmal nocturnal hemoglobinuria. N Engl J Med 355:1233–1243
41. Brodsky RA, Young NS, Antonioli E et al (2008) Multicenter phase 3 study of the complement inhibitor eculizumab for the treatment of patients with paroxysmal nocturnal hemoglobinuria. Blood 111:1840–1847
42. Kelly RJ, Hill A, Arnold LM et al (2011) Long-term treatment with eculizumab in paroxysmal nocturnal hemoglobinuria: sustained efficacy and improved survival. Blood 117:6786–6792
43. Socie G, Mary JY, de Gramont A et al (1996) Paroxysmal nocturnal haemoglobinuria: long-term follow-up and prognostic factors. French Society of Haematology. Lancet 348:573–577
44. Hillmen P, Lewis SM, Bessler M, Luzzatto L, Dacie JV (1995) Natural history of paroxysmal nocturnal hemoglobinuria. N Engl J Med 333:1253–1258
45. Yoshimi A, Strahm B, Baumann I et al (2014) Hematopoietic stem cell transplantation in children and young adults with secondary myelodysplastic syndrome and acute myelogenous leukemia after aplastic anemia. Biol Blood Marrow Transplant 20:425–429
46. Hussein AA, Halkes CM, Socie G et al (2014) Outcome of allogeneic stem cell transplantation for patients transformed to myelodysplastic syndrome or leukemia from severe aplastic anemia: a report from the MDS subcommittee of the chronic malignancies working party and the severe aplastic anemia working party of the European group for blood and marrow transplantation. Biol Blood Marrow Transplant 20:1448–1450

Chapter 20
Future Strategies of Complement Inhibition in Paroxysmal Nocturnal Hemoglobinuria

Antonio M. Risitano

Abstract The treatment of paroxysmal nocturnal hemoglobinuria (PNH) has dramatically changed since the availability of the first clinical complement inhibitor eculizumab. Eculizumab treatment has been proven terrifically effective in controlling intravascular hemolysis of PNH; however, unmet clinical needs are emerging, starting with the possible occurrence of C3-mediated extravascular hemolysis. Indeed, scientific and commercial reasons have triggered the development of a number of novel anticomplement agents. Different strategies are currently under investigation, which may target distinct steps and pathways of the complement system. Indeed, starting from the anti-C5 therapy that is already in the clinic, novel approaches are investigating the possibility of intercepting the complement cascade upstream, at the level of C3 and C3 convertase or of other initiating factors. Here we will review the majority of these strategies, focusing on available data in PNH and/or other preclinical models. The possible relevance for clinical application in PNH will be highlighted, based on well-established and emerging knowledge of molecular complement derangement in PNH.

Keywords PNH • C3 • C5 • CCP • CAP • CMP

20.1 Introduction

Paroxysmal nocturnal hemoglobinuria (PNH) [1–3] is a rare hematological disorder due to a somatic mutation in the *phosphatidylinositol glycan class A (PIG-A)* gene [4, 5], which impairs the biosynthesis of the glycosyl-phosphatidylinositol (GPI) anchor and the subsequent expression of a number of surface proteins on blood cells. Epidemiology, pathophysiology, clinical presentation, and treatment of PNH have been extensively described in other chapters of this book; thus they will not be

A.M. Risitano, M.D., Ph.D. (✉)
Hematology, Department of Clinical Medicine and Surgery, Federico II University of Naples, Via Pansini 5, 80131 Naples, Italy
e-mail: amrisita@unina.it

Y. Kanakura et al. (eds.), *Paroxysmal Nocturnal Hemoglobinuria*,
DOI 10.1007/978-4-431-56003-6_20

reviewed here. However, for a comprehensive discussion of anticomplement therapies, we feel appropriate a brief recall about some pathogenic mechanisms accounting for the clinical manifestations of PNH (which include hemolytic anemia, thrombophilia, and bone marrow failure). Indeed, among the several GPI-linked proteins which are lacking on PNH cells, two of them are physiological complement regulators and play a pivotal role in the pathophysiology of hemolytic anemia of PNH, possibly also contributing to the typical thrombophilia. CD55 (also known as decay accelerating factor, DAF) is a regulator of early complement activation [6], which physiologically inhibits the formation of C3 convertase (both C3bBb and C4b2a) and also promotes its decay [7]. CD59 (also known as membrane inhibitor of reactive lysis, MIRL) is rather a regulator of the terminal effector complement [8], which interacts with C8 and C9 inhibiting the incorporation of this latter onto the C5b-C8 complex, eventually preventing the assembly of the membrane attack complex (MAC) [9]. CD55 and CD59 are extremely important on red blood cell surface, which do not express other membrane complement inhibitors such as membrane cofactor protein (CD56), to prevent that harmful complement which may result in the destruction of cells. Thus, the concomitant lack of CD55 and CD59 renders PNH erythrocytes susceptible to complement activation, accounting for the chronic intravascular hemolysis which is the hallmark of PNH. The hierarchical contribution of CD55 and CD59 suggests that CD59 is the key protective molecule which, when absent, accounts for hemolysis [10]. Indeed, patients with an inherited isolated deficiency of CD55 (the so-called Inab phenotype) do not suffer from hemolysis [11, 12], and even in vitro data suggest that redundant mechanisms (possibly including CD59 itself) usually overcome the isolated deficiency of CD55 [13]. In contrast, anecdotic cases of inherited CD59 deficiency led to a clinical phenotype undistinguishable from PNH [14, 15], with susceptibility to hemolysis in vitro and in vivo.

20.2 The Need of Alternative Strategies of Complement Inhibition

The treatment of PNH has dramatically changed since the availability of the first complement inhibitor eculizumab (Soliris®, Alexion Pharmaceuticals), as discussed elsewhere in this book [16]. Eculizumab is a humanized monoclonal antibody (mAb) [17] which binds the terminal complement component 5 (C5), thereby inhibiting its cleavage to C5a and C5b and thus preventing the assembly of the MAC. The clinical efficacy of eculizumab has been demonstrated in two large multinational trials where it has been proven highly effective in controlling intravascular hemolysis of PNH patients, leading to reduced transfusional need, hemoglobin stabilization, and resolution of all hemolysis-related symptoms [18, 19]. Furthermore, eculizumab seems to reduce the risk of thromboembolic events in this patient cohort [20], possibly due to the pathogenic linkage between intravascular hemolysis and thrombosis (e.g., nitric oxide consumptions [21], pro-thrombotic microvesicles) or to any direct effect on complement-mediated thrombophilia (i.e., on PNH platelets) [22]. Preliminary data on survival seem to suggest that eculizumab may also improve survival in PNH [23], as expected given its effect on the main cause of death in PNH (i.e., thrombosis).

However, as usually in medicine, new therapies may also hide some pitfalls that emerge only once physicians became more familiar with such novel treatments. Eculizumab does not make an exception, even if in this case the pitfalls seem not related to the drug itself, but rather to pathogenic insights that we are learning, thanks to the eculizumab treatment. As discussed in Chap. 17 of this book [24], response to eculizumab is heterogeneous among patients: according to the registration trials, only about half of the patients actually achieve transfusion-independence during eculizumab treatment [18, 19]. In subsequent post-marketing experience, this percentage seems lower, but in any case around 25–40 % of patients continue to require some blood transfusions to sustain their hemoglobin levels [25, 26]. Different factors may be responsible for this insufficient hematological response to eculizumab. Bone marrow failure is the most obvious reason for a poor hematologic response, which is clearly identified by low/inadequate reticulocyte counts in patients who do not show any laboratory sign of hemolysis. For these patients eculizumab treatment might be considered sensu stricto effective, and it is rather the pertinence of anticomplement treatment that could be questioned, given that alternative or additional treatments specifically aiming to treat the bone marrow failure are appropriate (i.e., bone marrow transplantation or immunosuppression) [27]. Another possible reason for insufficient response is residual intravascular hemolysis, which appears recurrently in the few hours preceding the next dosing of eculizumab. This phenomenon is known as "breakthrough" intravascular hemolysis, and it has been described in about 10–15 % of PNH patients [28], potentially requiring increased dosages of eculizumab. However, irrespective of these two possibilities, the most common cause of residual anemia during eculizumab treatment is C3-mediated extravascular hemolysis, which mechanistically pertains to all PNH patients on eculizumab, even if its clinical impact is largely heterogeneous and unpredictable. This novel pathogenic mechanism has been described recently by our group and subsequently confirmed by other investigators [25, 26, 29–31]; Chap. 17 of this book provides a comprehensive overview of this phenomenon [24]. In brief, PNH erythrocytes, which are spared by hemolysis thanks to the C5-blockade provided by eculizumab, remain susceptible to membrane complement activation due to the lack of CD55. As a result, they progressively accumulate on their surface C3 fragments, which eventually work as opsonins leading to phagocytosis by professional cells like liver and spleen macrophages. This mechanism of extravascular hemolysis occurs through the recognition of C3 opsonins by specific complement receptors expressed on phagocytic cells, resulting in a selective destruction of PNH erythrocytes which have been exposed to threshold complement activation.

These observations demonstrate that complement may result harm to PNH erythrocytes irrespective of eculizumab, because of either residual intravascular hemolysis or supervening extravascular hemolysis, eventually accounting for insufficient response to eculizumab. Recently, it has been documented that individual genetic background may contribute or even determine the occurrence of these phenomena. The most terrific observation came from Japan, where some patients exhibited persistent massive intravascular hemolysis irrespective of eculizumab treatment [32]. Genetic and functional studies demonstrated that such intrinsic resistance to eculizumab was associated to a relatively common (in Japan) polymorphism of C5 gene, which codes for a protein that does not bind to eculizumab and thus continues to be cleaved by C5 convertase even in the presence of high levels of eculizumab [32]. Effects of polymorphisms of other complement genes are more subtle and may have a broader pathogenic effect. For instance, a common CR1 polymorphism determining lower CR1 surface expression (and thus impaired membrane-bound complement regulation) has been found associated with a lower hematological response to eculizumab [33]. Mechanistically, the impaired CR1 function on PNH erythrocytes (once added to CD55 deficiency) results in increased complement activation, which eventually leads to more pronounced C3 opsonization and subsequent extravascular hemolysis, in presence on pharmacological levels of eculizumab. However, this boosted complement activation might also contribute to residual intravascular hemolysis due to a breakthrough that is better described as harmacodynamics, possibly due to a huge amount of C5 convertases that may compete with eculizumab for the few free C5 molecules (newly synthesized or available from an on-off rate from eculizumab itself). In contrast, data on the effect of C3 polymorphism are still contradictory; indeed, it has been reported that a specific C3 polymorphism may be associated with poor response to eculizumab [34]. However, functional data are lacking, and these results are in conflict with previous observation from a different group [33]. Given the plethora of data dealing with the effect of other genetic variants (especially of complement factor H and complement factor H-related proteins) and complement activation in other diseases (atypical hemolytic-uremic syndrome, C3 glomerulopathy, dense deposit disease) [35, 36], it would not be surprising that in the near future additional polymorphisms with specific prognostic impact may be identified.

Thus, several reasons may limit the hematological benefit during eculizumab treatment, and there is an obvious unmet clinical need in the treatment of PNH. The development of novel strategies of complement inhibition and/or modulation will hopefully offer to patients and physicians treatment options to overcome this clinical issue.

20.3 Classification of Novel Complement Therapeutics

For the purpose of this review, novel complement therapeutics will be classified according to their specific target in the complement cascade (see also Fig. 20.1); indeed, based on this classification and on the recent pathogenic insights described above, one may anticipate the possible biological effects of these compounds, in vitro as well as possibly in vivo. An alternative classification might categorize

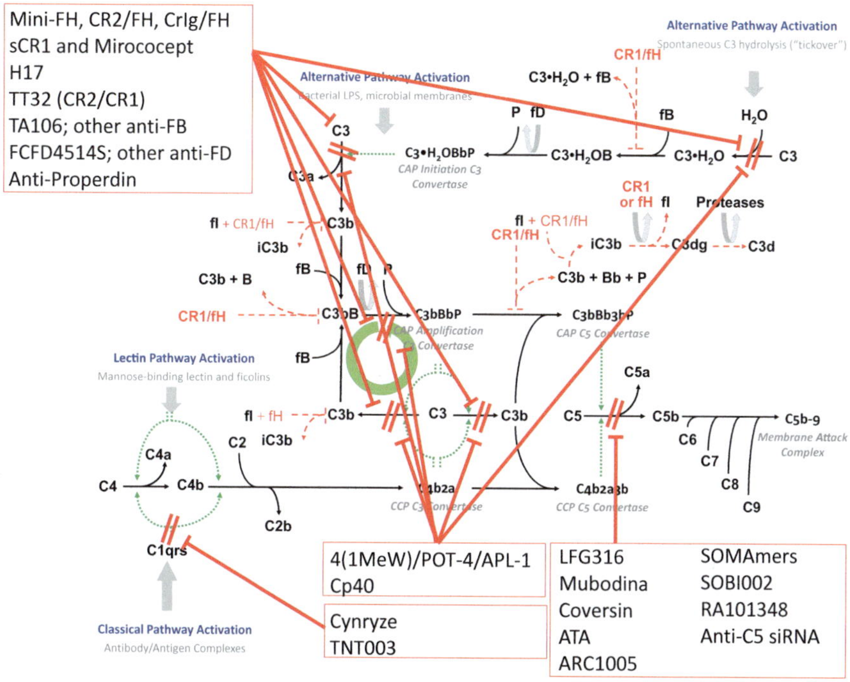

Fig. 20.1 Complement system and its targeted modulation. Overview of the complement cascade, including all main functional components and physiologic regulators. The three activating pathways (alternative, classical, and mannose/lectin) are individually depicted, together with the alternative pathway amplification loop. Candidate inhibitors are grouped according to their specific target; their modulatory effects are indicated by *red lines* intercepting specific steps of the complement cascade. See also main text for a more detailed description

these agents according to the class of the molecules, which includes monoclonal antibodies, other engineered large proteins, small peptides, chemicals, and even novel technology molecules (e.g., small interfering RNAs). Table 20.1 includes an updated list of the most relevant candidate complement inhibitors, for which public information or data are available; the status of development and the corresponding references are reported too, in addition to the specific target. Given the complexity of the complement cascade and the high number of proteins involved in its proper functioning, a simplified view may focus on the two key steps of this system, which are the initial complement activation and amplification and the subsequent tissue damage mediated by complement effector molecules. Indeed, a rough distinction among complement inhibitors may dissect between agents that inhibit the damage mediated by effector complement and agents which are able to prevent the arming of the terminal complement by inhibiting early complement activation. C5 and C3 are the key molecules that one may wish to target to inhibit terminal effector complement or early complement activation, respectively.

Table 20.1 Candidate complement inhibitors in the development for PNH and other complement-mediated diseases

Target	Name	Company	Class of molecule	Status of development	References
C5	LFG316	Novartis/Morphosys	Monoclonal antibody	Clinical (phase II, AMD)	[37]
C5	Mubodina®	Adienne	Monoclonal antibody (minibody)	Preclinical (non-PNH)	[38, 39]
C5	Coversin (OmCI)	Volution Immuno Pharmaceuticals	Small animal protein (recombinant)	Preclinical (PNH), clinical (phase I, healthy volunteers)	[45]
C5 (+ C3?)	Aurin tricarboxylic acid (ATA)	n.a.	Chemical	Preclinical (PNH)	[46]
C5	ARC1005	Novo Nordisk	Aptamers	Preclinical (non-PNH); clinical (phase I, AMD)	[50, 51]
C5	SOMAmers	SomaLogic	Aptamers (SELEX)	Preclinical (non-PNH)	[50, 52]
C5	SOBI002	Swedish Orphan Biovitrum (affibody)	Affibody (fused with albumin-binding domain)	Preclinical (non-PNH); clinical (phase I, healthy volunteers)	[50, 54, 55]
C5	RA101348	Ra Pharma	Small molecule (unnatural peptide)	Preclinical (unknown)	[56, 57]
C5	Anti-C5 siRNA	Alnylam	Si-RNA	Preclinical (non-PNH and PNH)	[58]
C3 (C3b/iC3b)	H17	Elusys Therapeutics	Monoclonal antibody	Preclinical (PNH and non-PNH)	[63, 64]
C3/C3b	4(1MeW)/POT-4	Potentia	Compstatin family	Preclinical (non-PNH); clinical (Phase I and II, AMD)	[67]
C3/C3b	4(1MeW)/APL-1, APL-2	Apellis	Compstatin family	Preclinical (PNH and non-PNH); clinical (PNH and non-PNH, planned)	[34]
C3/C3b	Cp40/AMY-101, PEG-Cp40	Amyndas	Compstatin family	Preclinical (PNH and non-PNH); clinical (PNH and non-PNH, planned)	[73]

AP C3 convertase	TT30 (CR2/FH)	Alexion	FH-based protein	Preclinical (PNH and non-PNH); clinical (phase I, PNH)	[83–85]
AP C3 convertase	Mini-FH	Amyndas	FH-based protein	Preclinical (PNH and non-PNH)	[86]
AP C3 convertase	Mini-FH	n.a.	FH-based protein	Preclinical (non-PNH)	[87]
AP C3 convertase	CRIg/FH	n.a.	FH-based protein	Preclinical	[88]
AP and CP C3 convertase	sCR1 (CDX-1135)	Celldex	CR1-based protein	Preclinical (non-PNH); clinical (phase I, DDD)	[94–96]
AP and CP C3 convertase	Mirococept (APT070)	n.a.	CR1-based protein	Preclinical (non-PNH); clinical (phase I, kidney transplantation)	[97–100]
AP and CP C3 convertase	TT32 (CR2/CR1)	Alexion Pharmaceuticals	CR1-based protein	Preclinical (non-PNH)	[102]
FB	TA106	Alexion Pharmaceuticals	Monoclonal antibody	Preclinical (unknown)	[103]
FD	FCFD4514S	Genentech/Roche	Monoclonal antibody	Preclinical (non-PNH); clinical (phase II, AMD)	[104]
FB	Anti-FB siRNA	Alnylam	Si-RNA	Preclinical (non-PNH)	[58]
FB and FD	SOMAmers	SomaLogic	Aptamers (SELEX)	Preclinical (non-PNH)	[50, 52]
FB and FD	n.a.	Novartis	Small molecules (chemicals)	Preclinical (non-PNH)	[105, 106]
Properdin	n.a.	Novelmed	Monoclonal antibody (and mAb derivatives)	Preclinical (unknown)	[107, 108]
C1r/C1s	Cinryze®	ViroPharma/Baxter	Human purified protein (C1-INH)	Clinical (approved for hereditary angioedema)	[109]
C1s	TNT003	True North Therapeutics	Monoclonal antibody	Preclinical (Ab-mediated hemolytic anemias)	[110]
MASP-3	n.a.	Omeros	n.a.	Preclinical (PNH and non-PNH)	[111]

20.3.1 Inhibitors of Terminal Effector Complement

The inhibition of the terminal effector complement has been pioneered by the anti-C5 monoclonal antibody eculizumab, which is currently the only complement inhibitor approved for the treatment of PNH. As discussed elsewhere in this book, the use of eculizumab demonstrated that a pharmacological inhibition at the level of C5 results in a sustained control of intravascular hemolysis of PNH, with the few caveats discussed above. For PNH, it is obvious that the pharmacological effect relies on the prevention of C5 cleavage by the C5 convertase, which eventually disables C5b from starting MAC assembly via its interaction with C6, C7, C8, and C9. Even if the anti-C5 eculizumab also prevents the release of C5a, this effect should not play any role in the control of hemolysis and other clinical manifestations of PNH, at least according to current knowledge. Thus, eculizumab is the paradigm of inhibition of the effector complement and the only approved drug with this mechanism of action. Nevertheless, there are several novel compounds which target C5 and may offer some alternative to eculizumab, or even differentiating from it because of their specific pharmacological properties.

Staying in the field of monoclonal antibodies (mAbs), there are at least two additional anti-C5 monoclonal antibodies which are currently in clinical or preclinical development. Even if they should not differ too much from eculizumab in their mechanism of action and thus in their clinical efficacy, the interest for alternative anti-C5 mAb has been strengthened by the recent description of the Japanese C5 polymorphism which impairs the C5 binding to eculizumab. In vitro data from the same group have demonstrated that this specific C5 polymorphism abolishes the binding of C5 to eculizumab, but not to other anti-C5 mAb specific for different C5 epitopes, such as N19-8 [32]. LFG316 (Morphosys®) is a fully human combinatorial antibody libraries of anti-C5 mAb produced by Novartis, which is under clinical development for age-related macular degeneration (AMD) and other ophthalmologic diseases. The agent is now in phase II, and after initial testing employing local administration, it is now under investigation as systemic treatment by intravenous injection (NCT01624636) [37]. An additional candidate agent is Mubodina® (Adienne Pharma & Biotech), an anti-C5 “minibody,” consisting of an engineered antibody fragment which includes the antigen-specific VL and VH domains of its parental anti-C5 mAb [38]. The original anti-C5 mAb was initially isolated as a single-chain variable fragment (scFv) from phage display library derived from rearranged V gene amplicons obtained from normal peripheral lymphocytes [39]. The minibody Mubodina® prevents the cleavage of C5 and inhibits the generation of inflammatory molecule C5a and of C5b and the subsequent lytic MAC [40]. Mubodina® has been approved as orphan drug for some kidney diseases by both FDA and EMA. Even if either Morphosys or Mubodina has not been tested in vivo for PNH yet, nor in vitro data are available, both agents can reasonably be considered alternative agents to be tested in PNH, especially in the few patients with intrinsic genetic resistance to eculizumab. In addition, further derivatives of the original anti-C5 scFv are pioneering the possibility of targeting the anti-C5 agent at specific sites; this strategy, which exploits anti-C5 scFv fused with specific tag peptides, has proven effective in an animal model of arthritis [41] and might be developed also for erythrocytes. Thinking about a possible clinical use of other anti-C5 mAbs in PNH, it is expected that efficacy and toxicity may parallel those of eculizumab, and in particular no benefit can be expected on possible C3-mediated extravascular hemolysis. However, it cannot be excluded that antibody-specific association and dissociation rates for C5 may result in differences of pharmacokinetic and/or harmacodynamics properties, with possible clinical consequences. For instance, different anti-C5 mAb may entail specific risk of breakthrough hemolysis, eventually requiring different treatment schedules. Compliance to frequent hospitalizations still represents a problem for some PNH patients on eculizumab; if any of these novel mAbs may allow a longer interval between dosing and different administration routes (i.e., subcutaneous), this would offer a possible clinical benefit over the current eculizumab treatment.

The spectrum of C5 inhibitors also includes agents other than mAbs. Among these, a novel complement inhibitor of the lipocalin family isolated from the tick of *Ornithodoros moubata* is emerging as an interesting candidate molecule [42]. This inhibitor is a small (16 kDa) protein named coversin (also known as OmCI, Volution Immuno Pharmaceuticals) which binds to human C5 and prevents its cleavage by C5 convertases [43, 44]; coversin exhibits also additional anti-inflammatory effect by binding to leukotriene B4 [43, 44]. Preliminary in vitro data in PNH suggest possible inhibitory effects on intravascular hemolysis, as well as some effect in preventing C3 opsonization [45]. Coversin has been recently investigated in vivo in a phase I study in healthy volunteers, which demonstrated amenable pharmacokinetic and pharmacodynamic profiles; indeed, complement inhibitory levels may be achieved after subcutaneous injections and retained for several hours after dosing [45]. Based on these data, a clinical translation plan for PNH patients has been announced [45]; further clinical trials will also have to rule out possible concerns about the immunogenicity of such evolutionary distant protein. Even if this agent might provide an effective alternative for terminal complement interception at the level of C5 (likely with cheap production cost), at the moment robust preclinical data in PNH are lacking (or unpublished); furthermore, it is not clear if this anti-C5 agent could also interfere with early complement activation and C3 opsonization on PNH erythrocytes. Similar concerns about an inexplicably broad anticomplement effect can be applied to another complement inhibitor recently reported potentially effective for PNH. Indeed, aurin tricarboxylic acid (ATA) has proven effective in protecting PNH erythrocytes in a CH50 assay employing zymosan as complement activation trigger [46]. According to the authors, ATA inhibited not only MAC-mediated hemolysis but also possible C3 deposition on surviving erythrocytes, consistent with a dual effect of ATA on both MAC assembly [48] and alternative pathway C3 convertase [47]. However, it is not clear whether these effects of ATA are actually target specific, or rather some broader inhibition of proteases which may impair the function of several unrelated proteins, not restricted to complement components. Furthermore, these data on PNH in vitro have not been confirmed by other groups (Risitano et al. unpublished data).

Four novel classes of compounds are currently exploiting new technologies for possible clinical application of C5 inhibition. Aptamers are large (either oligonucleic or peptide) compounds which selectively bind to specific molecules, eventually impairing their function [49]. They are usually created by using large random sequence pools, from where target-specific molecules are selected. ARC 1905 (Zimura™, Ophthotech Corp. Princeton, NJ) is a pegylated, stabilized oligonucleic aptamer targeting C5 [50]. ARC 1905 is currently in phase II clinical investigation for ophthalmologic disease (AMD) as topic agent (NCT00950638) [51]; however, ARC 1905 or other anti-C5 aptamers might also be considered in the future for systemic C5 inhibition. A further evolution of this technology by SELEX (systematic evolution of ligands by exponential enrichment) led to the discovery of SOMAmers (slow off-rate modified aptamers), which may have a more favorable PK/PD profile for therapeutic application. SOMAmers® specific for different key components of the complement cascade (C5, C3, FD, and FB) are currently under preclinical development by SomaLogic (Colorado, USA) [52]; they promise to increase the growing arsenal of complement inhibitors to be tested in PNH. A similar technology which exploits target-specific inhibition is developed by the Swedish company Affibody. Affibody molecules are small antibody mimetic proteins (about 6 kDa) consisting of a three-helix bundle domain with favorable folding and stability; from this original scaffold, a combinatorial protein engineering approach results in small non-immunoglobulin proteins displaying high affinity binding to a wide range of protein targets [53]. Affibodies specific for C5 have been developed; recently, a C5-targeting affibody fused to an albumin-binding domain has been created by Swedish Orphan Biovitrum (SOBI002; 12 kDa). SOBI002 has been shown binding to human C5 with low-nanomolar affinity (KD ~ 1 nM), resulting in effective prevention of its cleavage and thus of activation of the effector complement (downstream C5: C5a and C5b toward to MAC), with IC_{50} values in the low nM range. The fusion with the albumin-binding moiety led to an increase in its half-life and stability in both rodent and nonhuman primate (cynomolgus monkey) plasma, with terminal half-life above 2 weeks [54]. In addition, the compound showed excellent bioavailability (>79 %) by subcutaneous injection in cynomolgus monkeys, anticipating very favorable pharmacokinetic properties for sustained clinical inhibition [54]. SOBI002 has been shown effective in preclinical models of complement (C5)-mediated diseases, and a phase I study evaluating safety, tolerability, and PK/PD in healthy volunteers has recently started (NCT02083666) [55].

A different approach to identify candidate complement inhibitors has been exploited at Ra Pharma, where scientists have developed a method of ribosomal synthesis of unnatural peptides [56] to produce massive peptidomimetic libraries for further drug screening. This technology led to the identification of small, cyclic, peptide-like polymers with backbone and side-chain modifications, called Cyclomimetics. Cyclomimetics™ have unique, beneficial properties as compared with natural peptides, including a low risk of immunogenicity (due to poor MHC presentation) and increased cell permeability, stability, potency, and bioavailability (due to the structural modifications). RA101348 is the lead anti-C5 macrocyclic peptide which is currently in preclinical investigation [57].

Finally, also RNA therapeutics have been developed for clinical complement inhibition, targeting liver-expressed genes such as C5 [58]. Indeed, a GalNAc-conjugated anti-C5 siRNA duplex (developed by Alnylam Pharmaceuticals) showed robust (>95 %) silencing of C5 production in rodent as well as human hepatocytes. In animal models, C5 silencing was achieved after subcutaneous injections of the siRNA, resulting in sustained and durable (recovery started 2 weeks after single dose injection) complement inhibition as effective as 90 %. This agent is currently under preclinical investigations in nonhuman primates, as well as in PNH in vitro. In addition, Alnylam is exploiting the same technology to target other complement proteins such as factor B [58], with the aim to silence early complement activation and in particular the alternative complement pathway (see below). Even if siRNA-mediated complement inhibition is an elegant and promising novel therapeutic approach, further studies are needed to confirm its clinical feasibility (as well as efficacy, given that residual low activity might be a concern).

20.3.1.1 Other Terminal Effector Complement Inhibitors

After the development of eculizumab, C5 has been considered the best target to inhibit terminal effector complement. However, it has to be remarked that, at least for PNH, additional strategies may exploit the possibility to correct the deranged surface complement regulation by restoring CD59 function on PNH erythrocytes. For instance, a soluble, synthetically modified recombinant human CD59 has been shown effective in attaching to PNH erythrocytes, thereby protecting them from complement-mediated hemolysis in vitro [59]. Even if the clinical translation of this compound (Adprotech, Inflazyme Pharmaceuticals) has now been stopped, this approach might be reconsidered in the future, even with the development of CD59-based large engineered proteins (such as the complement receptor 2-CD59 fusion protein TT33, Alexion Pharmaceuticals).

20.3.2 Inhibitors of Initiating Complement

As discussed above, the early phases of complement activation have emerged as a relevant pathogenic event in PNH independently from the typical MAC-mediated intravascular hemolysis resulting from the terminal effector complement. Thus, different strategies to inhibit the initiation of the complement cascade are currently under investigation, with the dual aim of preventing C3-mediated initiating events as well as to potentiate the inhibition of terminal complement; this may result in a better clinical efficacy in PNH. A number of early complement inhibitors are currently under development (see Table 20.1); even if all of them eventually result in C3 inhibition (given that C3 activation is the key event in complement activation, needed for enabling its harmful effects), they may be classified according to their specific target (Fig. 20.1). Indeed, inhibitors of C3 itself exist and include antibodies (or antibody-derived proteins), small compounds, and novel technology molecules. However, several agents prevent C3 activation by acting even upstream, on the very initial events which eventually result in C3 activation. To note, given that these events involve different initiating pathways which may occur separately (and may have distinct role in different diseases), upstream complement inhibitors include agents which may selectively shut down each of the complement-initiating pathways – the alternative pathway (AP), the classical pathway (CP), and the mannose/lectin pathway (MP). Thus, for the sake of clarity, C3 inhibitors will be classified according to their mechanism of action, irrespective of the class of molecule to which they pertain; a brief recall of complement biology is also included (reviewed in Chap. 4 of this book) [60].

20.3.2.1 Broad C3 Inhibitors

As mentioned above, C3 is the pivotal molecule of the complement system and its cleavage to C3a and C3b by C3 convertases is the key event of complement activation; thus, the most obvious target for inhibiting C3 activation is C3 itself. However, C3 is a large protein (183 kDa) which is very abundant in the human plasma (~1 mg/mL). For this reason, C3 is not usually considered a druggable target by conventional strategies, and even mAbs specific for native C3 are not considered adequate for clinical development. However, given that C3 activation process includes several protein-protein interactions with subsequent structural transitions [61, 62], candidate inhibitors may also target specific binding sites of C3 and may work by affecting such protein-protein interactions. Indeed, a recent strategy attempted to target activated C3 fragments (C3b/iC3b) rather native C3 for therapeutic C3 inhibition, by using an anti-C3b/iC3b mAb (clone 3E7) [63]. This mAb, as well as its humanized (de-immunized) derivative H17 (Elusys Therapeutics), has been tested in PNH in vitro, showing a complete abrogation of hemolysis as well as of C3 deposition on surviving PNH erythrocytes [63]. Notably, these mAbs seem to be specific for C3b/iC3b included in the AP C3 convertase, given that hemolysis driven by the CP was not affected by the use of the either 3E7 or H17. Indeed, 3E7 and H17 bind to C3b and prevent its interaction with complement factor B (FB) for AP C3 convertase formation; thus, these mAbs might be better classified as AP inhibitors (see below) rather than broad C3 inhibitors. Albeit mechanistically intriguing, these results still do not provide a candidate agent for clinical translation for PNH. Indeed, by binding to C3 fragments which activate on PNH erythrocyte surface, these antibodies with their Fc moieties (IgG1 isotype) provide additional opsonins eventually worsening rather than reducing phagocyte-mediated extravascular hemolysis (which now would be mediated by Fc receptors in addition to that by C3 receptors). Nevertheless, H17 may represent a good starting step for further development; indeed, engineered modified derivatives lacking the Fc portion may circumvent this hurdle which has hampered further development in PNH. Recently, a Fab fragment of H17 has been described [64]; it has been tested in preclinical model of kidney diseases and might be worth of further investigation in PNH.

In additional to immunoglobulin-based compounds, as for C5 different classes of inhibitors may be thought to silence C3 activity, eventually interfering with specific sites which are pivotal for interaction with its activating proteins (e.g., FB and C4b). They may include agents developed by using the novel technologies exploited for C5 inhibition, such as aptamers, SOMAmers, and affibodies; however, at the moment this application remains conceptual and there are no available data.

However, the use of small molecules to inhibit C3 has been pioneered since the 1990s with the development of a peptide named compstatin. Compstatin is a 13-residue disulfide-bridged peptide (H-Ile-[Cys-Val-Val-Gln-Asp-Trp-Gly-His-His-Arg-Cys]-Thr-NH2) that selectively binds to human and nonhuman primate (NHP) native C3, as well as to its active fragment C3b [65]. As a consequence, compstatin inhibits both the cleavage of C3 into C3b and the incorporation of C3b to form C3/C5 convertases [66]. Compstatin family exerts its effect along all the three complement-initiating pathways, AP, CP, and MP, and also inhibits the AP amplification loop (see below and Fig. 20.1), resulting in a broad and effective abrogation of all terminal effector complements (C3a, C5a, and MAC). Since the initial description in the 1990s, several derivatives of the original compound have been developed as candidate agents for a number of complement-mediated diseases [62]. One compstatin analog named 4(1MeW) has demonstrated beneficial results in phase I clinical trials for the local treatment of age-related macular degeneration [67] and is still in clinical development by Potentia Pharmaceuticals with the name of POT-4. The same analog, under the name of APL-1, is developed by Apellis Pharmaceuticals for other diseases [62], based also on the promising results shown by compstatin analogs in several models of systemic complement-mediated diseases, including hemodialysis to sepsis [66, 68, 69]. With the aim of improving PK and PD properties of compstatin for systemic therapeutic application, structure-guided optimization and activity refinement studies have been conducted at the Penn University, leading to the identification of second-generation compstatin derivatives [70–72]. The current lead analog Cp40 [62] showed strong binding affinity for C3b (KD ~ 0.5 nM) and excellent solubility, and it has been selected under the name of AMY-101 for further preclinical development by Amyndas Pharmaceuticals. Cp40/AMY-101 has recently received the orphan status for the treatment of PNH by the EMA. Initial in vivo studies of systemic administration in nonhuman primates demonstrated excellent plasma stability and favorable PK profile, with plasma half-life longer than that usually seen with other peptide drugs [71]. In addition, long-acting polyethylene glycol (PEG) derivatives of Cp40/AMY-101 have been developed with the aim to sustain pharmacological complement inhibition for therapeutic use [73]. These second-generation compstatin analogs have been tested in PNH in vitro; both unmodified Cp40/AMY-101 and its N-terminally pegylated derivative (PEG-Cp40) exhibited full complement inhibition, resulting in full protection of PNH erythrocytes from hemolysis [73]. In addition, by affecting early complement activation, these compstatin derivatives also prevented deposition of C3 fragments on surviving PNH erythrocytes [73]. These findings provide strong evidence that compstatin family effectively intercepts both intravascular (MAC-mediated) and extravascular (C3-mediated) hemolysis in PNH, eventually entailing possible therapeutic benefit over standard anti-C5 treatment. Thus, compstatin family represents an excellent candidate for clinical development in PNH (and other systemic complement-mediated diseases); recently, a different group has confirmed these data even using one first-generation analog (APL-1) and its long-acting derivative APL-2 [34]. Additional preclinical studies in animal models (NHP) with compstatin analogs are currently ongoing to identify the best candidates for clinical translation. Recent data showed that PEG-Cp40 after subcutaneous injection in NHP exhibits a favorable PK profile, with excellent bioavailability, increased plasma stability, and a remarkably prolonged elimination half-life (> 5 days) [73]. On the other hand, even unmodified Cp40/AMY-101 was shown to have an excellent bioavailability after repeated subcutaneous injections into cynomolgus monkeys, with a half-life of ~12 h which allows sustained inhibitory levels with bi-daily (and possibly even daily) multidose treatment schedules [73]. Whereas clinical translation is just on its way to be started by Amyndas, it is conceivable that for safety concerns initial studies will prefer unmodified Cp40/AMY-101, which may allow for a quicker restoration of complement activity if clinically needed, for instance, in case of infectious complications. Indeed, the increased (>tenfold) plasma residence of PEG-Cp40 would require much longer time to regain complement activity. The preference for the unmodified Cp40/AMY-101 is also warranted by the need of further studies to investigate the meaning of increased plasma C3 level after administration of PEG-Cp40 (possibly secondary to changes in the clearance and turnover of C3, once bound to PEG-Cp40) [73], as well as the possible adverse effect of high in vivo level of pegylated compounds. Indeed, even generally considered safe, the high levels needed to saturate C3 might exert unexpected effects, such as immunogenicity [74, 75] or other adverse reactions. These concerns may be extended to other compstatin analogs under development by Apellis Pharmaceuticals; irrespective of their positive in vitro result on PNH erythrocytes [34], further preclinical in vivo data in NHP are warranted to fully understand PK and PD properties, especially for the long-acting pegylated derivative APL-2.

20.3.2.2 Pathway-Specific Inhibitors

C3 is the key component of the complement system because all the three initiating pathways merge on its cleavage (Fig. 20.1); C3 cleavage eventually leads to the generation of the earliest effector mediator, C3a, as well as to the progression toward the generation of additional C3 convertase molecules (amplification loop) and of C5 convertases, that activate the terminal effector complement arm, including the anaphylatoxin C5a and the membrane-bound C5b-C9 (MAC) complex. However, each of the initiating pathway may independently lead to a fully activation of the complement cascade, complete of all its harmful effector mechanisms. Thus, candidate inhibitors may also intercept complement activation at a very initial phase, specifically targeting one or more initiating pathways (Fig. 20.1). Remarkably, each initiating pathway includes several distinct proteins cooperating to achieve C3 activation, and all of them can be potential targets for therapeutic intervention; in addition, several other proteins exert a fine regulation (regulators of complement activation, RCA) of these events, potentially representing additional therapeutic targets. Obviously, the benefit of this selective approach may be particularly useful in diseases where the pathogenic mechanisms include the derangement of a single complement pathway; this may be the case of PNH, which is traditionally considered an AP-mediated disease (see below for therapeutic implications). This reason, together with the knowledge that the AP also plays a key role in amplifying complement activation irrespective of the initiating pathway, prompts us to start our discussion on candidate selective inhibitors with the AP.

Selective Inhibitors of the Alternative Pathway

The key molecule of the AP is complement factor B (FB), a single-chain plasma protein which binds to C3(H_2O) generated from the spontaneous cleavage of the thioester bond of C3 (the so-called C3 tickover). Once bound to C3(H_2O), FB becomes susceptible to cleavage by the complement factor D (FD), which yields the non-catalytic chain Ba, and the active catalytic subunit Bb. Together with C3(H_2O) (or with C3b), Bb forms the active C3 convertase, which needs to be stabilized by the binding of an additional serum protein, properdin. The addition of a further C3b molecule to this C3 convertase leads to the generation of a C5 convertase (analogously to the formation of CP/MP C5 convertases). As discussed below, all these complement components are candidate targets for therapeutic intervention; however, so far drug development has been based on some endogenous RCA which can be used for tuning complement activity [76]. They include complement factor H (FH) and complement receptor 1 (CR1).

FH is the main fluid-phase regulator of AP activation: indeed, it prevents the formation of the AP C3 convertase and accelerates the decay of existing ones [77]. In addition, FH also plays a major role in the regulatory effect of complement factor I, acting as its cofactor for the disabling of C3b into iC3b [78]. Thus, FH has a pleomorphic role in complement homeostasis, which is further increased by the fact that it regulates the AP amplification loop eventually starting regardless of the initial triggering pathway. In addition, the protective role of surface-bound FH has been clearly demonstrated in vitro on PNH erythrocytes [79]. Based on these assumptions, several strategies attempted to employ this complement regulatory effect for therapeutic intervention, possibly targeting it specifically at sites of complement activation. Indeed, FH-based recombinant proteins merging the complement regulatory domain of FH with a C3-specific recognizing domain from complement receptor 2 (CR2) have been initially developed in murine models, where they effectively reduced complement-mediated damage [80–82]. More recently, a human version of this fusion protein has been created with TT30 (Alexion Pharmaceuticals), a 65 kDa engineered protein consisting of the iC3b/C3dg-binding domain of CR merged with AP inhibitory domain of FH [83]. TT30 has been thought a perfect candidate inhibitor for PNH; indeed, it completely inhibits in a dose-dependent manner MAC-mediated hemolysis of PNH erythrocytes in vitro [84]. In addition, by acting on C3 convertase, TT30 also inhibits early complement activation on PNH erythrocytes, preventing the deposition of C3 fragments on their surface [84]. These observations reasonably anticipate that TT30 should inhibit MAC-mediated intravascular hemolysis typical of PNH and may also prevent C3-mediated extravascular hemolysis eventually emerging during anti-C5 therapies. The inhibitory effect of TT30 depends on an efficient membrane targeting of FH on erythrocyte surface, since only partial inhibition was achieved when CR2-mediated binding of TT30 to PNH cells was blocked, in vitro [84]. Based on these preclinical data (which also demonstrated excellent availability after subcutaneous injection) [83], a phase I clinical trial evaluating TT30 as a potential therapeutic option for treating PNH in humans has been started (NCT01335165) [85]. This study has recently been reported as terminated, and results are now awaited.

TT30 represented the first proof that the targeted delivery of FH function through the generation of C3-specific docking sites may provide an excellent strategy to rescue deficient complement regulation on PNH erythrocytes. Indeed, additional surface-targeted FH-based engineered proteins have been developed through the engineering of a miniaturized version of human FH (mini-FH). Mini-FH is a small (43 kDa) protein consisting of the regulatory complement control protein (CCP) 1–4 domains of FH fused with its CCP 19–20 domains, which are involved in the recognition of self-cell pattern (including C3) [86]. Mini-FH retains the regulatory function of FH (C3 convertase decay and cofactor activities), resulting even in an increased (almost tenfold) inhibitory effect on AP activation; in addition, thanks to an additional iC3b/C3dg binding site unmasked in CCP 19–20, mini-FH displays a triple-targeting profile which includes oxidative damage markers, polyanionic surfaces, and the full spectrum of C3-derived opsonins [86]. Once investigated in PNH in vitro, mini-FH effectively inhibited intravascular hemolysis of PNH erythrocytes, as well as their opsonization by C3 fragments [86]. These findings perfectly paralleled those of TT30, consistent with their common mechanism of action; however, although head-to-head comparison was not performed, fully inhibitory concentrations for mini-FH were about tenfold lower than TT30 (and even lower when compared with full-length nontargeted FH) [86]. Thus, mini-FH is another FH-based protein which may deserve further clinical development for PNH; like TT30 (and like another miniaturized version of FH [87]), all these FH-engineered proteins may prevent the development of C3-mediated extravascular hemolysis in addition to the control of intravascular hemolysis. Furthermore, very recently investigators from China have reported about another engineered fusion protein which exploits the complement receptor of the immunoglobulin superfamily (CRIg) as the targeting module; indeed, this CRIg/FH fusion seems to exhibit functional properties similar to those of TT30 and of mini-FH [88].

The approach of specifically targeting on the cell surface the inhibitory effect of endogenous AP C3 convertase inhibitors has been developed even beyond FH [76]; indeed, similar approaches have been attempted using CR1as the regulatory protein. CR1 is another inhibitor of the complement cascade with pleomorphic functions

[89]; indeed, similar to FH, CR1 binds to C3b and C4b, promoting the decay of C3 and C5 convertases of both the AP and the CP [90]. In addition, it parallels FH also in working as cofactor of FI to inactivate C3b and C4b. Thus, CR1 is a broad complement regulator which tunes both the AP and the CP (and as a consequence also the MP) of the complement system [91, 92]. The possible role of CR1 in PNH has recently emerged with the observation that patients carrying a hypofunctional polymorphism of CR1 have a lower chance of good clinical response to eculizumab, in vivo [33]. This observation was corroborated by robust in vitro data, showing that once exposed to complement activation in the presence of C5 inhibition, PNH erythrocytes carrying the hypomorphic CR1 allele exhibited a faster and increased surface deposition of C3 fragments [33]. Furthermore, there was an obvious quantitative effect, since erythrocytes from patients homozygous for the hypomorphic allele showed an even increased C3 opsonization [33], clearly supporting the concept that the density of CR1 modulates complement activation and C3 deposition on PNH erythrocytes (this effect may become evident just because of the lack of CD55). Thus, different attempts are currently under investigation trying to exploit CR1 for therapeutic inhibition [93]. Indeed, a soluble CR1 (sCR1, TP10) named CDX-1135 is currently under development by Celldex; CDX-1135 is a potent inhibitor of complement activation that, in vitro, inhibits all the classical, alternative, and lectin pathways of complement at both early (C3 convertase) and late (C5 convertase) stages by downregulating the activation of these cascades. Due to its mechanism of action, sCR1 affects only activated complement and is not consumed, but can recycle in the inhibitory process. CDX-1135 has previously been evaluated in more than 500 patients in different clinical trials which have demonstrated clear evidence of complement inhibition with acceptable tolerance. A pilot study of CDX-1135 has been initiated to explore the potential for clinical benefit in patients with earlier stage dense deposit disease (DDD), a kidney disorder where C3 consumption and deposition play an important role in disease progression (NCT01791686) [94]. In a mouse model of DDD, the administration of CDX-1135 was shown to control complement activation in vivo, restoring complement regulation and preventing the damaging deposition of C3 in the glomerular basement membranes [95]. Short-term compassionate use of CDX-1135 in a pediatric patient with end-stage renal failure secondary to DDD demonstrated its safety and ability to normalize activity of the terminal complement pathway [96].

Another candidate CR1-based protein is mirococept (APT070), which is currently under development for the treatment of rheumatoid ischemia/reperfusion injury [97]. Mirococept consists of the first three short consensus domains of CR1, which are targeted on the membranes by an amphiphilic peptide based on the naturally occurring membrane-bound myristoyl-electrostatic switch peptide [98]. Mirococept has been demonstrated effective in preventing complement-mediated ischemia/reperfusion injury of transplanted kidneys in rats [99] and is currently under investigation with the aim of improving both the immediate and the long-term function of transplanted kidney by reducing posttransplant complement-mediated inflammatory response [100]. A clinical randomized placebo-controlled trial investigating a method for coating the inner surface of donor kidneys with a protective layer of mirococept is ongoing [101]. Even if preclinical data are lacking, this agent represents another possible candidate for systemic complement inhibition in PNH, such as also another CR1-based fusion protein under development by Alexion Pharmaceuticals (TT32, a CR2-CR1 fusion protein) [102].

Therapeutic interception at the level of AP activation may also directly target the complement factors involved in the first initiating event of the AP, namely, the cleavage of FB into Ba and Bb operated by FD. Both FB and FD are ideal targets, but the development of specific inhibitors is in the early stages. An antibody-based inhibitor of FB (TA106, a Fab fragment which binds native FB preventing its cleavage by FD) has been initially developed by Taligen Therapeutics, and it is now under investigation by Alexion Pharmaceuticals [76, 103]; however, even preclinical data are not available yet. An anti-FD mAb fragment named FCFD4514S is under development by Genentech/Roche; a phase II trial is currently ongoing for local use in ophthalmologic indication (NCT01602120) [103, 104].

Other candidate FB and FD inhibitors are included in the pipeline of different companies, exploiting many of the novel technologies described to develop anti-C5 inhibitors; indeed, SomaLogic has announced the development of anti-FB and anti-FB SOMAmers which may completely block the AP activation [52]. In addition, Alnylam is attempting to exploit its siRNA technology to silence FB [58], which for PNH might be beneficial over anti-C5 siRNA. Small inhibitors of both FB and FD are also under preclinical investigation by Novartis [105, 106]. Finally, Novelmed has announced the development of a humanized anti-properdin mAb and anti-properdin antigen-binding portions [107, 108]; this would be another strategy to inhibit the AP complement activation which seems worth of additional investigation.

Selective Inhibitors of the Classical Pathway

The role of the complement classical pathway in the pathophysiology of PNH has not been fully elucidated; indeed, even if the AP is though the key mechanism accounting for intravascular hemolysis, CD55 deficiency on PNH erythrocytes also impairs the regulation of the CP. As for the AP, CP activation includes the interaction of several proteins which actually lead to the cleavage of C3 into C3a and C3b (Fig. 20.1). In brief, the formation of CP C3 convertase starts with the binding of antigen-bound antibodies to C1q, which activates the tetramer $C1r_2s_2$. The two activated C1s subunits cleave C4 into C4a and C4b, which then binds to C2, stimulating its cleavage by C1s; the resulting C4b2b complex constitutes the CP C3 convertase. As for the AP, endogenous inhibitors regulate the different steps of CP activation; they include C4bp, CR1, and CD55 (these latter two exert on CP C3 convertase effects similar to those observed on AP C3 convertase) and an upstream inhibitor of C1. C1 esterase inhibitor (C1-INH) is a serine protease inhibitor (SERPIN) with a broad inhibitory activity in the complement, contact, and coagulation pathways. C1-INH inhibits the CP activation by binding to C1r and C1s and preventing their catalytic effect on C4 and C2; in addition, C1-INH exerts a similar action on the mannose-binding lectin-associated serine proteases in the lectin pathway. C1-INH is the second complement inhibitor approved for clinical use; indeed, Cinryze® (ViroPharma/Baxter) is a nanofiltered human plasma-derived C1-INH which is used as substitutive therapy in patients with hereditary angioedema (HAE), a disease due to constitutional deficiency or dysfunction of endogenous C1-INH. This agent has been recently tested in vitro for PNH, showing a potential effect in preventing hemolysis and C3 fragment decoration of PNH erythrocytes [109]. Further mechanistic studies are needed to fully understand its actual mechanism of action (i.e., is C1-INH also an AP inhibitor, or is the CP involved in PNH pathophysiology?); however, its clinical translation for PNH seems hard, mostly because of the extremely high dose that would be needed to achieve pharmacological levels [109]. Recently, another CP inhibitor has been described which specifically targets C1s. TNT003 (True North Therapeutics) is a mouse IgG2a mAb which inhibits the catalytic effect of C1s; this agent has been tested in vitro in antibody-mediated hemolytic anemia (more specifically, in cold agglutinin disease, CAD) [110]. TNT003 has proven effective in preventing antibody-mediated surface complement activation, preventing possible hemolysis as well as C3 decoration of target erythrocytes [110]. TNT003 recapitulates in a CP-mediated disease the findings described using selective AP inhibitors in PNH: indeed, by blocking the very initial step of CP activation, TNT003 may prevent C3-mediated extravascular hemolysis (which in CAD is the dominant pathogenic mechanism) as well as possible intravascular hemolysis (which in CAD and other autoimmune anemias play a minimal role due to the presence of CD55 on normal erythrocytes) [110]. While this agent seems very promising for clinical development in CAD and other antibody-mediated hemolytic anemia, its role in PNH should be addressed starting from preclinical studies. The list of candidate agents potentially intercepting the CP should be completed by mentioning strategies exploiting RCAs acting at the level of the C3 convertase; indeed, given the dual effect of CR1 on both the AP and CP, CR1-based approach may be used also for tuning the activation of CP C3 and C5 convertases (see above).

Selective Inhibitors of the Mannose/Lectin Pathway

Quite recently, the role of the mannose/lectin pathway (MP) in complement activation has been revisited, and it has been emerging as more relevant than initially thought. This pathway is similar and someway overlapping to the CP; indeed, they merge at the level of C4 cleavage. In contrast to the CP, in the MP the catalytic action of $C1r_2s_2$ is exerted by some other proteins called mannose-binding lectin-associated serine proteases (MASPs), which are similar (and possibly evolutionarily related) to C1r and C1s. Different MASPs have been described (MASP-1, MASP-2, and MASP-3), which are triggered by mannan-binding lectin (MBL, also called mannose-binding protein), collectin, and ficolins. Different evidences are emerging supporting the concept that the MP may cross-talk with the other complement pathways through its different effector arms. Indeed, whereas MASP-2 seems involved in activation of the CP C3 and C5 convertases, MASP-3 might play a role in the proper functioning of the AP. Even if the role of the MP in complement-mediated diseases remains to be elucidated, the availability of selective MASP inhibitors (under development by Omeros) is triggering the interest for their use as novel candidate complement inhibitors. Some preliminary data are available in vitro for PNH: consistent with the pivotal role of the AP in PNH pathophysiology, MASP-2 inhibitors did not exert any protective effect on PNH erythrocytes (Risitano and Schwaeble, unpublished data), whereas novel MASP-3 inhibitors have been reported to be someway protective [111].

20.4 Therapeutic Complement Inhibition for PNH: Pros and Cons of Different Strategies and Molecules

Complement inhibition has been proven dramatically effective for the treatment of PNH, and nowadays the challenge moved to develop further treatments which aim to improve these excellent results. The main scientific goal of developing novel therapeutics is for sure the improvement of hematological response, eventually preventing C3-mediated extravascular hemolysis; however, clinical benefits may also consider a patient perspective. For instance, moving to easier administration routes or treatment schedules would represent a significant step forward for patient well-being and even their social productivity. On the other hand, these novel treatments should not expose patients to unacceptable risks of treatment-related complications; last but not least, any novel anticomplement agent (irrespective of its efficacy) should avoid the outrageous cost of eculizumab (which in the end may limit the access to the treatment for many PNH patients). We have discussed different strategies which exploit a number of candidate agents, entailing different advantages and disadvantages. Thus, what is the best strategy of complement inhibition for PNH? The anti-C5 approach, as clinically available with eculizumab, has been demonstrated effective, with minimal safety concerns. Indeed, the risk of infectious complications (and especially of meningococcal infection) resulted well controlled by active (vaccination) and possibly passive (antimicrobial agents) prophylaxis, and no further side effects have emerged. It is conceivable that such amenable safety profile may be shared by other novel anti-C5 approaches; however, in terms of efficacy, it is hard to hypothesize that different anti-C5 agents may improve the excellent results seen with eculizumab. However, these alternative anti-C5 agents might entail different kind of benefits over eculizumab. First of all, they look excellent candidates to overcome the genetic resistance to eculizumab demonstrated in PNH patients with C5 mutation. Another possible benefit of these alternative agents relies on the class of molecules, which might allow for different administration routes (i.e., subcutaneously or even orally) and possible self-administration, eventually sparing frequent hospitalization and making the treatment less burdensome for patients. Whether some of these molecules may also result in a more sustained C5 inhibition, preventing both possible pharmacokinetic and harmacodynamics breakthrough, it remains at the moment a theoretical hypothesis.

In contrast, the pattern of possible pros and cons may drastically chance once we deal with therapeutic strategies which intercept the complement cascade upstream, at the level of C3 or even of pathway-specific initiating events. Since PNH pathophysiology mainly reflects the uncontrollable activation of the AP, with an initial accumulation of C3 fragments followed by terminal complement activation, devising a strategy that targets the C3 generation is an attractive therapeutic approach. As C3 marks the point of convergence for all initiation pathways, interception of C3 activation is largely independent of underlying triggering mechanisms and should not be influenced by known polymorphisms of C5 and CR1 (which have been associated with poor response to eculizumab). All strategies targeting the C3 are expected to be effective in preventing all downstream terminal effector complement activation similar to the anti-C5, clinically resulting in inhibition of the intravascular hemolysis typical of PNH; thus, anti-C3 agents should be used as single agents, and no rational for combination with current anti-C5 agents exists. In addition, by inhibiting initial C3 fragment accumulation on PNH erythrocytes, C3-targeted therapies will also prevent possible C3-mediated extravascular hemolysis, possibly resulting in a substantial clinical benefit. Selecting C3 as a therapeutic target is therefore expected to lead to a more comprehensive treatment option for PNH; however, this likely benefit is counterbalanced by obvious concerns, since no data are available on clinical C3 inhibition. Anti-C3 therapies may have to deal with a theoretical impairment of microbial defense, possibly leading to increased risk of infections. Indeed, subjects with inherited C3 deficiency are known to be at risk of severe infections from encapsulated pyogenic organisms [112, 113] and possibly of immune-complex-mediated diseases; however, the clinical phenotype is not dramatic and tends to improve with age, when in the presence of a fully competent adaptive immunity, the complement system may become somehow redundant for the control of infections. While these safety concerns may be common to all anti-C3 agents, different molecules may have specific advantages, such as administration route, PK/PD profiles, and cost, which make all of them worth of future clinical investigation. At the moment, small molecules targeting the C3 seem the best candidates for clinical translation, and indeed plans for human studies have started, based on the idea that potential benefits should exceed potential risks entailed by these treatments. While a broad anti-C3 strategy may anticipate a better efficacy as compared with current anti-C5 treatment (with safety and toxicity to be investigated in vivo), a pathway-specific anti-C3 treatment might be considered as a possible alternative. Indeed, pathway-specific approaches may reduce the safety concerns by selectively inhibiting only the complement pathway(s) playing a pivotal role in PNH pathophysiology, leaving intact physiological functions essential for microbial defense and prevention of immune-mediated diseases. PNH is classically considered a complement AP-mediated disease, with initial C3 tickover and subsequent AP-mediated amplification eventually leading to hemolysis; thus, selective AP inhibitors are good candidates to be investigated in PNH. However, it has to be remarked that while intact CP and MP might preserve physiological protection from microbial agents, it has not been ruled out that the same pathways may also precipitate hemolysis in PNH independently from the AP, for instance, during infectious episodes (which are known to be associated with hemolytic paroxysms). On the other hand, given the pivotal role of AP components in the amplification of initial complement activation (irrespective of the initiating trigger), it is not known whether an in vivo blockade of the AP may also impair the proper functioning of other complement pathways (this possibility would be beneficial for control of hemolysis, but detrimental for infectious risk). Thus, looking for complement therapeutics which may be effective for C3-mediated extravascular hemolysis, AP-specific inhibitors are an excellent alternative to broad anti-C3 inhibitors. At the moment, the choice between the different classes of AP inhibitors is not easy; indeed, RCA-based approaches are extremely elegant leading to a quasi-physiological modulation of complement activity, but they seem challenging due to the regulatory implications of using large engineered proteins and to the possible high cost. On the other hand, specific inhibitors of key AP components (e.g., FB and FD) are an intriguing option, because the clinical development of small inhibitors may be easier and cheaper. At the moment, given that the role of the complement CP and MP in PNH is questionable, inhibitors of these pathways seem less intriguing for clinical investigation, at least until robust preclinical data will support their use in PNH.

20.5 Conclusions

The availability of the complement inhibitor eculizumab has changed the natural history of PNH. However, emerging scientific observations as well as pharmaceutical business have prompted the development of novel complement therapeutic. All these researches are more than welcome, since substantial unmet clinical needs remain in PNH; however, any attempt to interfere with the complement cascade must come to terms with the potential risks that the blockade of key components might entail. The search for best anticomplement agent for PNH has just started, with a dual challenge: first, to identify therapeutic agents that may lead to improved efficacy, without increasing the potential risks, and, second, to guarantee treatment options which will have reasonable costs, allowing a worldwide access to therapy for all PNH patients. However, given the plethora of candidate agents in preclinical and clinical investigation, it is conceivable that the next decade will bring us with one or more novel anticomplement agents which may extend the scenario of treatment options for PNH patients, possibly with improved clinical outcome. It would be of extraordinary importance that the scientific community will be able to drive this development, making sure that the most appropriate agents will be the ones to be investigated in the clinic, and that financial interests will not hinder the progress of medical science.

References

1. Risitano AM (2012) Paroxysmal nocturnal hemoglobinuria. In: Silverberg D (ed) Anemia. InTech, Rijeka
2. Luzzatto L, Notaro R (2003) Paroxysmal nocturnal hemoglobinuria. In: Handin RI, Lux SE, Stossel TP (eds) Blood, principles and practice of hematology, 2nd edn. Lippincot Williams & Wilkins, Philadelphia, pp 319–334
3. Parker CJ, Ware RE (2003) Paroxysmal nocturnal hemoglobinuria. In: Greer J et al (eds) Wintrobe's clinical hematology, 11th edn. Lippincott Williams & Wilkins, Philadelphia, pp 1203–1221
4. Miyata T, Takeda J, Iida Y et al (1993) The cloning of PIG-A, a component in the early step of GPI-anchor biosynthesis. Science 259:1318–1320
5. Takeda J, Miyata T, Kawagoe K et al (1993) Deficiency of the GPI anchor caused by a somatic mutation of the PIG-A gene in paroxysmal nocturnal hemoglobinuria. Cell 73:703–711
6. Nicholson-Weller A, Burge J, Fearon DT, Weller PF, Austen KF (1982) Isolation of a human erythrocyte membrane glycoprotein with decay-accelerating activity for C3 convertases of the complement system. J Immunol 129(1):184–189
7. Nicholson-Weller A (1992) Decay accelerating factor (CD55). Curr Top Microbiol Immunol 178:7–30
8. Holguin MH, Fredrick LR, Bernshaw NJ et al (1989) Isolation and characterization of a membrane protein from normal human erythrocytes that inhibits reactive lysis of the erythrocytes of paroxysmal nocturnal hemoglobinuria. J Clin Invest 84:7–17
9. Meri S, Morgan BP, Davies A, Daniels RH, Olavesen MG, Waldmann H, Lachmann PJ (1990) Human protectin (CD59), an 18,000-20,000 MW complement lysis restricting factor, inhibits C5b-8 catalysed insertion of C9 into lipid bilayers. Immunology 71(1):1–9
10. Wilcox LA, Ezzell JL, Bernshaw NJ, Parker CJ (1991) Molecular basis of the enhanced susceptibility of the erythrocytes of paroxysmal nocturnal hemoglobinuria to hemolysis in acidified serum. Blood 78:820–829
11. Telen MJ, Green AM (1989) The Inab phenotype: characterization of the membrane protein and complement regulatory defect. Blood 74(1):437–441
12. Merry AH, Rawlinson VI, Uchikawa M, Daha MR, Sim RB (1989) Studies on the sensitivity to complement-mediated lysis of erythrocytes (Inab phenotype) with a deficiency of DAF (decay accelerating factor). Br J Haematol 73(2):248–253
13. Holguin MH, Martin CB, Bernshaw NJ, Parker CJ (1992) Analysis of the effects of activation of the alternative pathway of complement on erythrocytes with an isolated deficiency of decay accelerating factor. J Immunol 148:498–502
14. Yamashina M, Ueda E, Kinoshita T, Takami T, Ojima A, Ono H, Tanaka H, Kondo N, Orii T, Okada N et al (1990) Inherited complete deficiency of 20-kilodalton homologous restriction factor (CD59) as a cause of paroxysmal nocturnal hemoglobinuria. N Engl J Med 323(17):1184–1189
15. Motoyama N, Okada N, Yamashina M, Okada H (1992) Paroxysmal nocturnal hemoglobinuria due to hereditary nucleotide deletion in the HRF20 (CD59) gene. Eur J Immunol 22(10):2669–2673
16. Kelly R, Hillmen P (2014) Clinical effects of Eculizumab in PNH. In: Yuzuru Kanakura Y, Kinoshita T, Nishimura J (eds) PNH; from bench to bedside (in press)
17. Rother RP, Rollins SA, Mojcik CF et al (2007) Discovery and development of the complement inhibitor eculizumab for the treatment of paroxysmal nocturnal hemoglobinuria. Nat Biotechnol 25:1256–1264
18. Hillmen P, Young NS, Schubert J et al (2006) The complement inhibitor eculizumab in paroxysmal nocturnal hemoglobinuria. N Engl J Med 355:1233–1243

19. Brodsky RA, Young NS, Antonioli E et al (2008) Multicenter phase III study of the complement inhibitor eculizumab for the treatment of patients with paroxysmal nocturnal hemoglobinuria. Blood 114:1840–1847
20. Hillmen P, Muus P, Duhrsen U et al (2007) Effect of the complement inhibitor eculizumab on thromboembolism in patients with paroxysmal nocturnal hemoglobinuria. Blood 110:4123–4128
21. Rother RP, Bell L, Hillmen P et al (2005) The clinical sequelae of intravascular hemolysis and extracellular plasma hemoglobin: a novel mechanism of human disease. JAMA 293:1653–1662
22. Helley D, de Latour RP, Porcher R, French Society of Hematology (2010) Evaluation of hemostasis and endothelial function in patients with paroxysmal nocturnal hemoglobinuria receiving eculizumab. Haematologica 95:574–581
23. Kelly RJ, Hill A, Arnold LM et al (2011) Long-term treatment with eculizumab in paroxysmal nocturnal hemoglobinuria: sustained efficacy and improved survival. Blood 117:6786–6792
24. Notaro R, Risitano AM, Luzzatto L (2014, In press) Clinical effects of Eculizumab in PNH; extravascular hemolysis after EculizumabTreatment. In: Yuzuru Kanakura Y, Kinoshita T, and Nishimura J (ed). PNH; from bench to bedside
25. Risitano AM, Notaro R, Marando L et al (2009) Complement fraction 3 binding on erythrocytes as additional mechanism of disease in paroxysmal nocturnal hemoglobinuria patients treated by eculizumab. Blood 113:4094–4100
26. Hill A, Rother RP, Arnold L et al (2010) Eculizumab prevents intravascular hemolysis in patients with paroxysmal nocturnal hemoglobinuria and unmasks low-level extravascular hemolysis occurring through C3 opsonization. Haematologica 95:567–573
27. Marotta S, Giagnuolo G, Basile S, Pagliuca S, Grimaldi F, Pane F, Risitano AM (2014) Excellent outcome of concomitant intensive immunosuppression and eculizumab in aplastic anemia/paroxysmal nocturnal hemoglobinuria syndrome. J Hematol Thromb Dis 2(1):128
28. Hillmen P, Muus P, Roth A et al (2013) Long-term safety and efficacy of sustained eculizumab treatment in patients with paroxysmal nocturnal haemoglobinuria. Br J Haematol 162(1):62–73
29. Luzzatto L, Risitano AM, Notaro R (2010) Paroxysmal nocturnal hemoglobinuria and eculizumab. Haematologica 95(4):523–526
30. Risitano AM, Marando L, Seneca E, Rotoli B (2008) Hemoglobin normalization after splenectomy in a paroxysmal nocturnal hemoglobinuria patient treated by eculizumab. Blood 112(2):449–451
31. Risitano AM, Notaro R, Luzzatto L, Hill A, Kelly R, Hillmen P (2010) Paroxysmal nocturnal hemoglobinuria–hemolysis before and after eculizumab. N Engl J Med 363(23):2270–2272
32. Nishimura J, Yamamoto M, Hayashi S et al (2014) Genetic variants in C5 and poor response to eculizumab. N Engl J Med 370(7):632–639
33. Rondelli T, Risitano AM, Peffault de Latour LR et al (2014) Polymorphism of the complement receptor 1 gene correlates with the hematologic response to eculizumab in patients with paroxysmal nocturnal hemoglobinuria. Haematologica 99(2):262–266
34. Kaudlay P, Hua H, He G, Newton DJ, Varghese AM, Munir T, Hill A, Kelly RJ, Richards SJ, Hillmen P (2013) Red cell complement loading in PNH patients on Eculizumab is associated with a C3 polymorphism which influences C3 function, predicts for increased extravascular hemolysis and provides a rationale for C3 inhibition. Blood 122(21):2466
35. Kavanagh D, Goodship T (2010) Genetics and complement in atypical HUS. Pediatr Nephrol 25(12):2431–2442
36. Licht C, Fremeaux-Bacchi V (2019) Hereditary and acquired complement dysregulation in membranoproliferative glomerulonephritis. Thromb Haemost 101(2):271–278
37. ClinicalTrials.gov. A service of the U.S. National Institutes of Health. http://clinicaltrials.gov/ct2/show/NCT01624636
38. Adienne Pharma & Biotech (2014) http://www.adienne.com/en/rd/pipeline/mubodina®.html

39. Marzari R, Sblattero D, Macor P, Fischetti F, Gennaro R, Marks JD, Bradbury A, Tedesco F (2002) The cleavage site of C5 from man and animals as a common target for neutralizing human monoclonal antibodies: in vitro and in vivo studies. Eur J Immunol 32(10):2773–2782
40. Woodruff TM, Nandakumar KS, Tedesco F (2011) Inhibiting the C5-C5a receptor axis. Mol Immunol 48(14):1631–1642
41. Macor P, Durigutto P, De Maso L, Garrovo C, Biffi S, Cortini A, Fischetti F, Sblattero D, Pitzalis C, Marzari R, Tedesco F (2012) Treatment of experimental arthritis by targeting synovial endothelium with a neutralizing recombinant antibody to C5. Arthritis Rheum 64(8):2559–2567
42. Nunn MA, Sharma A, Paesen GC et al (2005) Complement inhibitor of C5 activation from the soft tick Ornithodoros moubata. J Immunol 174(4):2084–2091
43. Roversi P, Lissina O, Johnson S et al (2007) The structure of OMCI, a novel lipocalin inhibitor of the complement system. J Mol Biol 369(3):784–793
44. Barratt-Due A, Thorgersen EB, Lindstad JK et al (2011) Ornithodoros moubata complement inhibitor is an equally effective C5 inhibitor in pigs and humans. J Immunol 187(9):4913–4919
45. Weston-Davies WH, Westwood JP, Nunn M et al (2014) Phase I clinical trial of coversin, a novel complement C5 and LTB4 inhibitor. Paper presented at: 7th international conference on complement therapeutics, Olympia, June 6–11, 2014. Aegean conferences 82, abs 31
46. Lee M, Narayanan S, McGeer EG, McGeer PL (2014) Aurin tricarboxylic acid protects against red blood cell hemolysis in patients with paroxysmal nocturnal hemoglobinemia. PLoS One 9(1), e87316
47. Lee M, Guo JP, McGeer EG, McGeer PL (2012) Aurin tricarboxylic acid self-protects by inhibiting aberrant complement activation at the C3 convertase and C9 binding stages. Neurobiol Aging 34(5):1451–1461
48. Lee M, Guo JP, Schwab C, McGeer EG, McGeer PL (2012) Selective inhibition of the membrane attack complex of complement by low molecular weight components of the aurin tricarboxylic acid synthetic complex. Neurobiol Aging 33(10):2237–2246
49. Cox JC, Rajendran M, Riedel T, Davidson EA, Sooter LY, Bayer TS, Schmitz-Brown M, Ellington AD (2002) Automated acquisition of aptamer sequences. Comb Chem High Throughput Screen 5(4):289–299
50. Leung E, Landa G (2013) Update on current and future novel therapies for dry age-related macular degeneration. Expert Rev Clin Pharmacol 6(5):565–579
51. ClinicalTrials.gov. A service of the U.S. National Institutes of Health. http://clinicaltrials.gov/ct2/show/NCT00950638
52. Drolet DW, Zhang C, O'Connell DJ, Gupta S, Janjic N (2014) SOMAmer inhibitors of the complement system. Paper presented at: 7th international conference on complement therapeutics, Olympia, June 6–11, 2014. Aegean conferences 82, abs 23
53. Feldwisch J, Tolmachev V (2012) Engineering of affibody molecules for therapy and diagnostics. Methods Mol Biol 899:103–126
54. Strömberg P (2014) Introducing SOBI002, a small Affibody-ABD fusion protein targeting complement component C5. Paper presented at: 7th international conference on complement therapeutics, Olympia, June 6–11, 2014. Aegean conferences 82, abs 30
55. ClinicalTrials.gov. A service of the U.S. National Institutes of Health. http://clinicaltrials.gov/ct2/show/NCT02083666
56. Josephson K, Ricardo A, Szostak JW (2014) mRNA display: from basic principles to macrocycle drug discovery. Drug Discov Today 19(4):388–399
57. Ricardo A, Arata M, DeMarco S, Dhamnaskar K, Hammer R, Josephson K, Seyb K, Tobe S, Wang Z, Zheng H, Treco D (2014) Development of RA101348, a potent cyclic peptide inhibitor of C5 for complement-mediated diseases. American Society of Hematology meeting 2014, submitted

58. Borodovsky A, Yucius K, Sprague A, Butler J, Fishman S, Nguyen T, Vaishnaw A, Maier M, Kallanthottathil R, Kuchimanchi S, Manoharan M, Meyers R, Fitzgerald K (2013) Development of RNAi therapeutics targeting the complement pathway. Blood 122(21):2471
59. Hill A, Ridley SH, Esser D, Oldroyd RG, Cullen MJ, Kareclas P, Gallagher S, Smith GP, Richards SJ, White J, Smith RA, Hillmen P (2006) Protection of erythrocytes from human complement-mediated lysis by membrane-targeted recombinant soluble CD59: a new approach to PNH therapy. Blood 107(5):2131–2137
60. Parker C (2014) Complement in PNH. In: Yuzuru Kanakura Y, Kinoshita T, Nishimura J (ed) PNH; from bench to bedside (in press)
61. Ricklin D, Hajishengallis G, Yang K, Lambris JD (2010) Complement: a key system for immune surveillance and homeostasis. Nat Immunol 11(9):785–797
62. Ricklin D, Lambris JD (2013) Complement in immune and inflammatory disorders: therapeutic interventions. J Immunol 190(8):3839–3847
63. Lindorfer MA, Pawluczkowycz AW, Peek EM, Hickman K, Taylor RP, Parker CJ (2010) A novel approach to preventing the hemolysis of paroxysmal nocturnal hemoglobinuria: both complement-mediated cytolysis and C3 deposition are blocked by a monoclonal antibody specific for the alternative pathway of complement. Blood 115(11):2283–2291
64. Paixao-Cavalcante D, Torreira E, Lindorfer MA et al (2014) A humanized antibody that regulates the alternative pathway convertase: potential for therapy of renal disease associated with nephritic factors. J Immunol 192(10):4844–4851
65. Sahu A, Kay BK, Lambris JD (1996) Inhibition of human complement by a C3-binding peptide isolated from a phage-displayed random peptide library. J Immunol 157(2):884–891
66. Ricklin D, Lambris JD (2008) Compstatin: a complement inhibitor on its way to clinical application. Adv Exp Med Biol 632:273–292
67. ClinicalTrials.gov. A service of the U.S. National Institutes of Health. http://clinicaltrials.gov/ct2/show/NCT00473928
68. Silasi-Mansat R, Zhu H, Popescu NI et al (2010) Complement inhibition decreases the procoagulant response and confers organ protection in a baboon model of Escherichia coli sepsis. Blood 116(6):1002–1010
69. Kourtzelis I, Markiewski MM, Doumas M et al (2010) Complement anaphylatoxin C5a contributes to hemodialysis-associated thrombosis. Blood 116(4):631–639
70. Qu H, Magotti P, Ricklin D et al (2011) Novel analogues of the therapeutic complement inhibitor compstatin with significantly improved affinity and potency. Mol Immunol 48(4):481–489
71. Qu H, Ricklin D, Bai H et al (2013) New analogs of the clinical complement inhibitor compstatin with subnanomolar affinity and enhanced pharmacokinetic properties. Immunobiology 218(4):496–505
72. Magotti P, Ricklin D, Qu H, Wu YQ, Kaznessis YN, Lambris JD (2009) Structure-kinetic relationship analysis of the therapeutic complement inhibitor compstatin. J Mol Recognit 22(6):495–505
73. Risitano AM, Ricklin D, Huang Y et al (2014) Peptide inhibitors of C3 activation as a novel strategy of complement inhibition for the treatment of paroxysmal nocturnal hemoglobinuria. Blood 123(13):2094–2101
74. Jevsevar S, Kunstelj M, Porekar VG (2010) PEGylation of therapeutic proteins. Biotechnol J 5(1):113–128
75. McDonnell T, Ioannou Y, Rahman A (2014) PEGylated drugs in rheumatology–why develop them and do they work? Rheumatology 53(3):391–396
76. Ricklin D, Lambris JD (2013) Progress and trends in complement therapeutics. Adv Exp Med Biol 735:1–22
77. Whaley K, Ruddy S (1976) Modulation of the alternative complement pathway by β1H globulin. J Exp Med 144:1147–1163
78. Ricklin D, Lambris JD (2013) Complement in immune and inflammatory disorders: pathophysiological mechanisms. J Immunol 190(8):3831–3838

79. Ferreira VP, Pangburn MK (2007) Factor H mediated cell surface protection from complement is critical for the survival of PNH erythrocytes. Blood 110(6):2190–2192
80. Huang Y, Qiao F, Atkinson C, Holers VM, Tomlinson S (2008) A novel targeted inhibitor of the alternative pathway of complement and its therapeutic application in ischemia/reperfusion injury. J Immunol 181(11):8068–8076
81. Rohrer B, Long Q, Coughlin B (2009) A targeted inhibitor of the alternative complement pathway reduces angiogenesis in a mouse model of age-related macular degeneration. Invest Ophthalmol Vis Sci 50(7):3056–3064
82. Song H, Qiao F, Atkinson C, Holers VM, Tomlinson S (2007) A complement C3 inhibitor specifically targeted to sites of complement activation effectively ameliorates collagen induced arthritis in DBA/1J mice. J Immunol 179(11):7860–7867
83. Fridkis-Hareli M, Storek M, Mazsaroff I et al (2011) Design and development of TT30, a novel C3d-targeted C3/C5 convertase inhibitor for treatment of human complement alternative pathway-mediated diseases. Blood 118(17):4705–4713
84. Risitano AM, Notaro R, Pascariello C et al (2012) The complement receptor 2/factor H fusion protein TT30 protects paroxysmal nocturnal hemoglobinuria erythrocytes from complement-mediated hemolysis and C3 fragment. Blood 119(26):6307–6316
85. ClinicalTrials.gov. A service of the U.S. National Institutes of Health. http://clinicaltrials.gov/ct2/show/NCT01335165
86. Schmidt CQ, Bai H, Lin Z et al (2013) Rational engineering of a minimized immune inhibitor with unique triple-targeting properties. J Immunol 190(11):5712–5721
87. Hebecker M, Alba-Domínguez M, Roumenina LT, Reuter S, Hyvärinen S, Dragon-Durey MA, Jokiranta TS, Sánchez-Corral P, Józsi M (2013) An engineered construct combining complement regulatory and surface-recognition domains represents a minimal-size functional factor H. J Immunol 191(2):912–921
88. Qiao Q, Teng X, Wang N, Lu R, Guo L, Zhang X, Du Y, Wang W, Chen S, Wu Q, He G, Wang Y, Hu W (2014) A novel CRIg-targeted complement inhibitor protects cells from complement damage. FASEB J 28(11):4986–4999 [Epub ahead of print]
89. Khera R, Das N (2009) Complement receptor 1: disease associations and therapeutic implications. Mol Immunol 46(5):761–772
90. Iida K, Nussenzweig V (1981) Complement receptor is an inhibitor of the complement cascade. J Exp Med 153(5):1138–1150
91. Ross GD, Lambris JD, Cain JA, Newman SL (1982) Generation of three different fragments of bound C3 with purified factor I or serum. I. Requirements for factor H vs CR1 cofactor activity. J Immunol 129(5):2051–2060
92. Medof ME, Nussenzweig V (1984) Control of the function of substrate-bound C4b-C3b by the complement receptor Cr1. J Exp Med 159(6):1669–1685
93. Pratt JR, Hibbs MJ, Laver AJ, Smith RA, Sacks SH (1996) Effects of complement inhibition with soluble complement receptor-1 on vascular injury and inflammation during renal allograft rejection in the rat. Am J Pathol 149(6):2055–2066
94. ClinicalTrials.gov. A service of the U.S. National Institutes of Health. http://clinicaltrials.gov/ct2/show/NCT01791686
95. Zhang Y, Nester CM, Holanda DG, Marsh HC, Hammond RA, Thomas LJ, Meyer NC, Hunsicker LG, Sethi S, Smith RJ (2013) Soluble CR1 therapy improves complement regulation in C3 glomerulopathy. J Am Soc Nephrol 24(11):1820–1829
96. Smith RJH, Xiao H, Nester CM, Holanda DG, Marsh HC, Meyer NC, Sethi S, Zhang Y (2014) Soluble CR1 therapy improves complement regulation in C3 glomerulopathy. Paper presented at: 7th international conference on complement therapeutics, Olympia, June 6–11, 2014. Aegean conferences 82, abs 37
97. Souza DG, Esser D, Bradford R, Vieira AT, Teixeira MM (2005) APT070 (Mirococept), a membrane-localised complement inhibitor, inhibits inflammatory responses that follow intestinal ischaemia and reperfusion injury. Br J Pharmacol 145(8):1027–1034
98. Smith RA (2012) Membrane-targeted complement inhibitors. Mol Immunol 38:249–255

99. Patel H, Smith RA, Sacks SH, Zhou W (2006) Therapeutic strategy with a membrane-localizing complement regulator to increase the number of usable donor organs after prolonged cold storage. J Am Soc Nephrol 17(4):1102–1111
100. Sacks S, Karegli J, Farrar CA, Asgari E, Schwaeble W, Zhou W, Smith RA (2013) Targeting complement at the time of transplantation. Adv Exp Med Biol 735:247–255
101. International Standard Randomised Controlled Trial Number Register (2104). http://www.controlled-trials.com/ISRCTN49958194
102. Holers M, Banda N, Mehta G, Fridkis. Hareli M, Or E, Storek M, Altman R, Johnson K, Katti S (2012) The human complement receptor 2 (CR2)/CR1 fusion protein TT32, a targeted inhibitor of the classical and alternative pathway C3 convertase, prevents arthritis in active immunization and passive transfer models and acts by CR2-dependent targeting of CR1 regulatory activity. In: XXIV international complement workshop, Chania, October 10–15, 2012: abs #230
103. Taube C, Thurman JM, Takeda K, Joetham A, Miyahara N, Carroll MC, Dakhama A, Giclas PC, Holers VM, Gelfand EW (2006) Factor B of the alternative complement pathway regulates development of airway hyperresponsiveness and inflammation. Proc Natl Acad Sci U S A 103(21):8084–8089
104. ClinicalTrials.gov. A service of the U.S. National Institutes of Health. http://clinicaltrials.gov/ct2/show/NCT01602120
105. Altmann E, Hommel U, Lorthiois ELJ, Maibaum JK, Ostermann N, Quancard J, Randl SA, Simic O, Vulpetti A, Rogel O, Novartis Ag (2012) Indole compounds or analogs thereof as complement factor D inhibitors useful for the treatment of age-related macular degeneration and their preparation. From PCT Int. Appl., WO 2012093101 http://www.google.com/patents/WO2012093101A1?cl=en&hl=it
106. Dechantsreiter MA, Grob JE, Mac Sweeney A, Miltz W, Randl S, Sedrani R, Sellner H, Sirockin F, Valeur E, Novartis Ag (2013) Preparation of quinazoline compounds as modulators of the complement alternative pathway for treating macular degeneration, diabetic retinopathy, and other diseases. From PCT Int. Appl., WO 2013192345 http://www.google.com.ar/patents/WO2013192345A1?cl=en&hl=it
107. Bansal R, Novelmed Therapeutics (2013) Anti-properdin antibodies. US Patent 8435512, 5 July 2013. http://www.freepatentsonline.com/8435512.html, https://www.google.com/patents/US20140186348
108. Novelmed Therapeutics. http://www.novelmed.com/ProductPipeline/ParoxysmalNocturnalHemoglobinuria(PNH).aspx
109. DeZern AE, Uknis M, Yuan X, Mukhina GL, Varela J, Saye J, Pu J, Brodsky RA (2014) Complement blockade with a C1 esterase inhibitor in paroxysmal nocturnal hemoglobinuria. Exp Hematol 42(10):857–861 [Epub ahead of print]
110. Shi J, Rose EL, Singh A, Hussain S, Stagliano NE, Parry GC, Panicker S (2014) TNT003, an inhibitor of the serine protease C1s, prevents complement activation induced by cold agglutinins. Blood 123(26):4015–4022
111. Scwaeble WJ (2014) The utility of lectin pathway inhibitors as modulators if inflammatory, thrombotic and haemolytic diseases. Paper presented at: 7th international conference on complement therapeutics, Olympia, June 6–11, 2014. Aegean conferences 82, abs 25
112. Botto M, Kirschfink M, Macor P, Pickering MC, Würzner R, Tedesco F (2009) Complement in human diseases: lessons from complement deficiencies. Mol Immunol 46(14):2774–2783
113. Lachmann PJ, Smith RA (2009) Taking complement to the clinic–has the time finally come? Scand J Immunol 69(6):471–478

Chapter 21
Pregnancy in Paroxysmal Nocturnal Hemoglobinuria

Naoyuki Miyasaka and Osamu Miura

Abstract In paroxysmal nocturnal hemoglobinuria (PNH), pregnancy is associated with increased risks of severe complications such as thromboembolic diseases like Budd-Chiari syndrome, hypertensive disorders like preeclampsia, and cerebrovascular diseases. Therefore, female PNH patients are generally discouraged from becoming pregnant. Recently, however, successful pregnancy outcomes have been reported for PNH patients with eculizumab treatment. Eculizumab, a humanized monoclonal antibody that specifically targets the terminal complement protein C5, inhibits intravascular hemolysis, thereby reducing the risk of complications, especially thrombosis, in pregnant patients. Although the available clinical data are limited, eculizumab is likely to improve pregnancy outcomes in patients with PNH. We propose management protocols for pregnancies in PNH. Patients are classified into four categories depending on previous eculizumab use and the history of venous thromboembolisms. Eculizumab and anticoagulant use is determined depending on risk severity. The importance of managing patients from preconception through pregnancy and until the postpartum stage is emphasized, along with cooperation between hematologists and obstetricians. A review of additional cases and reevaluation of outcomes is, nonetheless, required before a definitive recommendation for the management of pregnancy with PNH can be made.

Keywords Pregnancy • Paroxysmal nocturnal hemoglobinuria • Eculizumab • Anticoagulation

---

N. Miyasaka, M.D., Ph.D. (✉)
Department of Pediatrics, Perinatal and Maternal Medicine, Graduate School of Medical and Dental Sciences, Tokyo Medical and Dental University (TMDU), 1-5-45 Yushima, Bunkyo-ku, 113-5819 Tokyo, Japan
e-mail: n.miyasaka.gyne@tmd.ac.jp

O. Miura
Department of Hematology, Graduate School of Medical and Dental Sciences, Tokyo Medical and Dental University (TMDU), Tokyo, Japan

Y. Kanakura et al. (eds.), *Paroxysmal Nocturnal Hemoglobinuria*,
DOI 10.1007/978-4-431-56003-6_21

21.1 Introduction

Paroxysmal nocturnal hemoglobinuria (PNH) is a consequence of clonal expansion of hematopoietic stem cells that have an acquired somatic mutation in the *PIG-A* gene [1–3]. Because *PIG-A* encodes glycosyl phosphatidylinositol-anchored proteins (GPI-APs), which anchor the complement regulatory proteins CD55 and CD59, the affected hematopoietic cells are unusually susceptible to complement-mediated intravascular hemolysis [4–6]. The clinical manifestation of PNH is complex, primarily involving three sets of symptoms: hemolysis with acute exacerbation, cytopenia of varying severity, and a tendency for thrombosis [7–10]. The diagnosis of clinical PNH is based on the detection of GPI-AP-negative hematopoietic cells with clinical evidence of intravascular hemolysis [4]. For many years, female patients with PNH were generally discouraged from becoming pregnant because of the increased risk of life-threatening complications like thromboembolisms [4–6]. Recently, however, successful pregnancy outcomes have been reported for such individuals with use of eculizumab [11–13], a humanized monoclonal antibody that specifically targets the terminal complement protein C5 [14, 15]. In this chapter, pregnancy outcomes in patients with PNH are overviewed, and possible pathophysiological mechanisms of PNH during pregnancy are described. Additionally, possible management protocols for pregnancy with PNH are proposed.

21.2 Pregnancy in PNH Before the Introduction of Eculizumab

PNH is usually diagnosed in patients in their 30s and 40s [7–10], and this condition is now being increasingly diagnosed in female patients of childbearing age because of advances in diagnostic technology and improved disease understanding. However, pregnancy in PNH is associated with increased risks of severe complications.

21.2.1 Pregnancy Outcomes

A review by Fieni et al. [16] and a case series from France [17] reported pregnancy outcomes in patients with PNH before eculizumab came into clinical use (Table 21.1). Although there is a substantial difference in the prevalence of anticoagulant therapy between the two studies (Fieni et al. [16], 14 %; de Guibert et al. [17], 72 %), the complications and their incidences during pregnancy and in the postpartum period are similar. These studies reported that RBC and/or platelet transfusion for anemia and/or thrombocytopenia was required in 52–63 % cases. Additionally, thromboembolic events including Budd-Chiari syndrome, venous thrombosis, and pulmonary embolism occurred in 14–20 % cases; hypertensive

Table 21.1 Pregnancy outcomes in PNH before the introduction of eculizumab

	Fieni et al. [16]	de Guibert et al. [17]
Years	1965–2005	1978–2008
Number of cases	43	25
Number of patients who received anticoagulation therapy (%)	6 (14 %)	18 (72 %)
Complications during pregnancy and in the postpartum period		
RBC and/or platelet transfusion	27 (63 %)	13 (52 %)
Thromboembolisms (Budd-Chiari syndrome, venous thromboembolisms)	6 (14 %)	5 (20 %)
Hypertensive disorder (PIH, preeclampsia, eclampsia, HELLP synd.)	6 (14 %)	5 (20 %)
Cerebrovascular complications (cerebral hemorrhage, sinus thrombosis)	5 (12 %)	3 (12 %)
Infectious disease	3 (7 %)	0 (0 %)
Hemorrhagic delivery	2 (5 %)	3 (12 %)
Preterm delivery	16 (37 %)	7 (28 %)
Cesarean section	12 (28 %)	10 (40 %)
Maternal death	5 (12 %)	2 (8 %)
Fetal/neonatal death	3 (7 %)	1 (4 %)

RBC red blood cell, *PIH* pregnancy-induced hypertension, *HELLP synd.* hemolysis, elevated liver enzyme, low platelet count

disorders including preeclampsia, eclampsia, and HELLP (hemolysis, elevated liver enzyme and low platelet count) syndrome occurred in 14–20 % cases; cerebrovascular diseases including cerebral hemorrhage and sinus thrombosis occurred in 12 % cases; and abnormal intra- and/or postpartum uterine bleeding occurred in 5–12 % cases. Further, the preterm delivery and cesarean section rates were 28–37 % and 28–40 %, respectively. Finally, the maternal and fetal mortality rates were 8–12 % and 4–7 %, respectively.

21.2.2 Pathophysiology of PNH-Related Complications During Pregnancy

Possible pathophysiological mechanisms underlying PNH-related complications during pregnancy are illustrated in Fig. 21.1. In PNH patients, intravascular hemolysis is precipitated during pregnancy due to increased levels of complement factors [18], which results in accelerated hemolytic anemia and also platelet activation directly and/or via cell-free hemoglobin elevation and nitric oxide (NO) depletion [19]. As pregnancy itself is a physiological prothrombotic state, excessive platelet activation easily causes thromboembolic complications and thrombocytopenia during pregnancy and in the postpartum period. Hyper-thrombophilic conditions in

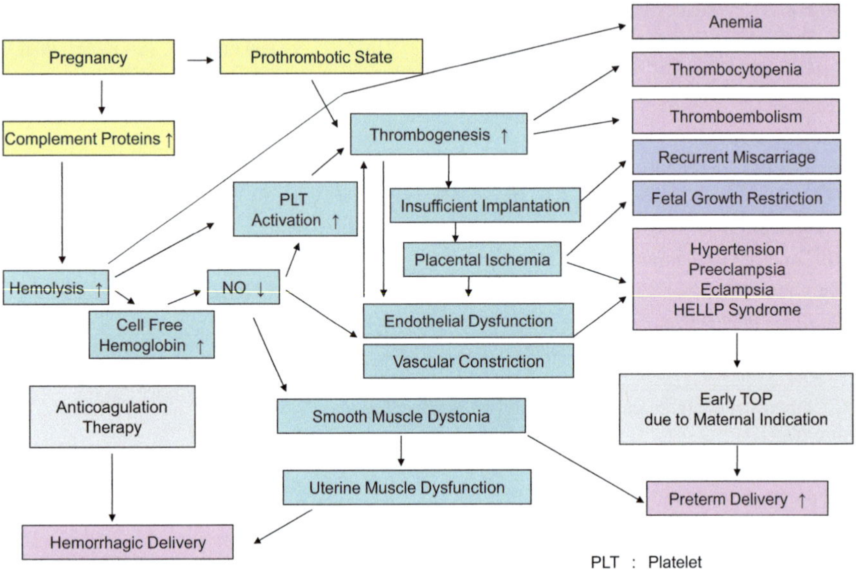

Fig. 21.1 Schematic representation of the pathophysiology of PNH-related complications during pregnancy. During pregnancy, intravascular hemolysis is precipitated because of increased levels of complement proteins, which results in accelerated hemolytic anemia and platelet (PLT) activation directly and/or via cell-free hemoglobin elevation and nitric oxide (NO) depletion. As pregnancy itself is a physiological prothrombotic state, excessive platelet activation causes thromboembolic complications and thrombocytopenia. As in the case of antiphospholipid syndrome (APS), thrombophilia in early gestation causes insufficient implantation and placental hypoxia/ischemia, resulting in recurrent miscarriage, fetal growth restriction (FGR), and pregnancy-induced hypertension (PIH). Endothelial dysfunction and vascular constriction due to NO depletion form a vicious circle with enhanced thrombophilia, causing pregnancy-associated hypertensive disorders like gestational hypertension, preeclampsia, eclampsia, and HELLP (hemolysis, elevated liver enzyme, low platelet count) syndrome. In addition, NO depletion also causes smooth muscle dystonia, which is associated with an increased incidence of preterm delivery, cesarean section, and hemorrhagic delivery because of cervical incompetence, dystocia, and uterine atony, respectively. *TOP* termination of pregnancy

early pregnancy, such as anti-phospholipid syndrome (APS), are associated with insufficient implantation and placental ischemia, which lead to recurrent miscarriage, fetal growth restriction (FGR), and pregnancy-induced hypertension (PIH) [20]. Thus, PNH patients may also have a risk of these complications. Endothelial dysfunction and vascular constriction caused by NO depletion [19] form a vicious circle with enhanced thrombophilia, resulting in pregnancy-associated hypertensive disorders, including gestational hypertension, preeclampsia, eclampsia, and HELLP syndrome. NO depletion has also been reported to cause smooth muscle dystonia [19]. As the uterus consists of smooth muscle, the incidence of preterm delivery and hemorrhagic delivery may increase because of uterine muscle dysfunction.

21.3 Pregnancy in PNH with Eculizumab Therapy

Eculizumab is a humanized monoclonal antibody directed against the terminal complement protein C5, and it inhibits complement-mediated cell lysis [21]. According to clinical trials in PNH patients, eculizumab stabilizes hemoglobin levels, reduces intravascular hemolysis and thrombotic events, decreases transfusion requirements, and improves quality of life [22, 23]. As eculizumab inhibits intravascular hemolysis itself, it can be expected to lower the risk of complications during pregnancy and in the postpartum period in women with PNH. Although available clinical data are still very limited, successful pregnancy outcomes of patients with PNH have been reported with eculizumab therapy [11–13].

21.3.1 Pregnancy Outcomes

The clinical characteristics and pregnancy outcomes of patients with PNH who have received eculizumab therapy during pregnancy are summarized in Table 21.2 [11–13]. Although the time and duration of eculizumab administration during pregnancy varied, no patient developed thromboembolic complications. However, preeclampsia occurred in one case, which may suggest that PNH is a risk factor for preeclampsia even with eculizumab therapy. Although the standard protocol of eculizumab infusion was 900 mg every 2 weeks, the interval between eculizumab infusions had to be reduced because of breakthrough hemolysis during pregnancy in two cases (every 12 days and weekly). These findings appear to be associated with the relative shortage of eculizumab because of increased complement levels and dilution because of the increased plasma volume during pregnancy. Therefore, it might be necessary to monitor lactate dehydrogenase (LDH) and/or CH50 levels and accordingly adjust the dosage and/or interval of eculizumab infusion.

Eculizumab is a hybrid of IgG4 and IgG2, and the latter is known to be less capable of crossing the placenta [24]. In previous studies, among three cases in which eculizumab concentration in the cord blood was measured, it was detected in one case and not in the remaining three. Although the possibility of maternal blood contamination cannot be completely excluded and the concentration was substantially lower than the therapeutic level, this level may not be negligible for the fetus. Therefore, long-term follow-up of the fetus and accumulation of clinical data are necessary. Nonetheless, it should be noted that no anomalies or adverse events have been reported thus far in neonates whose mothers have received eculizumab treatment, even in cases in which eculizumab was administered during the first trimester of pregnancy.

Table 21.2 Summary of the pregnancies in PNH treated with eculizumab

Case number	Author's names, year	Maternal age at pregnancy (years)	PNH granulocyte clone size (%)	LDH at baseline (IU/L)	Anticoagulation therapy		Eculizumab use in pregnancy	Complications in pregnancy	Gestational week at delivery (weeks)	Delivery method	Newborn status (birth weight [g])	Eculizumab level (μg/mL)		
					Before pregnancy	During pregnancy						Maternal blood	Cord blood (days after last dose)	Breast milk (days after last dose)
1	Danilov et al. 2009 [11]	34	30	1500	Thera peutic heparin	Therapeutic heparin	From 30 weeks and postpartum	Thrombo-cytopenia, RBC/PLT transfusion	36	C-section (twin, breech)	Healthy (2919 and 2199)	NM	NM	NM
2	Kelly et al. 2010 [12]	25	92.9	2376	Warfarin	Therapeutic heparin	Up to 5 weeks	None	Not stated	Not stated	Healthy (not stated)	NM	NM	NM
3	Kelly et al. 2010 [12]	22	95.8	2014	Not known	Not known	Up to 14 weeks	Postpartum pyrexia of unknown origin	Not stated	Not stated	Healthy (not stated)	NM	NM	NM
4	Kelly et al. 2010 [12]	26	87.5	1263	Not known	Therapeutic heparin	Up to 4 weeks	None	Not stated	Not stated	Healthy (not stated)	NM	NM	NM
5	Kelly et al. 2010 [12]	27	99.7	10,300	No	Prophylactic heparin	Entire pregnancy (increased from 28 weeks) and postpartum	Breakthrough hemolysis, RBC transfusion	Term	Normal vaginal	Healthy (not stated)	116.1	Undetected	Undetected

6	Kelly et al. 2010 [12]	35	97.6	1616	No	Therapeutic heparin	From 27 weeks (weekly) & postpartum	Postpartum hemorrhage	35	C-section (twin)	Healthy (2400 and 2000)	80.5	19.2/14.4	NM
7	Kelly et al. 2010 [12]	28	98.1	2642	Warfarin	Therapeutic heparin	Entire pregnancy and postpartum	Preeclampsia	28	C-section (preec-lampsia)	Healthy (900)	63.2	Undetected	NM
8	Marasca et al. 2010 [13]	34	69	Not stated	No	Prophylactic heparin	Entire pregnancy and postpartum	None	38	Normal vaginal	Healthy (3430)	NM	NM	NM

LDH lactate dehydrogenase, *C-section* cesarean section, *NM* not measured

21.3.2 Role of Anticoagulant Therapy in the Era of Eculizumab

The importance of anticoagulation therapy has been emphasized for the management of pregnancy with PNH. However, anticoagulation therapy alone might sometimes be inadequate, since severe maternal complications have been reported even in the patients who underwent prophylactic anticoagulation [17]. Theoretically, if intravascular hemolysis is completely inhibited by eculizumab, the risk of thromboembolic complications would become as low as that in non-PNH pregnancies. However, considering the fact that venous thromboembolism is a life-threatening complication, the use of anticoagulants should not be delayed for any reason. Although it is not clear whether the use of anticoagulants is mandatory for pregnant patients receiving eculizumab therapy, it has been administered to these patients, as shown in Table 21.2. Because the half-life of eculizumab is relatively long (10–12 days), subtle adjustment of its dosage or interval is not easy. Therefore, realistically, complementary anticoagulant therapy seems necessary, along with close monitoring of thrombotic markers such as the D-dimer. Conversely, eculizumab could reduce the need for anticoagulants, which will in turn help decrease heparin-associated complications such as hemorrhagic deliveries.

21.4 Management of Pregnant PNH Patients in the Era of Eculizumab

In patients with PNH, pregnancy places both the mother and fetus at high risk of severe complications. Combined use of eculizumab and anticoagulation therapies should be considered depending on the patient's condition, and cooperation between hematologists and obstetricians is consequently important.

21.4.1 Eculizumab and Anticoagulation Therapy

We propose the following protocol for the management of a pregnancy with PNH (Fig. 21.2), mainly based on the cases reported in the literature together with the additional four cases in which pregnancy was successfully managed with eculizumab in Japan (manuscript in preparation). Patients are classified into four categories depending on previous eculizumab use and their history of venous thromboembolisms (VTE) or anticoagulant use.

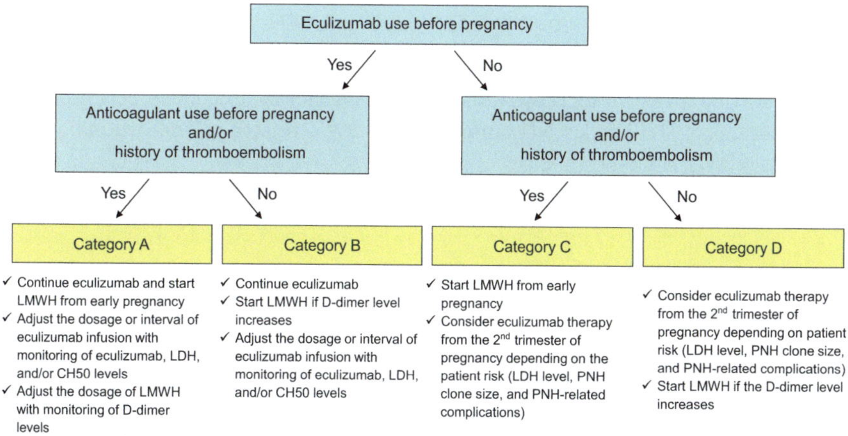

Fig. 21.2 Protocol for the management of a pregnancy with PNH. Patients are grouped into four categories depending on eculizumab use and the history of venous thromboembolisms or anticoagulant use. *LMWH* low molecular weight heparin

Category A Patients with a history of VTE or anticoagulant therapy who are receiving eculizumab therapy.

- Continue eculizumab therapy and start low molecular weight heparin (LMWH) from early pregnancy.
- Adjust the dosage or interval of eculizumab infusion, with continuous monitoring of eculizumab, LDH, and/or CH50 levels.
- Adjust the dosage of LMWH with continuous monitoring of the D-dimer level.

Category B Patients without a history of VTE or anticoagulant therapy who are receiving eculizumab therapy.

- Continue eculizumab therapy.
- Start LMWH if the D-dimer level increases.
- Adjust the dosage or interval of eculizumab infusion with continuous monitoring of eculizumab, LDH, and/or CH50 levels.

Category C Patients with a history of VTE or anticoagulant therapy who are not receiving eculizumab therapy.

- Start LMWH from early pregnancy.
- Consider eculizumab therapy depending on patient risk (LDH level, PNH close size, and PNH-related complications).

Category D Patients without a history of VTE or anticoagulant therapy who are not receiving eculizumab therapy.

- Consider eculizumab therapy from the 2nd trimester of pregnancy depending on patient risk (LDH level, PNH close size, and PNH-related complications).
- Start LMWH if the D-dimer level increases.

21.4.2 *Obstetrical Management*

Before pregnancy, information about possible complications should be explained to the patient and her partner. Scheduled pregnancy with folic acid supplementation is recommended in order to lower the risk of fetal neural tube defects, since patients with PNH have an increased need for folic acid. If the state of PNH is unstable or the patient has severe organ damage, such as renal dysfunction or liver dysfunction, it is not safe for her to become pregnant, and elective termination of pregnancy (TOP) should be considered in case of unexpected pregnancy.

An increased incidence of preterm delivery has been reported in the case of pregnancies with PNH. Although iatrogenic TOP because of maternal complications is the most probable reason, uterine cervical incompetence and abnormal uterine contraction caused by PNH-related smooth muscle dystonia [19] may also contribute to this outcome. Obstetricians must pay attention to ensure early detection of high-risk patients for preterm labor, which can be through cervical length measurement by transvaginal ultrasonography. In addition, it is also important to recognize PNH as a risk factor for pregnancy-induced hypertensive disorders such as preeclampsia and HELLP syndrome. Fetal well-being should be evaluated more closely than usual using ultrasound examination and fetal heart rate monitoring.

With regard to the mode of delivery, vaginal delivery is preferable because cesarean section increases the risk of infectious, hemorrhagic, and venous thromboembolic complications. In order to control prophylactic anticoagulant therapy during delivery, a scheduled delivery is preferable. Obstetricians should keep in mind that PNH-related smooth muscle dystonia may cause not only dystocia because of weak labor pains but also massive bleeding because of postpartum uterine inertia. Further, postpartum anticoagulation is very important because life-threatening thromboembolic events are reported to most likely occur in this period.

Although eculizumab is promising for the management of PNH during pregnancy and increases the chances of women with PNH to have children, clinical experience and evidence of its use during pregnancy remain insufficient. A review of additional cases and reevaluation of outcomes is required before a definitive recommendation can be made.

References

1. Miyata T, Takeda J, Iida Y, Yamada N, Inoue N, Takahashi M et al (1993) The cloning of PIG-A, a component in the early step of GPI-anchor biosynthesis. Science 259(5099):1318–1320
2. Takeda J, Miyata T, Kawagoe K, Iida Y, Endo Y, Fujita T et al (1993) Deficiency of the GPI anchor caused by a somatic mutation of the PIG-A gene in paroxysmal nocturnal hemoglobinuria. Cell 73(4):703–711
3. Miyata T, Yamada N, Iida Y, Nishimura J, Takeda J, Kitani T et al (1994) Abnormalities of PIG-A transcripts in granulocytes from patients with paroxysmal nocturnal hemoglobinuria. N Engl J Med 330(4):249–255
4. Parker C, Omine M, Richards S, Nishimura J, Bessler M, Ware R et al (2005) Diagnosis and management of paroxysmal nocturnal hemoglobinuria. Blood 106(12):3699–3709
5. Brodsky RA (2009) How I, treat paroxysmal nocturnal hemoglobinuria. Blood 113(26):6522–6527
6. Luzzatto L, Gianfaldoni G, Notaro R (2011) Management of paroxysmal nocturnal haemoglobinuria: a personal view. Br J Haematol 153(6):709–720
7. Hillmen P, Lewis SM, Bessler M, Luzzatto L, Dacie JV (1995) Natural history of paroxysmal nocturnal hemoglobinuria. N Engl J Med 333(19):1253–1258
8. Socie G, Mary JY, de Gramont A, Rio B, Leporrier M, Rose C et al (1996) Paroxysmal nocturnal haemoglobinuria: Long-term follow-up and prognostic factors. french society of haematology. Lancet 348(9027):573–577
9. Nishimura J, Kanakura Y, Ware RE, Shichishima T, Nakakuma H, Ninomiya H et al (2004) Clinical course and flow cytometric analysis of paroxysmal nocturnal hemoglobinuria in the united states and japan. Medicine 83(3):193–207
10. de Latour RP, Mary JY, Salanoubat C, Terriou L, Etienne G, Mohty M et al (2008) Paroxysmal nocturnal hemoglobinuria: natural history of disease subcategories. Blood 112(8):3099–3106
11. Danilov AV, Smith H, Craigo S, Feeney DM, Relias V, Miller KB (2009) Paroxysmal nocturnal hemoglobinuria (PNH) and pregnancy in the era of eculizumab. Leuk Res 33(6):e4–e5
12. Kelly R, Arnold L, Richards S, Hill A, Bomken C, Hanley J et al (2010) The management of pregnancy in paroxysmal nocturnal haemoglobinuria on long term eculizumab. Br J Haematol 149(3):446–450
13. Marasca R, Coluccio V, Santachiara R, Leonardi G, Torelli G, Notaro R et al (2010) Pregnancy in PNH: another eculizumab baby. Br J Haematol 150(6):707–708
14. Rother RP, Rollins SA, Mojcik CF, Brodsky RA, Bell L (2007) Discovery and development of the complement inhibitor eculizumab for the treatment of paroxysmal nocturnal hemoglobinuria. Nat Biotechnol 25(11):1256–1264
15. Parker C (2009) Eculizumab for paroxysmal nocturnal haemoglobinuria. Lancet 373(9665):759–767
16. Fieni S, Bonfanti L, Gramellini D, Benassi L, Delsignore R (2006) Clinical management of paroxysmal nocturnal hemoglobinuria in pregnancy: a case report and updated review. Obstet Gynecol Surv 61(9):593–601
17. de Guibert S, de Latour RP, Varoqueaux N, Labussiere H, Rio B, Jaulmes D et al (2011) Paroxysmal nocturnal hemoglobinuria and pregnancy before the eculizumab era: the french experience. Haematologica 96(9):1276–1283
18. Tedder RS, Nelson M, Eisen V (1975) Effects on serum complement of normal and pre-eclamptic pregnancy and of oral contraceptives. Br J Exp Pathol 56(5):389–395
19. Rother RP, Bell L, Hillmen P, Gladwin MT (2005) The clinical sequelae of intravascular hemolysis and extracellular plasma hemoglobin: a novel mechanism of human disease. JAMA 293(13):1653–1662

20. Kwak-Kim J, Agcaoili MS, Aleta L, Liao A, Ota K, Dambaeva S et al (2013) Management of women with recurrent pregnancy losses and antiphospholipid antibody syndrome. Am J Reprod Immunol 69(6):596–607
21. Thomas TC, Rollins SA, Rother RP, Giannoni MA, Hartman SL, Elliott EA et al (1996) Inhibition of complement activity by humanized anti-C5 antibody and single-chain fv. Mol Immunol 33(17–18):1389–1401
22. Brodsky RA, Young NS, Antonioli E, Risitano AM, Schrezenmeier H, Schubert J et al (2008) Multicenter phase 3 study of the complement inhibitor eculizumab for the treatment of patients with paroxysmal nocturnal hemoglobinuria. Blood 111(4):1840–1847
23. Hillmen P, Young NS, Schubert J, Brodsky RA, Socie G, Muus P et al (2006) The complement inhibitor eculizumab in paroxysmal nocturnal hemoglobinuria. N Engl J Med 355(12):1233–1243
24. Hashira S, Okitsu-Negishi S, Yoshino K (2000) Placental transfer of IgG subclasses in a japanese population. Pediatr Int 42(4):337–342

MIX
Papier aus verantwortungsvollen Quellen
Paper from responsible sources
FSC® C105338

If you have any concerns about our products,
you can contact us on
ProductSafety@springernature.com

In case Publisher is established outside the EU,
the EU authorized representative is:
Springer Nature Customer Service Center GmbH
Europaplatz 3, 69115 Heidelberg, Germany

Printed by Libri Plureos GmbH
in Hamburg, Germany